Essentials of Patient Education

Susan B. Bastable, EdD, RN
Professor and Director of Nursing
Nursing Program
Le Moyne College
Syracuse, New York

JONES AND BARTLETT PUBLISHERS
Sudbury, Massachusetts
BOSTON   TORONTO   LONDON   SINGAPORE

World Headquarters

Jones and Bartlett Publishers
40 Tall Pine Drive
Sudbury, MA 01776
978-443-5000
info@jbpub.com
www.jbpub.com

Jones and Bartlett Publishers
Canada
6339 Ormindale Way
Mississauga, ON L5V 1J2
Canada

Jones and Bartlett Publishers
International
Barb House, Barb Mews
London W6 7PA
United Kingdom

Jones and Bartlett's books and products are available through most bookstores and online book-sellers. To contact Jones and Bartlett Publishers directly, call 800-832-0034, fax 978-443-8000, or visit our website www.jbpub.com.

Substantial discounts on bulk quantities of Jones and Bartlett's publications are available to corporations, professional associations, and other qualified organizations. For details and specific discount information, contact the special sales department at Jones and Bartlett via the above contact information or send an email to specialsales@jbpub.com.

Library of Congress Cataloging-in-Publication Data

Essentials of patient education / [edited by] Susan B. Bastable.
   p. ; cm.
 Includes index.
 ISBN 0-7637-4842-0 (pbk. : alk. paper)
 1. Patient education. 2. Nursing.
 [DNLM: 1. Education, Nursing—methods. 2. Learning. 3. Patient Education—methods.
 4. Teaching. WY 18 E785 2005] I. Bastable, Susan Bacorn.
 RT90.E85 2005
 615.5'071—dc22

                         2004026030

Production Credits
Acquisitions Editor: Kevin Sullivan
Associate Editor: Amy Sibley
Production Director: Amy Rose
Associate Production Editor: Carolyn F. Rogers
Marketing Manager: Emily Ekle
Manufacturing and Inventory Coordinator: Amy Bacus
Composition: Paw Print Media
Cover Design: Timothy Dziewit
Printing and Binding: Malloy, Inc.
Cover Printing: Malloy, Inc.

Printed in the United States of America
09 08 07 06 05   10 9 8 7 6 5 4 3 2 1

Dedication

To the past and present students in my education courses and to my professional colleagues, who have shared insights, ideas, and perspectives stemming from their teaching experiences in the practice of delivering nursing care to the clients they serve.

Contents

Preface

This textbook, a simplified version of the second edition of *Nurse as Educator: Principles of Teaching and Learning for Nursing Practice*, was written as a primary resource for undergraduate nursing students as well as for staff nurses in practice, for whom the role of teacher is a significant component of their daily caregiving activities. Like *Nurse as Educator*, this text is comprehensive in its scope of content. However, it was scaled down to focus on patients and their family members as the audience of learners and with just enough depth of information necessary to provide the essentials of patient teaching.

Teaching patients and their family members has been a responsibility of professional nurses at all levels of education for many years. Although nurses recognize their legal, ethical, and moral responsibility to teach clients, most of us acknowledge that we have not had the formal preparation to successfully and securely carry out this role. Every nurse must be prepared with the knowledge and skills to competently and confidently educate clients in a variety of settings. We must be able to do so with efficiency and effectiveness based on a solid understanding of the principles of teaching and learning.

The focus of this text is on the nurse's role in teaching patients, well or ill, to maintain optimal health and prevent disease and disability by assisting them to become as independent as possible in self-care activities. However, teachers are not born with an innate ability to teach nor to understand the ways in which people learn. The act of teaching takes special knowledge and skills about how to best communicate information and how that information is most successfully acquired. Patient teaching is essential to the delivery of high quality nursing care and we must be able to capture this domain as an important and unique aspect of our holistic approach to practice.

Thus, the chapters of this text address the basic foundations of the education process, the needs and characteristics of the learner, and the instructional techniques and strategies appropriate for teaching and learning. Emphasis is on the nurse functioning in partnership with the learner, as a "guide by the side" and as a "facilitator" of learning, rather than on the traditional and outmoded role of the nurse as primarily the "giver of information." Also of particular relevance is the focus on health literacy, especially with the recent surge of interest in how literacy levels affect the consumer's ability to comply with treatment regimens and how nurses can select and design printed education materials to match the reading and comprehension skills of their learners.

Online instructor's materials accompany this *Essentials* text as a unique resource for faculty to assist them with instruction of content as well as with assessment and evaluation of students learning the role of the nurse as teacher. It contains multiple choice and essay test items, learning activities, and instructional materials, including PowerPoint slides, which coincide with the respective chapters of the textbook. All test items were critiqued by an expert in item analysis to ensure consistency in format and adherence with the highest standards and protocols for test construction.

Contributors

Susan B. Bastable, EdD, RN
Professor and Director of Nursing
Nursing Program
Le Moyne College
Syracuse, New York

Margaret M. Braungart, PhD
Professor of Bioethics and Humanities
Center for Bioethics and Humanities
State University of New York
Upstate Medical University
Syracuse, New York

Richard G. Braungart, PhD
Professor Emeritus
Maxwell School of Citizenship and
    Public Affairs
Syracuse University
Syracuse, New York

Michelle A. Dart, MS, RN, PNP
Joslin Diabetes Center
State University of New York
Upstate Medical University
Syracuse, New York

Julie A. Doody, RN
Matriculated Student
College of Nursing
State University of New York
Upstate Medical University
Syracuse, New York

Kathleen Fitzgerald, MS, RN, CDE
Patient Educator
St. Joseph's Hospital Health Center
Syracuse, New York

Diane S. Hainsworth, MS, RN, ANP
Clinical Case Manager: Oncology
University Hospital
State University of New York
Upstate Medical University
Syracuse, New York

Sharon Kitchie, PhD, MS, RNCS
Patient Education Coordinator
University Hospital
State University of New York
Upstate Medical University
Syracuse, New York

M. Janice Nelson, EdD, RN
Professor and Dean Emeritus
College of Nursing
State University of New York
Upstate Medical University
Syracuse, New York

Eleanor Richards, PhD, RN
Associate Professor
Department of Nursing
State University of New York at
    New Paltz
New Paltz, New York

Wendy R. Sayward, MS, RN, CNS
Assistant Professor
State University of New York at
    Plattsburgh
Plattsburgh, New York

Deborah L. Sopczyk, MS, RN
    (Doctoral Candidate)
Director of Health Sciences Programs
School of Health Sciences
Excelsior College
Albany, New York

Kay Viggiani, MS, RNCS
Associate Professor, Coordinator of
    Gerontology Programs
Nursing Division
Keuka College
Keuka Park, New York

Priscilla Sandford Worral, PhD, RN
Coordinator of Nursing Research
University Hospital
State University of New York
Upstate Medical University
Syracuse, New York

Acknowledgments

The ability to complete this text could never have been achieved without the encouragement and understanding of my family, who endured the many long months I spent on writing and editing these chapters. Deep appreciation is extended to my husband, Jeffrey, to our two children, Garrett and Leigh, both serving as officers in the U.S. Navy, to my parents, Robert and Dorrie Bacorn, and to my "other" mother, Gerry Bastable, all of whom have always been my source of inspiration and support.

A most sincere thank you is expressed to each and every one of my contributors for their knowledge and expertise in the principles of teaching and learning and for their loyalty and steadfastness during the editing of their respective chapters. A special recognition is paid to Julie A. Doody, a former nursing student of mine, who edited and condensed the content on behavioral objectives in Chapter 10 and on instructional settings in Chapter 11.

Also, utmost gratitude is extended to three of my colleagues at Le Moyne College: Dr. John Smarrelli, Jr., Provost and Vice President for Academic Affairs, and Dr. Linda M. LeMura, Dean of Arts and Sciences, for providing me with flexibility in scheduling needed to complete this project as well as for demonstrating interest in my scholarly endeavors, and Jackie Utton, Nursing Program Assistant, who willingly spent the time to copy and mail chapter materials and manage the office affairs in my absence.

Finally, praise must be given to the editorial staff of Jones and Bartlett Publishers, in particular Kevin Sullivan, Amy Sibley, and Carolyn Rogers, for their consistent guidance and expert advice throughout every step of the publication process.

About the Author

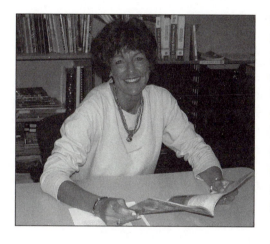

Susan Bacorn Bastable earned her MEd in community health nursing and her EdD in curriculum and instruction in nursing at Teachers College, Columbia University, in 1976 and 1979 respectively. She received her diploma from Hahnemann Hospital School of Nursing (now known as Drexel University of the Health Sciences) in Philadelphia in 1969 and her bachelor's degree in nursing from Syracuse University in 1972.

Dr. Bastable, currently Professor and founding Director of the Nursing Program at Le Moyne College in Syracuse, New York, began her academic career in 1979 as Assistant Professor at Hunter College, Bellevue School of Nursing, in New York City where she remained on the faculty for two years. From 1987 to 1989, she was Assistant Professor in the College of Nursing at the University of Rhode Island. In 1990, she joined the faculty of the College of Nursing at Upstate Medical University of the State University of New York (SUNY) in Syracuse, where she was Associate Professor and Chair of the Undergraduate Program for 14 years. In 2004, she assumed her present leadership position at Le Moyne College and has successfully established an RN-to-BSN completion program and an innovative 4-year undergraduate dual degree program in nursing.

Dr. Bastable has taught undergraduate courses in nursing research, community health, and the role of the nurse as educator, and courses at the master's and post-master's level on the nursing faculty role and on educational evaluation. For the past 24 years, she has been a consultant and external faculty member for Excelsior College (formerly known as Regents College of the University of the State of New York). Her clinical practice includes experience in community health, oncology, rehabilitation and neurology, occupational health, and medical–surgical nursing. Dr. Bastable has been recognized with the 1996 President's Award for Excellence in Teaching at Upstate Medical University, the SUNY 1999 Chancellor's Award for Excellence in Teaching, and the 2001 Nursing Education Alumni Association Award, and with induction in 2001 into the nursing education's Hall of Fame at Teacher's College, Columbia University.

PART I

Perspectives on Teaching and Learning

CHAPTER 1

Overview of Education in Health Care

Susan B. Bastable

CHAPTER HIGHLIGHTS

Historical Foundations for the Teaching
  Role of Nurses
Social, Economic, and Political Trends
  Affecting Health Care
Purpose, Goals, and Benefits of Patient
  Education

The Education Process Defined
The Teaching Role of the Nurse
Barriers to Teaching and Obstacles
  to Learning
Questions to Be Asked About Teaching and
  Learning

KEY TERMS

barriers to teaching
education process
learning

obstacles to learning
patient education

OBJECTIVES

After completing this chapter, the reader will be able to

1. Discuss the evolution of the teaching role of nurses.
2. Recognize trends affecting the healthcare system in general and nursing practice in particular.
3. Identify the purpose, goals, and benefits of patient education.
4. Compare and contrast the education process to the nursing process.
5. Define the terms *education process*, *learning*, and *patient education*.
6. Identify reasons why patient education is an important duty for professional nurses.
7. Discuss barriers to teaching and obstacles to learning.
8. Formulate questions that nurses in the role of patient teachers should ask about the teaching-
   learning process.

Today, patient education is a topic of significant interest to nurses in every setting in which they practice. Teaching is a major aspect of the nurse's professional role. The current trends in health care are making it essential that patients and their families be prepared to assume responsibility for self-care management. The focus of care is on outcomes that demonstrate the extent to which patients and their significant others have learned the knowledge and skills necessary for independent living.

The need for nurses to teach others and to help others learn will continue to increase in this era of healthcare reform. With changes rapidly occurring in the system of healthcare delivery, nurses will find themselves in increasingly demanding, constantly fluctuating, and highly complex positions (Jorgensen, 1994). Nurses in the role of teachers must understand the forces, both historical and present-day, that have influenced and continue to influence their responsibilities in practice.

One purpose of this chapter is to shed light on the historical evolution of teaching as part of the professional nurse's role. Another purpose is to offer a perspective on the current trends in health care that make patient teaching a highly visible and required function of nursing care delivery. In addition, this chapter clarifies the broad purpose, goals, and benefits of the teaching-learning process; focuses on the philosophy of the nurse–patient partnership in teaching and learning; compares the education process to the nursing process; and identifies barriers to teaching and obstacles to learning. Nurses must have a basic understanding of the principles and processes of teaching and learning to carry out their practice responsibilities with efficiency and effectiveness.

HISTORICAL FOUNDATIONS FOR THE TEACHING ROLE OF NURSES

Patient education has long been considered a major function of standard care given by nurses. The role of the nurse as teacher is deeply entrenched in the growth and development of the profession. Since the mid-1800s, when nursing was first recognized as a unique discipline, the responsibility for teaching has been a focus of efforts by nurses as caregivers.

Florence Nightingale, the founder of modern nursing, not only taught nurses, physicians, and health officials about the importance of proper conditions in hospitals and homes to improve health care, but also emphasized the importance of teaching patients the need for adequate nutrition, fresh air, exercise, and personal hygiene to improve their well-being. By the early 1900s, public health nurses in this country clearly understood the significance of the role of the nurse as teacher in preventing disease and in maintaining the health of society (Chachkes & Christ, 1996).

For decades, then, patient teaching has been recognized as an independent nursing function. Nurses have always educated patients and their family members, and it is from these roots that nurses have expanded their practice to include the broader concepts of health and illness (Glanville, 2000).

As early as 1918, the National League of Nursing Education (NLNE) in the United States (now the National League for Nursing [NLN]) observed the importance of health teaching as a function within the scope of nursing practice. This organization recognized nurses as agents for the promotion of health and the prevention of illness in all settings in which they practiced (National League of Nursing Education, 1937). By 1950, the NLNE had identified course content in nursing school curricula to prepare nurses to assume the role as teacher of others. Also, the American Nurses Association (ANA) has for many years put forth statements on the functions, standards, and qualifications for nursing practice, of which patient teaching is a key element. In addition, the International Council of Nurses (ICN) has long supported teaching as an essential element of nursing care delivery.

Today, all state nurse practice acts (NPAs) include teaching within the scope of nursing practice responsibilities. Nurses, by legal mandate of the NPAs, are expected to provide instruction to consumers to assist them to maintain optimal levels of wellness, prevent disease, and manage illness. Nursing career ladders often incorporate teaching effectiveness as a measure of excellence in practice (Rifas, Morris, & Grady, 1994). By teaching patients and families, nurses can achieve the professional goal of providing cost-effective, safe, and high-quality care.

In recognition of the importance of patient education by nurses, the Joint Commission on Accreditation of Healthcare Organizations (JCAHO) established nursing standards for patient education as early as 1993. These standards, known as mandates, describe the type and level of care, treatment, and services that must be provided by an agency or organization to receive accreditation. The JCAHO standards emphasize improving nursing care interventions to achieve expected client outcomes (McGoldrick, Jablonski, & Wolf, 1994). Positive outcomes of patient care are to be achieved, in part, through teaching activities that must be patient- and family-oriented, include an interdisciplinary team approach, and provide evidence that patients and their significant others understand what they have been taught. This requirement means that providers must consider the literacy level, educational background, language skills, and culture of every client during the education process (Davidhizar & Brownson, 1999).

In addition, the Patient's Bill of Rights, first developed in the 1970s by the American Hospital Association, has been adopted by hospitals nationwide. It establishes the guidelines to ensure that patients receive complete and current information concerning diagnosis, treatment, and prognosis in terms they can reasonably be expected to understand.

In 1995, the Pew Health Professions Commission, influenced by the dramatic changes currently surrounding health care, published a broad set of competencies it believed would mark the success of the health professions in the 21st century. More recently, the Pew Health Professions Commission (1998) released a follow-up report on health professional practice in the new millennium. Numerous recommendations specific to the nursing profession have been proposed by this Commission. More than one-half of them directly or indirectly address the importance of patient education and the role of the nurse as teacher. These recommendations for the practice of nursing include the need to:

- Provide clinically competent and coordinated care to the public
- Involve patients and their families in the decision-making process regarding health interventions
- Provide clients with education and counseling on ethical issues
- Expand public access to effective care
- Ensure cost-effective and appropriate care for the consumer
- Provide for prevention of illness and promotion of healthy lifestyles for all Americans

Accomplishing the goals and meeting the expectations of these organizations calls for a shift in patient education efforts. Since the 1980s, the role of the nurse as teacher has evolved from what once was a disease-oriented approach to a more prevention-oriented approach. In other words, the focus is on teaching for the promotion and maintenance of health. Patient teaching, once done as part of discharge planning at the end of hospitalization, has expanded to become part of a comprehensive plan of care (Davidhizar & Brownson, 1999).

As described by Grueninger (1995), this transition toward wellness has progressed "from disease-oriented patient education (DOPE) to prevention-oriented patient education (POPE) to ultimately become health-oriented patient education (HOPE)" (p. 53). This new approach has changed the role of the nurse from one of wise healer to expert advisor/teacher to facilitator of change. Instead of the traditional aim of simply imparting information, the emphasis is now on empowering patients to use their potentials, abilities, and resources to the fullest (Glanville, 2000). It is essential for nurses to be prepared to effectively perform teaching services that meet the needs of many individuals and groups in different circumstances across a variety of practice settings.

SOCIAL, ECONOMIC, AND POLITICAL TRENDS AFFECTING HEALTH CARE

In addition to the professional and legal standards put forth by various organizations and agencies, many social, economic, and political trends nationwide have led to increased attention to the role of the nurse as teacher and the importance of patient education. The following are some of the significant forces influencing nursing practice in particular and the healthcare system in general (Birchenall, 2000; Glanville, 2000; Jorgensen, 1994; Latter, Clark, Wilson-Barnett, & Maben, 1992; McGinnis, 1993; Wilkinson, 1996):

- The federal government has published *Healthy People 2010: Understanding and Improving Health* (Department of Health and Human Services, 2000), a document that establishes national health goals and objectives for the future. These goals and objectives include the development of effective health education programs to help individuals to recognize and change risky behaviors, to adopt or maintain healthy practices, and to make appropriate use of available services for health care. Achieving these national priorities would dramatically cut the cost of health care, prevent the early onset of disease and disability, and help all Americans lead healthier and more productive lives. Nurses, as the largest group of health professionals, play an important role in making a real difference by teaching people to attain and maintain healthy lifestyles.
- The growth of managed care has resulted in shifts in reimbursement for health services. Greater emphasis has been placed on outcome measures, many of which can be achieved through patient education efforts.
- Health providers are recognizing the economic and social values of reaching out to communities, schools, and workplaces to provide education for disease prevention and health promotion.
- Politicians and healthcare administrators are beginning to recognize the importance of health education to accomplish the economic goal of reducing the high costs of health services.
- Consumers are demanding increased knowledge and skills about how to care for themselves and how to prevent disease. As people are becoming more aware of their needs and desire a greater understanding of treatments and goals, the demand for patient information services is expected to intensify. Emphasis on consumer rights and responsibilities, which began in the 1990s, will continue into the twenty-first century.
- As the percentage of the U.S. population over 65 years climbs dramatically in the next 20 to 30 years, the health needs of the baby boom generation of the

post-World War II era will become greater as members deal with degenerative illnesses and other effects of the aging process. Education of older adults will allow them to maintain a healthy status over an extended lifespan.

- Among the major causes of morbidity and mortality are those diseases now recognized as being lifestyle-related that can be prevented through educational interventions.
- The increase in chronic and incurable conditions requires that individuals and families become informed participants to manage their own illnesses. Patient teaching can facilitate an individual's adaptive responses to illness.
- Advanced technology is increasing the complexity of care and treatment in the home setting. Earlier hospital discharge is forcing patients and their families to be more self-reliant while managing their own illnesses. Patient education is necessary to help them to independently follow through with self-care activities.
- An increasing number of self-help groups exist that support clients in meeting their physical and psychosocial needs. The success of these support groups depends on the nurse's role as teacher and advocate.

Nurses recognize the need to develop their expertise in teaching to keep pace with the demands of patient education. As they continue to define their own role, body of knowledge, scope of practice, and professional expertise, nurses realize more than ever before that patient education is central to the practice of nursing and should be included as part of their domain. Nurses are in a key position to carry out health education. They are the healthcare providers who have the most continuous contact with patients and families, are usually the most accessible source of information for the consumer, and are the most highly trusted of all health professionals. In one Gallup poll, nurses were ranked first in honesty and ethics among 45 occupations (Mason, 2001). Patient teaching is becoming an increasingly important function within the scope of nursing practice.

PURPOSE, GOALS, AND BENEFITS OF PATIENT EDUCATION _____

The purpose of patient education is to increase the competence and confidence of clients for self-management. The role of the nurse is to support patients through the transition from being invalids to being independent in care; from being dependent recipients to being involved participants in the care process; and from being passive listeners to active learners. Interactive patient education efforts provide clients the opportunity to explore and expand their self-care abilities.

The most important goal of patient education is to prepare patients and their families for independence. If clients cannot maintain or improve their health status when on their own, we have failed to help them reach their potential (Glanville, 2000; McGoldrick et al., 1994).

The benefits of patient education are many. Effective teaching by the nurse has demonstrated the potential to:

- Increase consumer satisfaction
- Improve quality of life
- Ensure continuity of care
- Decrease patient anxiety
- Effectively reduce the complications of illness and the incidence of disease
- Promote adherence to treatment plans
- Maximize independence in the performance of activities of daily living
- Energize and empower consumers to become actively involved in the planning of their care

In turn, the role of nurses in patient education enhances their job satisfaction when they recognize that their teaching actions allow them to forge therapeutic relationships with patients, enhance patient–nurse autonomy, increase their accountability for practice, and create change that really makes a difference in the lives of others.

Because an estimated 80% of all health needs and problems are handled at home, there truly does exist a need to teach people how to care for themselves—both to get well and to stay well (Health Services Medical Corporation, 1993). Illness is a natural life process, but so is mankind's ability to learn. Along with the ability to learn comes a natural curiosity that allows people to view new and difficult situations as challenges rather than as defeats. As Robin Orr (1990) noted, "Illness can become an educational opportunity . . . a 'teachable moment' when ill health suddenly encourages [patients] to take a more active role in their care" (p. 47).

Numerous studies have documented the fact that informed patients are more likely to comply with medical treatment plans and find unique ways to cope with illness, and are less likely to experience complications. Overall, patients are more satisfied with care when they receive adequate information about how to manage for themselves. One of the most frequently cited complaints by patients in malpractice cases is that they were not adequately informed.

THE EDUCATION PROCESS DEFINED

The *education process* is a systematic, sequential, logical, planned course of action consisting of two major interdependent operations, teaching and learning. This process forms a continuous cycle that also involves two interdependent players, the teacher and the learner. Together, the teaching and learning activities lead to outcomes of mutually desired behavior changes. Thus, the education process is a framework for a participatory, shared approach to teaching and learning.

The education process has always been compared to the nursing process—rightly so, because the steps of each process run parallel to one another, although they have different goals and objectives. The education process, like the nursing process, consists of the basic elements of assessment, planning, implementation, and evaluation. The two are different in that the nursing process focuses on the planning and implementation of care based on the assessment of the physical and psychosocial needs of the patient. The education process, on the other hand, focuses on the planning and implementation of teaching based on an assessment of the client's learning needs, readiness to learn, and learning styles. The outcomes of the nursing process are achieved when the physical and psychosocial needs of the client are met. The outcomes of the education process are achieved when changes in knowledge, attitudes, and skills occur. Both processes are ongoing, with assessment and evaluation redirecting the planning and implementation phases of the processes (Figure 1-1).

The success of the nurse's efforts at teaching depends not on how much information has been imparted, but rather on how much the person has learned. *Learning* is

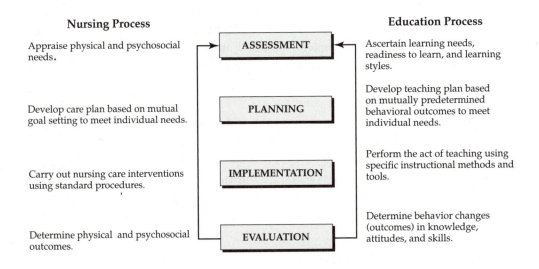

FIGURE 1-1 Education Process Parallels Nursing Process

defined as a change in behavior (knowledge, attitudes, and skills) that can be observed or measured and that can occur at any time or in any place (see Chapter 3). Specifically, *patient education* is a process of assisting people to learn health-related behaviors so that they can incorporate those behaviors into everyday life. As stated previously, the purpose of patient education is to help clients to achieve the goal of optimal health and independence in self-care. It involves establishing a relationship between the teacher and learner so that the information needs (cognitive, affective, and psychomotor) of a client can be met through the process of education (see Chapter 10).

A useful paradigm that helps nurses to organize and carry out the education process is the ASSURE model (Rega, 1993). The acronym stands for:

- **A**nalyze learner.
- **S**tate objectives.
- **S**elect teaching methods and instructional materials.
- **U**se teaching methods and instructional materials.
- **R**equire learner performance.
- **E**valuate the teaching plan and revise as necessary.

THE TEACHING ROLE OF THE NURSE

For many years, organizations governing and influencing nurses in practice have identified teaching as an essential responsibility of all registered nurses in caring for both well and ill clients. Legal and accreditation mandates as well as professional nursing standards of practice include patient education as an important activity expected to be carried out in the delivery of high-quality care. For nurses to fulfill the role of teacher of patients and family members, they must have a solid foundation in the principles of teaching and learning.

The role of the nurse as teacher is not just to be the "giver of information," but to promote learning and provide for an environment conducive to learning—to create the "teachable moment" rather than just waiting for it to happen (Wagner & Ash, 1998). A learner cannot be made to learn, but an effective approach to teaching others is to actively involve learners in the education process. The nurse should act as a facilitator, creating situations that motivate individuals to want to learn and that make it possible for them to learn. The assessment of learning needs, the planning and designing of a teaching plan, the implementation of teaching methods and instructional materials, and the evaluation of teaching and learning should include participation by both the nurse and the patient/family (Knowles, Holton, & Swanson, 1998).

Instead of the teacher teaching, the new educational paradigm focuses on the learner learning; that is, the nurse becomes "the guide on the side," assisting the learner in his or her effort to determine objectives and goals for learning, with both parties being active partners in decision making throughout the education process. To increase comprehension, recall, and application of information, patients and their family members must be actively involved in the learning experience (London, 1995). Glanville (2000) describes this move toward assisting learners to use their own abilities and resources as "a pivotal transfer of power" (p. 58).

Certainly patient education requires a collaborative effort among healthcare team members, all of whom play more or less important roles in teaching. However, physicians are first and foremost prepared "to treat, not to teach" (Gilroth, 1990, p. 30). Nurses, on the other hand, are prepared to provide a holistic approach to care delivery. The teaching role is a unique part of our professional domain. Because consumers have always respected and trusted nurses to be their advocates, nurses are in an ideal position to clarify confusing information and make "sense out of nonsense." With a fragmented healthcare delivery system involving many providers, the nurse serves as coordinator of care. By ensuring consistency of information, nurses can support patients and family members in their efforts to achieve the goal of optimal health (Donovan & Ward, 2001).

BARRIERS TO TEACHING AND OBSTACLES TO LEARNING

Unfortunately, nurses must overcome many barriers in carrying out their responsibilities for patient education. Also, clients face a variety of potential obstacles that can get in the way of their learning. For the purposes of this text, *barriers to teaching* are defined as those factors that interfere with the nurse's ability to deliver educational services. *Obstacles to learning* are defined as those factors that negatively affect the ability of the learner to pay attention to and process information.

Barriers to Teaching

The major barriers interfering with the ability of nurses to carry out their role as teachers include the following (Casey, 1995; Chachkes & Christ, 1996; Duffy, 1998; Gilroth, 1990; Glanville, 2000; Honan, Krsnak, Petersen, & Torkelson, 1988; Lipetz, Bussigel, Bannerman, & Risley, 1990):

1. Lack of time to teach is cited by nurses as the greatest barrier to being able to carry out their teaching role effectively. Early discharge from inpatient and

outpatient settings often results in nurses and patients having fleeting contact with one another. In addition, the schedules and responsibilities of nurses are very demanding. Finding time to allocate to teaching is very challenging in light of other work demands and expectations. Nurses must know how to adopt an abbreviated, efficient, and effective approach to patient education by first adequately assessing the learner and then using appropriate teaching methods and instructional tools at their disposal.

2. Many nurses admit that they do not feel competent or confident with their teaching skills. Although nurses are expected to teach, few have ever taken a specific course on the principles of teaching and learning. Kruger (1991) surveyed 1,230 nurses about their perceived responsibility and ability to carry out patient education. Although most of those surveyed believed that patient education is a primary responsibility of nurses, they also rated their ability to perform patient education activities as unsatisfactory. The findings of this research study indicate that the role of the nurse as teacher needs to be strengthened.

3. Low priority is often assigned to patient education by administrators and physicians. They tend to recognize the time spent by nurses in doing direct physical care tasks as more important than time spent devoted to patient teaching. With the new JCAHO mandates, the level of attention paid to the learning needs of consumers is changing. However, budget allocations for educational resources are often not enough to support new and time-saving teaching approaches to enhance the effectiveness of teaching and learning.

4. The environment in the various settings where nurses are expected to teach and learners are expected to learn is not always conducive to carrying out patient education. Lack of space, lack of privacy, noise, and frequent interruptions due to treatment schedules are just some of the factors that interfere with the ability of nurses and patients to concentrate and to interact with one another for patient education to be effective.

5. An absence of third-party reimbursement to support patient education relegates teaching and learning to less than high-priority status. Nursing services within healthcare facilities are part of hospital room costs and, therefore, are not specifically reimbursed by insurance payers. In fact, patient education in some settings, such as home care, often cannot be incorporated as a legitimate aspect of routine nursing care delivery unless specifically ordered by a physician.

6. Some nurses and physicians question whether patient education is effective as a means to improve health outcomes. Unless all healthcare members buy into the "utility of patient education" (that is, they believe it can lead to significant

behavioral changes and increased compliance to therapeutic regimens), some professionals may not devote the time and energy necessary to provide adequate and appropriate patient education.

7. The type of documentation system used by healthcare agencies influences the quality and quantity of patient teaching. Both formal and informal teaching are often done but not written down because of insufficient time, inattention to detail, and inadequate forms on which to record the extent of teaching activities. In addition, most nurses do not recognize the scope and depth of teaching that they perform on a daily basis. Communication among healthcare providers regarding what has been taught needs to be coordinated and appropriately delegated so that teaching can proceed in a timely, smooth, organized, and thorough fashion.

Obstacles to Learning

The following are some of the major obstacles interfering with a learner's ability to attend to and process information (Gilroth, 1990; Glanville, 2000; Lipetz et al., 1990; Seley, 1994):

1. Lack of time to learn due to rapid patient discharge from care can discourage and frustrate the learner, interfering with the ability and willingness to learn.

2. The stress of acute and chronic illness, anxiety, sensory deficits, and low literacy in patients are just a few of the problems that can diminish learner motivation and interfere with the process of learning.

3. The negative influence of the hospital environment itself, resulting in loss of control, lack of privacy, and social isolation, can interfere with a client's active role in health decision making and involvement in the teaching-learning process.

4. Personal characteristics of the learner have major effects on the degree to which behavioral outcomes are achieved. Readiness to learn, motivation and compliance, developmental stage characteristics, and learning styles are some of the prime factors influencing the success of educational endeavors.

5. The extent of behavioral changes needed, both in number and in complexity, can overwhelm learners and discourage them from attending to and accomplishing learning objectives and goals.

6. Lack of support and lack of ongoing positive reinforcement from the nurse and significant others serve to block the potential for learning.

7. Denial of learning needs, resentment of authority, and lack of willingness to take responsibility (locus of control) are some psychological obstacles to accomplish-

ing behavioral change.

8. The inconvenience, complexity, inaccessibility, and fragmentation of the health-care system often result in frustration and abandonment of efforts by the learner to participate in and comply with the goals and objectives for learning.

It should be noted that the lack of time to teach and the lack of time to learn serve as both a barrier to teaching and an obstacle to learning. Because time is scarce, the following chapters address ways in which nurses can wisely use the time they have to spend on teaching and the time the patient has for learning.

QUESTIONS TO BE ASKED ABOUT TEACHING AND LEARNING

To maximize the effectiveness of patient education by the nurse, it is necessary to examine the elements of the education process and the role of the nurse as teacher. Many questions arise related to the principles of teaching and learning. The following are some of the important questions that the chapters in this book address:

- How can members of the healthcare team work together more effectively to coordinate patient education?
- What are the ethical, legal, and economic issues involved in patient education?
- How can learning theories be applied to change the behaviors of learners?
- What assessment methods can be used to determine learning needs, readiness to learn, and learning styles?
- What learner attributes negatively and positively affect an individual's ability and willingness to learn?
- Which elements need to be taken into account when developing teaching plans?
- Which teaching methods and instructional materials are available to support patient education?
- Under which conditions should certain teaching methods and instructional tools be used?
- How can teaching be tailored to meet the needs of specific population groups?
- What common mistakes are made when teaching patients and their families?
- How are teaching and learning best evaluated?

SUMMARY

The role of nurses as information brokers significantly influences how patients and families cope with their illnesses, benefit from education directed at prevention of disease and promotion of health, and gain competency and confidence in self-care management. Historically, nurses have provided education to patients and their families as part of their standard care-giving functions. However, the teaching role is becoming even more important and more visible as nurses respond to the social, economic, and political trends impacting on health care today.

Many challenges and opportunities lie ahead for nurses in the delivery of health care as this nation moves forward in the 21st century. The foremost challenge for nurses is to overcome barriers to teaching and reduce the obstacles that interfere with learning. This requires nurses to have a solid understanding of the education process and be able to apply the principles of teaching and learning to meet the needs of individuals in a variety of practice settings. A definite link exists between patient education and positive behavioral outcomes of the learner.

For patient education to be effective and efficient, nurses must work in partnership with patients and their families to achieve mutually established goals. The responsibility and accountability of nurses for the delivery of high quality care to the consumer can be demonstrated through an ongoing commitment to carrying out their role in patient education.

REVIEW QUESTIONS

1. For how far back in history has teaching been a part of the professional nurse's role?
2. Which nursing organization was the first to recognize health teaching as an important function within the scope of nursing practice?
3. What legal mandate includes teaching as a responsibility of nurses?
4. How have the JCAHO, ANA, AHA, and Pew Commission influenced the responsibilities of the nurse for patient education?
5. What current social, economic, and political trends have led to an increased emphasis on patient education?
6. What are the similarities and differences between the education process and the nursing process?
7. How are barriers to teaching different from obstacles to learning?
8. What are three major barriers to teaching and three major obstacles to learning?
9. What common factor serves as both a barrier to teaching and an obstacle to learning?

REFERENCES

Birchenall, P. (2000). Nurse education in the year 2000: Reflection, speculation and challenge. *Nurse Education Today, 20,* 1–2.

Casey, F. S. (1995). Documenting patient education: A literature review. *Journal of Continuing Education in Nursing, 26*(6), 257–260.

Chachkes, E. & Christ, G. (1996). Cross cultural issues in patient education. *Patient Education & Counseling, 27,* 13–21.

Davidhizar, R. E. & Brownson, K. (1999). Literacy, cultural diversity, and client education. *Health Care Manager, 18*(1), 39–47.

Department of Health and Human Services. (2000). *Healthy people 2010: Understanding and improving health* (2nd ed.). Washington, DC: U.S. Government Printing Office.

Donovan, H. S. & Ward, S. (2001). A representational approach to patient education. *Journal of Nursing Scholarship,* Third Quarter, 211–216.

Duffy, B. (1998). Get ready—Get set—Go teach. *Home Healthcare Nurse, 16*(9), 596–602.

Gilroth, B. E. (1990). Promoting patient involvement: Educational, organizational, and environmental strategies. *Patient Education and Counseling, 15,* 29–38.

Glanville, I. K. (2000). Moving towards health oriented patient education (HOPE). *Holistic Nursing Practice, 14*(2), 57–66.

Grueninger, U. J. (1995). Arterial hypertension: Lessons from patient education. *Patient Education and Counseling, 26,* 37–55.

Health Services Medical Corporation, Inc. (1993). Wealth in wellness begins "selfwise." *Worksite Wellnews, 1*(3), 1.

Honan, S., Krsnak, G., Petersen, D., & Torkelson, R. (1988). The nurse as patient educator: Perceived responsibilities and factors enhancing role development. *Journal of Continuing Education in Nursing, 19*(1), 33–37.

Jorgensen, C. (1994). Health education: What can it look like after health care reform? *Health Education Quarterly, 21*(1), 11–26.

Knowles, M. S., Holton, E. F., & Swanson, R. A. (1998). *The adult learner: The definitive classic in adult education and human resource development* (5th ed.). Chapter 11. Houston, TX: Gulf.

Kruger, S. (1991). The patient educator role in nursing. *Applied Nursing Research, 4*(1), 19–24.

Latter, S., Clark, J. M., Wilson-Barnett, J., & Maben, J. (1992). Health education in nursing: Perceptions of practice in acute settings. *Journal of Advanced Nursing, 17,* 164–172.

Lipetz, M. J., Bussigel, M. N., Bannerman, J., & Risley, B. (1990). What is wrong with patient education programs? *Nursing Outlook, 38*(4), 184–189.

London, F. (1995). Teach your patients faster and better. *Nursing 95,* 68, 70.

Mason, D. (2001). Promoting health literacy: Patient teaching is a vital nursing function. *American Journal of Nursing, 101*(2), 7.

McGinnis, J. M. (1993). The role of patient education in achieving national health objectives. *Patient Education and Counseling, 21,* 1–3.

McGoldrick, T. K., Jablonski, R. S., & Wolf, Z. R. (1994). Needs assessment for a patient education program in a nursing department: A delphi approach. *Journal of Nursing Staff Development, 10*(3), 123–130.

National League of Nursing Education. (1937). *A curriculum guide for schools of nursing*. New York: Author.

Orr, R. (1990). Illness as an educational opportunity. *Patient Education and Counseling, 15,* 47–48.

Pew Health Professions Commission. (1995). *Critical challenges: Revitalizing the health professions for the twenty-first century. The third report of the Pew Health Professions Commission*. San Francisco: University of California.

Pew Health Professions Commission. (1998). *Recreating health professional practice for a new century. The Fourth Report of the Pew Health Professions Commission, Center for the Health Professions*. San Francisco: University of California.

Pohl, M. L. (1965). Teaching activities of the nursing practitioner. *Nursing Research, 14*(1), 4–11.

Rega, M. D. (1993). A model approach for patient education. *MEDSURG Nursing, 2*(6), 477–479, 495.

Rifas, E., Morris, R., & Grady, R. (1994). Innovative approach to patient education. *Nursing Outlook, 42*(5), 214–216.

Seley, J. J. (1994). Ten strategies for successful patient teaching. *American Journal of Nursing, 94*(11), 63–65.

Wagner, S. P. & Ash, K. L. (1998). Creating the teachable moment. *Journal of Nursing Education, 37*(6), 278–280.

Wilkinson, J. M. (1996). The C word: A curriculum for the future. *Nursing & Health Care, 17*(2), 72–77.

CHAPTER 2

Ethical, Legal, and Economic Foundations of the Educational Process

M. Janice Nelson

CHAPTER HIGHLIGHTS

An Introduction to Ethics, Morality, and
the Law
Ethical and Legal Principles in
Health Care
Application of Ethical Principles to
Patient Teaching
  Autonomy
  Veracity
  Nonmalfeasance
  Confidentiality
  Beneficence
  Justice

Patients' Rights to Information
The Importance of Documentation
Economic Factors of Patient Education
  Direct Costs
  Indirect Costs
  Cost Savings, Cost Benefit, and Cost
    Recovery
  Program Planning and Implementation
  Cost-Benefit Analysis and
    Cost-Effectiveness Analysis

KEY TERMS

autonomy
beneficence
confidentiality
cost benefit ratio
cost-benefit analysis
cost-effectiveness analysis
cost recovery

cost savings
ethical
justice
legal
moral
nonmalfeasance
veracity

OBJECTIVES

After completing this chapter, the reader will be able to

1. Define the terms *ethical*, *moral*, and *legal*.
2. Recognize ethical and legal aspects of health care.
3. Identify the six major ethical principles related to patient teaching.
4. Describe the impact of nurse practice acts on legal responsibilities of nurses to teach.

5. Discuss the impact of federal, state, professional, and accrediting body regulations and standards on the delivery of patient education services.
6. Explain the legal importance of documentation.
7. Distinguish between the financial terms associated with the development, implementation, and evaluation of patient education programs.

Today as never before in the healthcare field, there is increased awareness of individual rights that come from both natural law and the legal system. Healthcare organizations are heavily regulated to ensure patients' rights to a quality standard of care, to informed consent, and to the right of self-determination.

Although the physician is primarily responsible for the patient's medical care, the nurse is usually responsible for teaching the patient about his or her medical condition. Because of the close relationship between nurse and patient, the nurse's role in educating the patient is required by state nurse practice acts.

Today, the public is more aware than ever before of individual legal rights regarding freedom of choice and making one's own decisions. It may seem odd to some that the federal government, state governments, and organizations, such as the American Hospital Association (AHA), the American Nurses Association (ANA), and the Kennedy Institute for Bioethics in Washington, D.C., all find it necessary to legislate, regulate, or provide guidelines to ensure the protection of people's rights when it comes to matters of health care.

The issue of individual rights is basic to the delivery of quality healthcare services. An understanding by the nurse of these rights is very important when teaching patients to assist themselves in making choices based on correct information and to be able to deal with the consequences of those choices regardless of the outcome. In examining the role of the nurse as teacher, it is important to remember that legal and ethical principles apply to any teaching-learning situation. Also, the nurse must balance how much it costs the hospital or other healthcare facilities to offer these services with people's right to good health care.

The purpose of this chapter is to provide the nurse with basic knowledge about the ethical, legal, and economic principles that justify patient education and the rights and responsibilities of the nurse as provider. This chapter explores the differences among the definitions of the terms *ethical*, *moral*, and *legal*; covers the ethical and legal principles of human rights; reviews the ethical and legal principles of health care; highlights the importance of documenting what has been taught; and examines the economic impact of providing patient education in various healthcare settings.

AN INTRODUCTION TO ETHICS, MORALITY, AND THE LAW _____

Ethics is a branch of philosophy that has been studied for many years. In the past the study of ethics was left primarily to philosophers and members of religious communities. However, in more recent times, when life choices are more complicated and the public is better educated, ethical issues in health care have become a major concern of both those who provide health care and those who receive it. In the end, individual rights of clients take precedence (whether this refers to diagnosis, treatment, interventions, or educating people about their medical condition) so that they can make the best choices about options for care with the support of nurses, physicians, and other providers.

Ethical principles of human rights come from natural laws that govern society. Within these natural laws are the rules that relate to, for example, respect for others, truth telling, honesty, and regard for life. As a special area of study, ethics defines the meaning of these rules of behavior in a very broad way and offers several points of view that are sometimes in conflict with one another. There are many opinions on the rightness or wrongness of how people behave. The most common of these opinions were expressed many years ago by Immanuel Kant, who believed in the "golden rule" (treat others as you would have them treat you), and John Stuart Mill, who believed that behavioral choices should be made that will result in the greatest good for the greatest number of people.

Our legal system and its laws are based on ethical and moral principles that have, over time, been accepted by society (Lesnick & Anderson, 1962). This partly explains why the words *ethical, moral,* and *legal* are so often thought to have the same meaning. Although these words are closely related, they are, by definition, not the same thing. *Ethical* refers to standards of acceptable behavior. Although it is not unusual for the word moral to be interchanged with ethical, *moral* refers to a person's inner value system expressed through external behaviors. Moral values, because they cannot be directly measured, are not enforceable by law. Ethical behaviors, however, can be recognized in laws, but ethical principles are not laws in and of themselves. For example, making a decision for someone else about his or her health care may be unethical, but it is not necessarily against the law. What is *legal*, on the other hand, refers to rules of behavior that are enforceable under threat of punishment or penalty, such as a fine, imprisonment, or both. The very close relationship between ethics and the law explains why ethics terminology, such as informed consent, confidentiality, nonmalfeasance (do no harm), and justice, can be found within the language of the legal system. A good example of the interplay of these three words is patient teaching. Nurses might say that they are morally and ethically obligated to teach patients about their illness. The truth is that nurses are required by law to teach patients. The nurse practice act in each state where nurses live, are licensed, and are employed requires them to do patient teaching. The nurse practice act is not only legally binding on nurses, but also regulated by the police authority of the state for the purpose of protecting the public.

ETHICAL AND LEGAL PRINCIPLES IN HEALTH CARE

For centuries, health care was considered to be a work of charity, usually provided by nuns and religious brothers. As a result, the early hospitals were considered to be charitable institutions and, thus, were not subject to lawsuits "because it would force the charity to use its money for a purpose never intended" (Lesnik & Anderson, 1962, p. 211). Also, in the not too distant past, physicians and nurses were usually regarded as "Good Samaritans" who acted in "good faith" and, therefore, were rarely accused of wrong-doing. However, this began to change when Supreme Court Justice Benjamin Cardozo in 1914 determined that every adult of sound mind has a right to protect his or her own body and to decide how it shall be treated (Boyd, Gleit, Graham, & Whitman, 1998).

Nevertheless, for many years federal and state governments continued to hold physicians and nurses immune in issues of biomedical research and treatment of patients. It was not until the horrible human atrocities committed during World War II were discovered that the world was shocked into an awareness of unspeakable violations of human rights. But these abuses did not just happen in wartime Germany and did not stop after World War II ended. In the United States, physicians neglected to treat Black men for syphilis, even though antibiotics were available; they injected live cancer cells into elderly adults without their consent at the Brooklyn Chronic Disease Hospital; and they tested hepatitis vaccines on mentally retarded children who were institutionalized at Willowbrook Developmental Center on Long Island, N.Y., all in the name of research. Such activities made the public aware of disturbing breaches in the physician–patient relationship (Weisbard & Arras, 1984).

In 1974, the U.S. Congress took action by creating the National Commission for the Protection of Human Subjects of Biomedical and Behavioral Research. This led to the development of Institutional Review Boards for the Protection of Human Subjects (IRBPHS) at hospitals, community health centers, and academic institutions across the country that conduct human research. Over the past three decades, these local boards, known as IRBs for short, have focused on issues of informed consent, confidentiality, and truth telling, with special concern for infants, children, students, prisoners, and the mentally ill. Every biomedical research proposal that involves human subjects must be submitted to a local IRB for intensive review and approval before any study can be conducted. Also, because of concern about the many ethical issues associated with medical practice and the need to regulate biomedical research,

Congress established the President's Commission for the Study of Ethical Problems in Medicine and Biomedical and Behavioral Research (Weisbard & Arras, 1984).

With remarkable foresight, the American Nurses Association (ANA), as early as 1950, developed and adopted a *Code of Ethics for Nurses with Interpretative Statements*, which was revised in 1976, in 1985, and again in 2001. This code serves as a guide for nurses in practice when caring for patients; it also speaks to professional values and obligations that support nursing's mission. A provision worth noting in the ANA *Code of Ethics for Nurses* addresses the need for nurses to collaborate "with members of the health professions and other citizens in promoting community and national efforts to meet the health needs of the public" (ANA, 2001, #8). This provision justifies patient teaching within healthcare facilities as well as in the community. It supports the ethical basis for providing health education classes to audiences in need of information on childbirth, smoking cessation, weight reduction, women's health issues, child abuse prevention, and many more topics.

In 1975, the American Hospital Association (AHA) published a document entitled *Patient's Bill of Rights* (Boyd et al., 1998). A copy of these patient rights are framed and posted in a public place in every hospital and healthcare agency across the United States. Also, federal standards of the Health Care Financing Administration (HCFA) require every patient to be provided with a personal copy of these rights either at the time of admission to the hospital or long-term care facility or prior to the initiation of treatment when admitted to a health maintenance organization, home care, or hospice. Many states have adopted the statement of patient rights as part of the state health code, which places these rights under the jurisdiction of the law. This means that neglect of these rights can result in fines, prison sentences, or both for any guilty party.

APPLICATION OF ETHICAL PRINCIPLES TO PATIENT TEACHING

Six major ethical principles are woven through the ANA's *Code of Ethics for Nurses* and the AHA's *Patient's Bill of Rights*. These principles support the federal government's concern for ethical behavior practices. They are autonomy, veracity, nonmalfeasance, confidentiality, beneficence, and justice.

Autonomy

Autonomy refers to an individual's right to make his or her own decisions regarding medical treatment and healthcare services. Laws have been passed at the federal level to protect the patient's right to personal decision making based on the principle of informed consent. This means that the patient must be fully informed about his or her condition and be fully aware of what to expect as a result of medical treatment. Federal laws regarding informed consent are found in every application submitted for federal dollars to support biomedical research. The local IRBs are responsible for making sure that those conducting research involving human subjects are observing these regulations. The Patient Self-Determination Act (PSDA) passed by the U.S. Congress on December 1, 1991, is a good example of a law mandating autonomy. Any healthcare facility, such as a hospital or nursing home, HMO, hospice, or home care agency, receiving Medicare and/or Medicaid funds must adhere to regulations spelled out in the PSDA. The law requires, either at the time of hospital admission or before the initiation of treatment, "that every individual receiving health care be informed in writing of the right under state law to make decisions about his or her health care, including the right to refuse medical and surgical care and the right to initiate advance directives" (Mezey, Evans, Golub, Murphy, & White, 1994, p. 30). These authors point out that it is the nurse's responsibility to guarantee informed decision making by patients, which includes living wills and health care proxies. Documentation of such instruction must be noted in the patient record, which is the legal document guaranteeing that informed consent took place.

Although health teaching is not directly mentioned in the principle of autonomy, it is an important part of the ethical concept of assisting people to gain more independence, to avoid illness, and to keep themselves well. In fact, all nurse practice acts address patient teaching as a legal responsibility of the registered nurse.

Veracity

Veracity, or truth telling, is closely connected to informed decision making and informed consent. The Cardozo decision (*Schloendorff v. Society of New York Hospitals* [Smith, 1987]) legally protects an individual's basic right to make decisions about his or her own body. It provides a basis in law for patient teaching regarding invasive medical procedures requiring surgery, insertion of needles, or insertion of an instrument into a body cavity, such as the throat or colon. This includes being truthful about risks or benefits involved in these procedures (Boyd et al., 1998; Rankin & Stallings, 2001).

Nurses are often faced with ethical dilemmas related to truth telling. For example, the *Tuma* case (Rankin & Stallings, 1990) involved a nurse who gave a patient full information about choices in her medical treatment. Contrary to physician instruction, Nurse Tuma informed the patient of additional treatment options. She was eventually found innocent of professional misconduct charges, but the case emphasized a significant point of law found in the New York State Nurse Practice Act (1972). This law states, "A nursing regimen shall be consistent with and shall not vary any existing medical regimen." Such language in the law can create a problem for the nurse because the failure or omission to properly instruct the patient relative to invasive procedures is equivalent to inflicting physical harm on the patient (Creighton, 1986).

Truth telling also pertains to the role of the nurse as an expert witness. Professional nurses who are recognized for their skill or expertise in a particular area of nursing practice may be called on to testify in court on behalf of either the plaintiff (the one who is suing) or the defendant (the one being sued). The concept of truth telling in expert testimony speaks for itself—the requirement under oath to tell the truth.

Nonmalfeasance

Nonmalfeasance means "do no harm." This principle is at the heart of legal decisions concerning malpractice or negligence. In 1962, Lesnik and Anderson stated, "The term *negligence* refers to the doing or non-doing of an act, pursuant to a duty, that a reasonable person in the same circumstances would or would not do and the acting or the non-acting is the proximate cause of injury to another person or his property" (p. 234). In other words, Brent (2001) explains negligence as "conduct which falls below the standard established by law for the protection of others against unreasonable risk of harm" (p. 54).

The term *malpractice*, on the other hand, "refers to a limited class of negligent activities committed within the scope of performance by those pursuing a particular profession involving highly skilled and technical services" (Lesnik & Anderson, 1962, p. 234). This means that malpractice is limited to those whose profession requires special education and training, whereas negligence involves all improper or wrongful behavior by anyone resulting from any activity.

The concept of *duty* is closely related to the meaning of malpractice and negligence. Nurses' duties are spelled out in job descriptions at places of employment. Policy and procedure manuals exist to protect the patient, but they also exist to protect the employee (nurse) and the facility against lawsuits. Policies are more than guidelines. Policies and procedures contain standards of behavior (duties) expected of employees of a particular institution and can be used in court when there is a question of negligence or malpractice. Expectations of professional nursing performance are also measured against the nurse's level of education and skills, standing orders and protocols of an agency, standards of care published by the profession (ANA), and standards of care published by various clinical specialty organizations of which the nurse may be a member (Yoder Wise, 1995). If the nurse is certified in a clinical specialty or identifies him- or herself as a "specialist" although not certified, he or she will be held to the standards of that specialty (Smith, 1987).

When there is a lawsuit, an important point to remember is that the nurse is not necessarily held to the highest of professional standards of performance. Rather, the nurse is evaluated by the acceptable practice of what a prudent and reasonable nurse would do under the same circumstances in a given community. This means that the nurse's duty of patient teaching (or lack of it) must be compliant with the policy of the employing institution and it must also be compliant with acceptable practice in the geographical area in which the nurse practices.

Confidentiality

Confidentiality means protection of privileged information. In legal terms, confidentiality refers to a social contract or a covenant between the nurse and the patient. The nurse–patient relationship is considered privileged in most states. This means that the nurse may not reveal personal information gained in a professional capacity from a patient without the consent of the patient ". . . unless the patient has been the victim or subject of a crime, the commission of which is the subject of legal proceedings in which the nurse is a witness" (Lesnik & Anderson, 1962, p. 48). For example, the diagnosis of acquired immune deficiency syndrome (AIDS) has been protected as privileged and confidential information by state laws, regardless of the fact that AIDS is a communicable disease. Only in some states is it legal under certain conditions, such as death or impending death, for members of the family or a spouse to be told of the patient's diagnosis if it is not already known. The question of the moral obligation of the person with AIDS to tell others about his or her condition for their own protection has not yet been resolved.

Beneficence

Beneficence, which means "do good," is the requirement to perform critical tasks and duties in care of patients as specified in job descriptions, policies and procedures published and distributed by the healthcare facility, and standards and codes of ethics published and distributed by professional nursing organizations. These various performance standards include providing adequate and up-to-date patient teaching. The act of beneficence validates the nurse's commitment to do what is in the best interest of the patient, emphasizing patient safety and providing sufficient information to allow for optimal independence in self-care.

Justice

Justice refers to fairness and equality when distributing goods and services. Justice is intended to provide equal treatment for all in legal matters. Laws are intended to protect society. The focus of health law is the protection of the patient. The *Patient's Bill of Rights* is enforced as law in most states. That is, the nurse or any other health professional can be fined or sued for discrimination in the provision of care.

When a nurse is employed by a healthcare facility, that nurse enters into a contract, either written or understood, to provide nursing services in accordance with the policies of that facility. Failure to provide nursing care or providing less than quality care (including sufficient patient teaching) based on patient diagnosis or discriminating on the basis of someone's culture, national origin, sexual orientation, and the like can result in being liable for breaking a contract with the employing institution.

PATIENTS' RIGHTS TO INFORMATION

The patient's right to proper information regarding his or her physical condition, medications, risks, and access to information regarding other available treatments is published in the AHA's *Patient's Bill of Rights* (1975). As stated earlier, states have adopted these rights as part of their health code, which makes these rights legal and enforceable by law. Also, patients' rights to education are regulated in standards published by accrediting bodies such as the Joint Commission on Accreditation of Healthcare Organizations (JCAHO). Although these standards are not laws, lack of compliance with the standards by institutions or agencies can lead to loss of accreditation, which in turn places the facility in danger of losing reimbursement by insurance companies. State regulations pertaining to patient education are published and enforced under threat of penalty (fine, citation, or both) by the Department of Health in many states. Federal regulations also are enforceable as laws, and require patient education in those healthcare facilities that receive Medicare and Medicaid funding. The federal government also requires that the patient be well informed when participating in biomedical research or in any federally funded project involving human subjects.

Although federal authorities have tended to hold physicians responsible and accountable for proper patient education, particularly as this pertains to issues of informed consent (*Scakia v. St. Paul Fire and Marine Ins. Co.*, 1975 [Smith, 1987]), this task usually falls to the nurse. Despite the fact that from a professional and legal perspective, physicians are responsible for patient teaching, nurses also are required by their respective nurse practice acts to teach the patient. Often, the issue regarding patient education is not that the nurse failed to teach, but rather that proper documentation was lacking to indicate that appropriate teaching did occur.

THE IMPORTANCE OF DOCUMENTATION

The 89th Congress passed the Comprehensive Health Planning Act into law in 1965 (Public Law 89-97, 1965), establishing the programs of Medicare and Medicaid, which totally changed the provision of health care for the elderly and the poor. Provisions in the act stress the importance of prevention and rehabilitation. To qualify for Medicare and Medicaid reimbursement, "a hospital has to show evidence that patient teaching has been a part of patient care" (Boyd et al., 1998, p. 21). For a number of years, JCAHO has supported the federal law of requiring evidence through documentation of patient and/or family teaching in the patient record. The doctrine of *respondeat superior*, or the "master–servant" rule, holds the employer responsible for neglect, bodily harm, unauthorized use of body restraints, violating a patient's good name (possibly through a breach of confidentiality), or any other wrong-doing committed by an employee (Lesnik & Anderson, 1962). The critical case upholding the doctrine of *respondeat superior* in the healthcare field was the 1965 case of *Darling v. Charleston [S.C.] Memorial Hospital*. In brief, although the *Darling* case dealt with negligence in the performance of professional duties by the physician, it also brought to light the professional obligation of nurses to ensure the well-being of the patient.

Haggard (1989) points out that of all omissions in documentation, patient teaching "is probably the most undocumented skilled service because nurses do not recognize the scope and depth of the teaching they do" (p. 144). Lack of documentation also shows neglect in carrying out the role of the nurse as specified in nurse practice acts. Appropriate documentation can be the critical factor in the outcome of a lawsuit. An old rule of thumb is "if the instruction isn't documented, instruction didn't occur!" Also, documentation is a means of communication that provides critical information to other healthcare professionals involved with the patient's care. Failure to document not only puts other staff at risk for a lawsuit, but also puts the facility at risk of losing accreditation, as well as possibly losing Medicare and Medicaid reimbursement. In any lawsuit where the doctrine of *respondeat superior* is applied, the organization responsible for damages must pay money to those who won the lawsuit. It is, therefore, very important that nurses provide patient education and document it appropriately. It is also vitally important that nurses are aware of the legal and financial consequences to the healthcare facility in which they are employed.

Table 2-1 outlines the connections between ethical principles and the law. Note that the *Patient's Bill of Rights* (1975) is linked to or associated with every ethical principle. The *Patient's Bill of Rights* specifies conditions of participation in Medicare set forth under federal standards of the Center for Medicare/Medicaid Services (CMS). These rights are further emphasized in the accreditation standards published by JCAHO. All serve to ensure the fundamental rights of every person who receives healthcare services.

TABLE 2-1   Links between Ethical Principles and the Law

Principle	Law
Autonomy (self-determination)	Cardozo decision regarding informed consent Institutional review boards Patient Self-Determination Act *Patient's Bill of Rights* JCAHO/CMS standards
Veracity (truth telling)	Cardozo decision regarding informed consent *Patient's Bill of Rights* *Tuma* decision JCAHO/CMS standards
Confidentiality (privileged information)	*Patient's Bill of Rights* JCAHO/CMS standards
Nonmalfeasance (do no harm)	Malpractice/negligence rights and duties Nurse practice acts *Patient's Bill of Rights* *Darling v. Charleston Memorial Hospital* State health codes JCAHO/CMS standards
Beneficence (do good)	*Patient's Bill of Rights* State health codes Job descriptions Standards of practice Policy and procedure manuals JCAHO/CMS standards
Justice (equal distribution of benefits and burdens)	*Patient's Bill of Rights* Antidiscrimination/affirmative action laws Americans with Disabilities Act

ECONOMIC FACTORS OF PATIENT EDUCATION

In addition to the legal aspects of complying with regulations in health care no matter how much it costs, there are also ethical aspects of justice and duty related to quality of care issues. The client, as a unique person, has a right to good care regardless of ability to pay or attributes of gender, religion, or sexual orientation. Health professionals have a duty to see to it that these services are provided. The principle of justice must be applied to the delivery of patient education, the purpose of which is to help clients reach an optimal level of self-care. Rapid changes in the modern healthcare system seem to go against the humanitarian and charitable traits that have been the hallmark of healthcare services in this country for many years. Organizations providing such services find themselves caught between the reality of shrinking income, which in turn requires shorter patient stays in hospitals, and the expectation of providing more services for less money, as well as extending clinical services into outpatient and home care.

Any healthcare organization has the right to expect that it will receive its fair share of reimbursable revenues (money) for services rendered. However, to receive Medicare and Medicaid funding and to maintain accreditation by JCAHO, these organizations are also required to comply with the same standards of care addressed in the *Patient's Bill of Rights* (AHA, 1975). Although there are some exceptions (e.g., home healthcare agencies), accreditation of hospitals is a necessary requirement in both the public and private sectors to be eligible to receive third-party reimbursement.

These same "charitable," not-for-profit organizations are not immune to lawsuits as they were in the past. The potential for one or more lawsuits can pose a significant financial burden for any institution. In a Supreme Court decision regarding *Abernathy v. Sisters of St. Mary's* in 1969, the court stated that "a non-governmental charitable institution is liable for its own negligence and the negligence of its agents and employees acting within the scope of their employment" (Strader, 1985, p. 364). The nurse, as an employee, has a duty to carry out organizational policies and procedures in an accountable and responsible manner. This includes showing fiscal accountability for patient education activities, whether these are offered on an inpatient basis or as a service to the community.

At a time of shrinking healthcare dollars, nursing shortages, and shortened lengths of stay, the facility is still obligated to ensure the competency of nursing staff to provide educational services and to do so in the most efficient and cost-effective manner possible.

Understanding costs of educational programs within any healthcare facility requires an overview of financial terminology. Patient education is not a free service.

The expenses associated with personnel hours, equipment, and supplies must be taken into consideration. In general, costs are divided into two categories: direct and indirect.

Direct Costs

Direct costs include personnel salaries, employment benefits, and equipment (Gift, 1994). This portion of an organizational budget is always the largest and usually accounts for up to 80% of the total projected expenditure of any healthcare facility.

The department of nursing, as a labor-intensive division of any hospital, often uses up to 50% of its total budget to pay for nurses' salaries and benefits. The higher the educational level of the nursing staff, the higher the cost in salaries and benefits to the institution.

Although the purpose of a salary is to buy employee time and expertise, it is often difficult to predict how long it will take to plan, carry out, and evaluate the various educational programs being offered. For example, if patient teaching exceeds the time allocated and the nurse draws overtime pay, the extra cost may not have been planned for in the budget planning process. In addition, no organization can function without proper equipment and the need to replace it when necessary. Teaching requires such equipment as overhead projectors, slide projectors, blackboards, and copying machines. Although there may be times when renting or leasing equipment is less expensive than purchasing it, rental and leasing costs are still categorized as direct costs.

Time is a direct cost, and is a major factor considered in a cost-benefit analysis. This means that if it costs more to offer patient education programs than the facility planned, the organization may look for other ways of providing this service, such as computerized instruction or a patient television channel.

Direct costs are divided into two categories: fixed and variable. Fixed costs are those that remain the same over time and can be controlled. Salaries, for example, are fixed costs because they remain relatively stable and are also manipulated. Annual decisions are made by facilities to give employee raises, to freeze salaries, or to cut positions, thereby influencing the budget for direct cost expenditures. Also, mortgages, loan repayments, and the like are included as fixed costs.

Variable costs are those that depend on volume, in the case of healthcare organizations. The number of meals prepared, for example, depends on the patient census. From an educational perspective, the demand for patient teaching depends on the number and type of hospitalized patients. For example, if the volume of diabetic patients is low, educational costs may be high due to the fact that intensive one-to-one teaching would need to be offered for each patient admitted to the facility. If the volume of diabetic patients is high, it is less expensive to standardize programs and provide instruction for the diabetic clientele. Supplies, also a direct cost, can vary depending on volume. Variable costs can become fixed costs when volume remains consistently high or low.

Indirect Costs

Indirect costs are those not directly related to the actual delivery of an educational program. These include, but are not limited to, institutional overhead such as heating and air conditioning, lighting, and space, as well as support services of maintenance, housekeeping, and security (Gift, 1994).

Hidden costs, another type of indirect cost, can be neither expected nor accounted for until after the fact. Budgets are prepared on the basis of what is known, with variability of patient census included. Personnel budgets are based on levels of staff needed to accommodate expected patient census. This is determined by an annual projection of patient days and how many patients an employee can effectively care for on a daily basis. Low productivity of one or two people on the nursing unit can have a direct impact on the workload of others, which, in turn, can lead to low morale and employee turnover. Turnover increases recruitment and new employee orientation costs. These unexpected costs are appropriately identified as "hidden."

Cost Savings, Cost Benefit, and Cost Recovery

Although patient teaching is required by state laws and professional and institutional standards, unless it is ordered by a physician, these costs are generally not directly covered by insurance. The cost of patient teaching by nurses is usually included in the hospital room rate, and in this way is absorbed by the facility. Under diagnosis related groupings (DRGs), as a result of the managed care movement, reimbursement is based on a certain projected length of stay for each type of patient diagnosis. How long patients remain hospitalized and how often they are readmitted depends, to a large extent, on the effectiveness of patient teaching. Patients' understanding of how to care for themselves so that they can be discharged safely within a designated DRG time frame is a critical factor in reducing costs to the agency.

Hospitals realize *cost savings* when patient lengths of stay are shortened or fall within the allotted DRG time frame. Patients who have fewer complications and use less expensive services will yield a cost savings for the institution. In an ambulatory care setting such as an HMO, cost savings are realized when patient education keeps people healthy and independent longer, which prevents high use of expensive diagnostic testing and services.

Cost benefit occurs when patient satisfaction with an institution is increased as a result of the services it renders, including the educational programs it provides such as childbirth classes, stress reduction sessions, and cardiac fitness and rehabilitation programs. This is an opportunity for an institution to "capture" a patient population for lifetime coverage. Patient satisfaction is critical for the individual's return for future services.

Cost recovery results when an educational program charges a fee for its services. No matter whether a client is charged in full or pays on a sliding scale basis for the services, the American mentality is "if it costs something, it must be worth something." Thus, fee for service programs usually are well attended and result in revenues for the institution.

To control costs to realize cost savings, cost benefit, or cost recovery, healthcare organizations have developed other ways to deliver patient education. For example, a preoperative teaching program for surgical patients given prior to admission to the hospital has been found to lower patient anxiety, increase patient satisfaction, and decrease nursing care hours during hospitalization (Wasson & Anderson, 1993).

Program Planning and Implementation

The key elements to consider when planning a patient education program include an accurate assessment of direct costs such as paper supplies, printing of program brochures, publicity, rental space, and the time (based on an hourly rate) required of professional personnel to prepare and offer the service. However, indirect costs such as housekeeping and security, if needed, should be included as a legitimate cost of the program. Fees for the program should be set at a level high enough to cover all the costs of program preparation and delivery. If the goal is for cost savings to the facility, such as provision of diabetic education classes in the community to reduce the number of costly hospital admissions, then the aim may be to break even on costs. The price is set by dividing the number of anticipated participants attending into the estimated cost. If the goal is for cost benefit to the institution, success can be measured by increased patient satisfaction (as determined by questionnaires) or by an increase in the use of the sponsor's services (as determined by record keeping). If the intent is to offer a series of classes for smoking cessation or childbirth education to improve the wellness of the community and to increase income for the facility, then the price is set higher than cost so that a profit is made (cost recovery). Usually, it is necessary to give an annual report to administration of time and money spent and whether such expenditures were profitable to the institution in terms of cost savings, cost benefit, or cost recovery.

Cost-Benefit Analysis and Cost-Effectiveness Analysis

Cost-benefit analysis refers to determining the relationship between costs and outcomes that are easily measured. Outcomes can be the actual amount of money earned from providing an educational program, or can be the length of patient stays or the number of hospitalizations for particular diagnostic groups of patients. If the program costs less than the money that was earned in running the program, if costs can be recovered by insurance, or if savings to the institution are greater than the costs, the program is considered a cost benefit. The measurement of costs against monetary gain is commonly referred to as the *cost-benefit ratio* (Kelly, 1985).

Cost-effectiveness analysis refers to the impact an educational program has on patient behavior. If program objectives are achieved, as evidenced by positive and sustained change in the behavior of the participants over time, the program is said to be cost-effective. Although behavioral changes are highly desirable, many times they are less observable and not easily measured. For example, a lessening of patient anxiety cannot be converted into a gain in real dollars. Therefore, it is wise to analyze the outcome of teaching interventions by comparing behavioral outcomes between two or more programs to identify the one that is most cost-efficient and cost-effective.

SUMMARY

Ethical and legal aspects of human rights justify patient teaching, particularly as teaching relates to self-determination and informed consent. These rights are enforced through federal and state regulations and through performance standards put forth by accrediting bodies and professional nursing organizations. The role of the nurse as teacher is evident through the definition of nursing found in the nurse practice acts in the states where nurses reside and practice. In this respect, patient teaching is a nursing duty that is grounded in justice. The nurse has a legal responsibility to provide patient education to each and every patient regardless of their beliefs and values, socioeconomic status, or educational background. All patients have a right to learn about their medical condition. Patient education programs must be designed to meet the needs of patients to be informed, capable of self-direction, and in control of their own health.

REVIEW QUESTIONS _____

1. What are the definitions of the terms *ethical, moral,* and *legal?*
2. How do the terms identified in Question 1 differ from one another?
3. Which national, state, professional, and private sector organizations legislate, regulate, and provide standards to ensure the protection of human rights in matters of health care?
4. How does the American Hospital Association's *Patient's Bill of Rights* compare to the American Nurses Association's *Code of Ethics for Nurses with Interpretive Statements* with respect to ethical, moral, and legal obligations of the nurse?
5. What are the six ethical principles that dictate the actions of healthcare providers in delivering services to clients?
6. Why are nurse practice acts so important to nurses in carrying out their roles and responsibilities to the public?
7. What is the difference between the terms *negligence* and *malpractice?*
8. What is the nurse's role in situations involving informed consent?
9. What is meant by the legal term *respondeat superior,* and how does this term apply to professional nursing practice?
10. Why is documentation of professional nursing duties, particularly patient education, so important in the delivery of care by nurses?
11. What are the two categories of costs, and how are they defined? Give examples.
12. What are the definitions of these terms: *fixed direct costs, variable direct costs, indirect costs, cost savings, cost benefit, cost recovery, cost-benefit analysis,* and *cost-effectiveness analysis?*

REFERENCES _____

Abernathy v. Sisters of St. Mary's, 446 SW2d 559 (MO 1969).

American Hospital Association. (1975). *Patient's Bill of Rights.* Chicago: Author.

American Nurses Association. (1976, 1985). *Code for Nurses with Interpretive Statements.* Kansas City, MO: Author.

American Nurses Association. (2001). *Code of Ethics for Nurses with Interpretive Statements.* Washington, DC: Author.

Boyd, M. D., Gleit, C. J., Graham, B. A., & Whitman, N. I. (1998). *Health teaching in nursing practice: A professional model* (3rd ed.). Stamford, CT: Appleton & Lange.

Brent, N. J. (2001). *Nurses and the law* (2nd ed.). Philadelphia: Saunders.

Creighton, H. (1986). Informed consent. *Nursing Management, 17*(10), 11–13.

Darling v. Charleston Memorial Hospital, 211 NE2d 253 (IL 1965).

Gift, A. E. (1994). Understanding costs. *Clinical Nurse Specialist, 8*(2), 90.

Haggard, A. (1989). *Handbook of patient education*. Rockville, MD: Aspen.

Health Care Financing Administration. (1997). *The Balanced Budget Act of 1997*. (P.L. 105-33). Washington, DC: Office of Legislation.

Kelly, K. J. (1985). Cost-benefit and cost-effectiveness analysis: Tools for the staff development manager. *Journal of Nursing Staff Development, 6*(2), 9–15.

Lesnick, M. J. & Anderson, B. E. (1962). *Nursing practice and the law*. Philadelphia: Lippincott.

Mezey, M., Evans, L. K., Golub, Z. D., Murphy, E., & White, G. B. (1994). The patient self-determination act: Sources of concern for nurses. *Nursing Outlook, 42*(1), 30–38.

New York State Nurses' Association. (1972). New York State Nurse Practice Act. Albany, NY: Author.

Rankin, S. H. & Stallings, K. D. (1990). *Patient education: Issues, principles, practices*. Philadelphia: Lippincott.

Rankin, S. H. & Stallings, K. D. (2001). *Patient education: Principles & practices* (4th ed.). Philadelphia: Lippincott.

Smith, C. E. (1987). *Patient education: Nurses in partnership with other health professionals*. Philadelphia: Saunders.

Strader, M. K. (1985). Malpractice and nurse educators: Defining legal responsibilities. *Journal of Nursing Education, 24*(9), 363–367.

Thomas, S. B. & Quinn, S. C. (1991). Public health then and now. The Tuskegee syphilis study, 1932 to 1972: Implications for HIV education programs in the Black community. *American Journal of Public Health, 81*(11), 1498–1505.

Wasson, D. & Anderson, M. A. (1993). Hospital-patient education: Current status and future trends. *Journal of Nursing Staff Development, 10*(3), 147–151.

Weisbard, A. J. & Arras, J. D. (1984). Commissioning morality: An introduction to the symposium. *Cardozo Law Review, 6*(4), 223–241.

Whitman, N. I., Graham, B. A., Gleit, C. J., & Boyd, M. D. (1992). *Teaching in nursing practice: A professional model*. Norwalk, CT: Appleton & Lange.

Yoder-Wise, P. S. (1995). *Leading and managing in nursing*. St. Louis: Mosby.

CHAPTER 3

Applying Learning Theories to Health Care

Margaret M. Braungart
Richard G. Braungart

CHAPTER HIGHLIGHTS

Learning Theories
   Behaviorist Learning Theory
   Cognitive Learning Theory
   Social Learning Theory
   Psychodynamic Learning Theory
   Humanistic Learning Theory

Applying Learning Theories to Health Care
   How Does Learning Occur in the
     Healthcare Setting?
   What Kinds of Experiences Help or
     Hinder Learning?
   What Helps Learning Become Relatively
     Permanent?

KEY TERMS

behaviorist learning theory
cognitive development
cognitive learning theory
gestalt perspective
humanistic learning theory
information processing
learning

operant conditioning
psychodynamic learning theory
respondent conditioning
social cognition
social learning theory
spontaneous recovery
theories of learning

OBJECTIVES

After completing this chapter, the reader will be able to

1. Discuss the major differences in how teaching and learning are approached in the five learning theories.
2. Describe the role of the teacher according to each theory.
3. Identify at least three ways to motivate learners based on the learning theories.
4. Outline how to teach patients new information using different learning theories.
5. Indicate how learning theories are used to change attitudes and behaviors.

*L*earning is defined in this chapter as a relatively permanent change in thinking, emotional functioning, and/or behavior as a result of experience. It is the process by which individuals gain new knowledge and skills or change their attitudes and behaviors. Although people in every culture have beliefs about how teaching and learning should occur, psychologists have developed several major *theories of learning* that have been tested with research. Each theory describes or explains how learning occurs and has its own vocabulary, perspective on learning, and generalizations about teaching and learning. These learning theories are widely applicable and provide the foundation for primary and secondary education, health education, psychological and psychiatric counseling, and workplace organization and human resource management, as well as marketing and advertising.

Used singly or in combination, learning theories have much to offer the practice of health care and medicine—whether teaching patients information about their health and self-care, trying to improve communication and interpersonal relationships, struggling to become a more effective learner yourself, or endeavoring to change behavior and break bad habits. Increasingly, health professionals must demonstrate that they employ sound methods and clear reasons when they attempt to teach health information or encourage changes in patients' health attitudes and behavior. Beyond professional use, however, knowledge of the learning process relates to nearly every aspect of daily life. Psychological principles of learning can be applied at the individual, group, organizational, and community levels to understand people's behavior, learn and teach more effectively, solve problems, manage emotions, and build constructive relationships.

The purpose of this chapter is to review five major psychological theories of learning. The behaviorist, cognitive, and social learning theories are most often applied to patient education and healthcare practice (Redman, 2001). In addition, it is argued in this chapter that emotions and feelings are critical to understanding learning, especially in a healthcare setting. Emotional reactions are often learned as a result of experience, they play a significant role in the learning process, and they are an important consideration when dealing with health, disease, stress, relapse prevention, wellness, medical treatment, recovery, and healing. Although not always treated as learning theories in psychology (Hilgard & Bower, 1966), the psychodynamic theory and the humanistic theory are included in this review because they add much to our understanding of human motivation, emotions, and the learning process.

The chapter is organized as follows. First, the learning theories are each described and illustrated with examples from health care. Next, the theories are applied to healthcare practice by discussing how learning occurs, the kinds of experiences that encourage learning, and ways to ensure that learning lasts and is relatively permanent.

The goals of this discussion are to provide a framework for understanding subsequent chapters in this book and to offer a toolbox of approaches that can be used to encourage learning and change in patients, oneself, and others. After completing the chapter, readers should be able to describe basic principles of learning, discuss various ways in which teaching and learning can be approached, and develop alternative strategies to increase knowledge and change attitudes and behaviors in different settings.

LEARNING THEORIES

This section summarizes some of the basic principles of the behaviorist, cognitive, social learning, psychodynamic, and humanistic theories. While reviewing these theories, readers are asked to consider the following questions:

- What is the basic focus of each theory in explaining how learning and motivation occur?
- What motivates individuals to learn?
- What is the role of the teacher in the learning process?

Behaviorist Learning Theory

According to the *behaviorist theory*, learning is the result of connections made between the stimulus conditions in the environment (S) and the individual's responses (R)—sometimes termed the S-R model of learning. Whether dealing with animals or people, the learning process is relatively simple. Generally ignoring what goes on inside the individual, behaviorists closely observe a person's responses to the environment and then manipulate stimuli in the environment to bring about learning and behavior change (Bigge & Shermis, 1992; Hilgard & Bower, 1966).

To encourage people to learn new information or to change their attitudes and responses, behaviorists recommend altering conditions in the environment and reinforcing positive behaviors after they occur. Motivation is explained as the need to reduce some drive, such as the desire for food, security, recognition, or money. This is why individuals who are satisfied or have what they want may have little motivation to learn new behaviors or change old behaviors. Getting behavior to transfer from the initial learning situation to other settings is largely a matter of practice and making sure there is a similarity in the stimuli and responses in the initial learning situation and future situations where the behavior is expected to occur. Essentially, there are two ways to change behavior and encourage learning using behaviorist principles: respondent conditioning and operant conditioning.

First identified and demonstrated by the Russian physiologist Ivan Pavlov, *respondent conditioning* emphasizes the importance of stimulus conditions in the environment and the associations formed in the learning process (Klein & Mowrer, 1989). Although it may seem complicated at first, the explanation for learning or conditioning is really quite simple. A neutral stimulus (NS)—a stimulus that has no particular value or meaning to the learner—is paired with a naturally occurring unconditioned or unlearned stimulus (UCS) and unconditioned response (UCR) (Figure 3-1). After a few such pairings, the neutral stimulus alone, without the unconditioned stimulus, will elicit the same response. Often without thought or awareness, learning occurs when the newly conditioned stimulus (CS) becomes associated with the conditioned response (CR).

Consider an example from health care. Someone without much experience with hospitals (NS) may visit a sick relative (see Figure 3-1). While in the relative's room, the

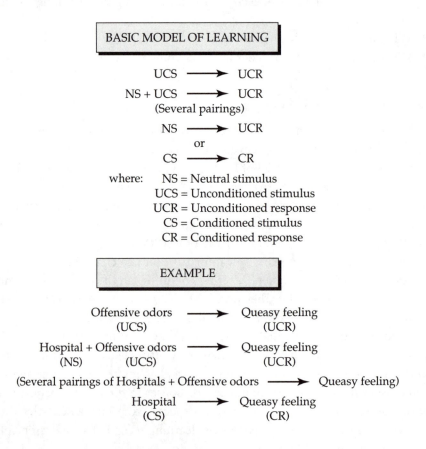

FIGURE 3-1   Respondent Conditioning Model of Learning

visitor may smell odors (UCS) that make him feel queasy and light-headed (UCR). After his first visit, his subsequent visits to hospitals (now the CS) may become associated with feeling anxious and nauseated (CR), especially if the visitor smells odors similar to those encountered during the first experience. Respondent conditioning highlights the importance of what is going on in the environment in health care. Patients and visitors form associations as a result of their hospital experiences, which may well provide the basis for long-lasting attitudes toward medicine, healthcare facilities, and health professionals.

Principles of respondent conditioning also may be used to get rid of or extinguish a previously learned response, which has been found to be especially useful in teaching people to reduce their anxiety or break bad habits. In this case, old responses or habits can be weakened if the presentation of the conditioned stimulus is not accompanied by the unconditioned stimulus at different times. Thus, if the visitor who became dizzy in one hospital (CS) then goes to other hospitals to see relatives or friends without smelling offensive odors (UCS), then his discomfort and anxiety about hospitals may lessen after several such experiences, and he has learned—or been conditioned to—a new response to hospitals (CR).

In respondent conditioning, the teacher works with the conditions in the environment to encourage the learner to build new associations for learning. The techniques of respondent conditioning are used often in advertising to get people to buy a particular product and in counseling to alter people's reactions and get them to respond in a different way to a particular situation. No thinking is required. Drug companies, for example, use principles of respondent conditioning to foster brand name recognition and to get people to associate their drug with feeling better, feeling more energetic, and having a better life.

In health care, respondent conditioning has been used to treat addictions, phobias, and tension. For example, taking the time to help patients relax and reduce their anxiety when applying some medical treatment lessens the likelihood that patients will build up negative and anxious reactions to medicine and health care. It is worth noting that although a response may appear to be extinguished, it may "recover" and reappear at any time (even years later), especially when stimulus conditions are similar to those in the initial learning experience. This is called *spontaneous recovery*, which helps us understand why it is so difficult to completely eliminate unhealthy habits and addictive behaviors such as smoking, alcoholism, or drug abuse.

Operant conditioning is another behaviorist approach to learning, which was developed primarily by B. F. Skinner (1974). Operant conditioning focuses on the behavior of the individual and the reinforcement that occurs after a response. A reinforcer is something that happens after a response occurs that strengthens the probability that the response will be performed again under similar circumstances. Praise, hugs, money, and prizes are examples of positive reinforcers. When specific responses are reinforced on the proper schedule, behaviors can be either increased or decreased.

The best way to increase the probability that a response will occur again is to apply positive reinforcement or rewards after the behavior occurs. As an illustration, although a patient moans and groans as she attempts to get up and walk for the first time after an operation, praise and encouragement (reward) for her efforts at walking (response) will improve the chances that she will continue struggling toward independence.

Decreasing a response, such as breaking a bad habit, is accomplished by using either nonreinforcement or punishment. The simplest way is not to provide any kind of reinforcement (nonreinforcement) for some unwanted action. For example, unpleasant jokes in the workplace may be handled by showing no reaction. After several such experiences, the joke teller, who more than likely wants attention, may stop his or her use of obnoxious humor. Keep in mind, however, that desirable behavior that is ignored may lessen as well.

If nonreinforcement does not work, then punishment may be employed as a way to decrease responses. For example, if the obnoxious joke teller does not respond to nonreinforcement, then someone might announce that the joke is offensive to the group, which might serve as a punishment—unless, of course, the joke teller most wants attention, and to some people, negative attention is preferable to no attention. However, there are risks in using punishment, especially because the learner may become so emotionally upset (ashamed, sad, or angry) that he does not even remember why he is being punished. The purpose of punishment is not to do harm or to serve as a release for anger. The goal is to get someone's attention to decrease a specific behavior and teach self-discipline. If punishment is used as a last resort, it should be immediate, reasonable, and focused clearly on the behavior, not the person.

For operant conditioning to be effective, it is necessary to assess what kinds of reinforcements are likely to increase or decrease behaviors for each individual. Not every client, for example, finds health practitioners' terms of endearment rewarding. Comments such as "Very nice job, dear," may be offensive to some clients. A second issue involves the timing of reinforcement. The success of operant conditioning partially depends on when the reinforcement is applied. In the early stages, learning needs to be reinforced every time it occurs. Once a response is well established, however, behavior needs to be reinforced only every so often, because the goal is for the learner to internalize the response and build good habits without being supervised.

Operant conditioning techniques provide relatively quick and effective ways to change behavior. Carefully planned programs using behavior modification procedures have been applied to health care. For example, the families of chronic back pain patients have been taught to minimize their attention to the patients when they complain of pain and behave in dependent, helpless ways, but to pay a lot of attention when the patients attempt to function independently, express a positive attitude, and try to live as normal a life as possible. Some patients respond so well to operant conditioning that they report experiencing less pain as they become more active and involved. Operant conditioning has been found to work well with some nursing home and long-term care residents and with patients who are not very verbal or do not engage in much thought or reflection.

The behaviorist theory is simple and easy to use. It requires careful analysis of what is happening in the environment that affects people's behavior and what factors influence a person's responses. There are, however, some criticisms and cautions to consider. For one thing, learners are assumed to be relatively passive and easily manipulated, which raises the ethical question: Who is to decide what the "desirable" behavior should be? Too often the desired response is conformity and cooperation to make someone's job easier or more profitable. In addition, the theory's emphasis on rewards and incentives promotes materialistic values and doing things only for some personal gain. Another shortcoming of behaviorist techniques is that clients' changed behavior may weaken over time, especially once they are back in the environment that may have caused their problems in the first place. The basic principles of behaviorist learning are summarized as follows:

- Focus on the learner's drives, the external factors in the environment that influence a learner's associations, and on reinforcements that increase or decrease responses.
- The teacher's task is first to assess conditions in the environment that lead to specific responses, the learner's past habits and history of S-R connections, and what is reinforcing for a learner. Then teachers must effectively manipulate conditions to build new associations, provide appropriate reinforcement, and allow for practice to strengthen connections between stimuli in the environment and a person's responses or behavior.

We now move from focusing on responses and behavior to the role of mental processes in learning.

Cognitive Learning Theory

In contrast to behaviorist theory, *cognitive learning theory* focuses on what goes on "inside" the learner, especially learners' perceptions, thoughts, memory, and ways of processing and structuring information (Brien & Eastmond, 1994). According to this perspective, for individuals to learn, they must change their perceptions and thoughts and form new understandings and insights. The individual largely directs the learning process by organizing information based on what is already known, and then reorganizing the information into a new understanding. Cognitive theory currently is enjoying considerable popularity in education, counseling, and management.

Unlike behaviorism, cognitive psychologists maintain that rewarding people for their behavior is not necessary for learning. More important are the learner's goals and expectations, which create tensions that motivate them to act. Teachers and those trying to influence the learning process must recognize that any learning situation is affected by learners' past experiences, perceptions, and ways of incorporating and thinking about information in relation to their goals, expectations, and the social influences on the situation. To promote remembering, the learner must think about or "act on" the information. Similarities in the initial learning situation and subsequent situations aid memory and the ability to transfer learning from one situation to the next.

Within cognitive learning theory are several approaches to learning, such as gestalt, cognitive development, information processing, and social cognition. When pieced together these approaches indicate much about what goes on inside the learner. Each approach is briefly described.

The *gestalt perspective* is one of the oldest in psychology and emphasizes the importance of perception in learning. *Gestalt* is a German word that means configuration or pattern. A key assumption is that each person perceives, interprets, and responds to any situation in his or her own way (Kohler, 1969). Several gestalt principles will be discussed here as they apply to health care.

A basic gestalt principle is that people strive for simplicity, balance, and familiarity in organizing information and experiences. For example, consider the bewildered faces of some patients listening to a detailed, unclear explanation about their disease, when what they desire most is a simple explanation that settles their uncertainty and relates directly to them and their past experiences. Another central gestalt principle is that perception is selective, which has several implications. First, because no one can attend to all the surroundings at any given time, individuals pay attention to certain features of an experience while screening out or ignoring other features. As an illustration, patients in severe pain or worried about their hospital bills may not attend to medical information, no matter how well presented. Second, what people "select" to pay attention to and what they ignore are influenced by a host of factors, such as past experiences, needs, motives and attitudes, and the particular structure of the information and the situation. Because individuals vary widely with regard to these and other characteristics, they will perceive, interpret, and respond to the same event in different ways, perhaps distorting information to fit their goals, expectations, and what they want to hear. This tendency helps explain why an approach that is effective with one client may not work with another client. The gestalt perspective has had a strong influence on more recent cognitive approaches to learning.

A second approach involves *cognitive development*, which focuses on advancements and changes in perception, thought, and reasoning as individuals grow and mature. This approach is especially useful to know when working with children and teenagers. How information and experiences are perceived and represented depends on an individual's stage of development and readiness to learn. A principal assumption is that learning is a sequential and active process that occurs as the child interacts with the environment and makes discoveries, which are interpreted in keeping with what she knows and is capable of understanding.

Jean Piaget is the best-known cognitive development theorist, and his observations of children's perception and thought processes at different ages have contributed much to our understanding of the special ways that youngsters reason, the changes in their ability to reason, and the limitations in their ability to understand, communicate, and perform (Piaget & Inhelder, 1969). By watching, asking questions, and listening to children, Piaget identified and described four successive stages of cognitive development (sensorimotor, preoperational, concrete operations, and formal operations) that unfold sequentially over the course of infancy, early childhood, middle childhood, and adolescence. (See Chapter 5 for more on developmental stages.) According to his theory, children take in information as they interact with people and the environment. They may make their experiences fit with what they already know, or they may change their perceptions and interpretations in keeping with the new information.

According to Piaget (Piaget & Inhelder, 1969) there are four sequential stages of cognitive development: (1) the sensorimotor stage during infancy, where infants explore their environments and attempt to coordinate sensory information with motor skills; (2) the preoperational stage during early childhood, where youngsters are able to mentally represent the environment, regard the world from their own egocentric perspective, and come to grips with symbolization; (3) the concrete operations stage during the elementary school years, where children are able to attend to more than one dimension at a time, conceptualize relationships, and operate on the environment; and (4) the formal operations stage during adolescence, where teenagers begin to think abstractly, are able to deal with the future, and can see alternatives and criticize. Thus, health professionals and family members need to understand children's perceptions and reasoning in a given situation. As an illustration, young children usually do not really understand that death is final. They react to the experience in their own way, perhaps asking God to give back the dead person, or they may believe that if they act like a good person, the person who died will return soon to them (Gardner, 1978).

What does the cognitive development research indicate about adult learning? First, some adults never reach a formal operations stage of reasoning where they can think abstractly. These adults may learn better from simple, concrete approaches to health education. In addition, although some older adults may demonstrate an advanced level of judgment, others may reflect lower stages of thinking due to lack of education, disease, depression, stress, or the effects of medications. The implication is that whether dealing with children or adults, teachers must assess each person's level and style of cognitive reasoning as a first step in communicating and being effective in educating patients and their family members (or one's own children).

Information processing is a third cognitive approach, which emphasizes thought, reasoning, the way information is approached and stored, and memory functioning (Sternberg, 1996). How people store and recall information is useful for health professionals to know, especially in relation to learning in older adults. An information-processing model of memory functioning is illustrated in Figure 3-2.

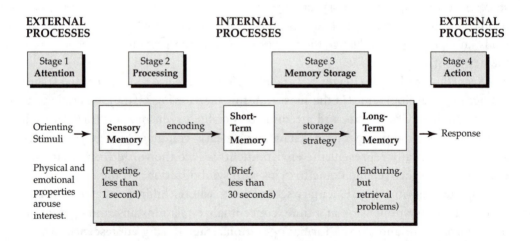

FIGURE 3-2 Information-Processing Model of Memory

The stages are described as follows:

- **Attention:** Certain information is focused on while other information in the environment is ignored. Attention is viewed as the key to learning. Thus, if a client is not concentrating on what a nurse is saying, it would be wise to try the explanation at another time when he or she is more receptive and attentive.
- **Sensory processing:** Information is processed by using one or more of the senses. Here it becomes important to consider the client's preferred mode of sensory learning (visual, hearing, or by using touch and motor skills). It is also important to determine whether there are sensory deficits, such as an older person whose hearing or sight is poor.
- **Short-term memory storage:** Information is briefly transferred into short-term memory (encoded), after which it is either disregarded and forgotten or stored for a longer period in long-term memory. Older adults may require extra effort and more time to process information through short-term memory.
- **Long-term memory storage:** Information is stored in long-term memory by using a strategy, such as forming a mental picture (visual imagery), associating the information with what is already known, repeating or rehearsing the information, or breaking the information into smaller units or chunks. Although long-term memories are enduring, a central problem is retrieving the stored information at a later time.
- **Action and response:** The action or response that the individual makes is based on how information was processed and stored. Responses need to be observed carefully in case corrections need to be made, although there is always a question as to whether any performance is a true indicator of someone's learning and competence. People may not really know the answer but guess correctly, or they may know the answer but do not perform correctly for some reason.

From this perspective, teaching involves assessing the ways that a learner attends to, processes, and stores the information that is presented as well as finding ways to encourage remembering and being able to recall the information. In general, cognitive psychologists note that memory is helped by organizing the information and making it meaningful. The instructor's job is to get in touch with the learner's cognitive style or ways of processing information and to appreciate and respect the different styles of thinking reflected among the many players in the healthcare setting (see Chapter 4 for more on learning styles).

The *social cognition* approach is a fourth perspective in cognitive psychology, which emphasizes the effects of social factors on perception, thought, and motivation (Berliner & Calfee, 1996; Fiske & Taylor, 1991). According to this view, the players in any healthcare setting would be expected to have differing perceptions, interpretations, and responses to a situation, which are strongly colored by their social and cultural experiences. For example, patients with certain religious views or a particular parental upbringing may believe that their disease is a punishment for their sins, whereas other patients may blame their disease on the actions of others. From this perspective, the route to changing health behaviors is to change distorted beliefs and explanations. It also has been argued that learning is a social process and that learning is encouraged by sharing beliefs, by discussing differing conceptions of a situation, and by negotiating to reach new levels of understanding (Marshall, 1998). Cooperative learning and self-help groups are examples of applying the social cognition approach to altering behavior. With America's rapidly changing age and ethnic composition, the social cognition approach will become especially useful in the healthcare setting.

When applied to health care, cognitive learning theory encourages an appreciation of the individuality and rich diversity in how people learn and process experiences. The challenge in teaching is to identify a learner's level of cognitive development, his or her goals and expectations, ways of perceiving and processing information, and the social influences that affect learning. Once identified, teachers can find ways to encourage new insights and to solve problems. To summarize, the basic principles of cognitive learning theory are as follows:

- Focus on internal factors within learners, such as their developmental stage of reasoning, perceptions, thoughts, ways of processing and storing information in memory, and the influence of social factors on attitudes, thoughts, and actions. Realize that learning is motivated by the learner's goals and expectations as well as a feeling of imbalance, tension, and a desire to restore equilibrium.
- The role of the teacher is first to assess each learner's developmental stage, goals and expectations, preferred style of learning, and ways of processing, storing, and retrieving information. The next steps are to foster curiosity (imbalance); organize learning experiences and make them meaningful; encourage understanding, insight, problem solving, and creativity in learners; and keep learning simple and at an appropriate level.

The next learning theory combines principles from both the behaviorist and cognitive theories.

Social Learning Theory

Most learning theories assume the individual must have direct experiences in order to learn. According to *social learning theory*, much of learning occurs by observation—watching other people and determining what happens to them. Learning is often a social process, and other individuals, especially "significant others," provide compelling examples or role models for how to think, feel, and act. While Miller and Dollard (1941) viewed social learning as a mixture of behaviorist and psychodynamic influences, Bandura (1977, 2001) is credited with outlining the behaviorist, cognitive, and, more recently, the social cognition dimensions of this theory. Figure 3-3 illustrates the dynamics of social learning based on Bandura's work.

Role modeling is a central concept of the theory. As an example, a more experienced nurse who demonstrates desirable professional attitudes and behavior sometimes is used as a mentor for a less experienced nurse, while medical students, interns, and residents are mentored by attending physicians. Vicarious reinforcement is another concept from the social learning theory and involves viewing other people's emotions and determining whether role models are rewarded or punished for their behavior. The behavior of a role model may be imitated, even when no reward is involved for either

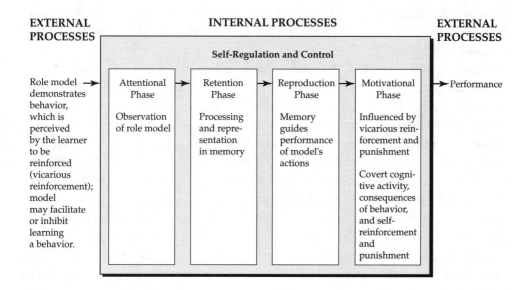

FIGURE 3-3 Social Learning Theory
Source: Based on Bandura (1977).

the role model or the learner. In many cases, however, whether the model is perceived by the observer to be rewarded or punished may have a direct influence on learning. This may be one reason why it is difficult to attract health professionals to geriatric care. Although some highly impressive role models work in the field, geriatric health care is often accorded low status within the health professions and may pay less than other specialty areas.

Although social learning theory is based partially on behaviorist principles, the self-regulation and the control that the individual exhibits in the learning process is critical and reflects cognitive principles. Bandura (1977) outlined a four-step, largely internal process that directs social learning. As seen in Figure 3-3, the first phase is the attentional phase, a necessary condition for any learning to occur. Research indicates that role models with high status and competence are more likely to be observed, although the learner's own characteristics (needs, self-esteem, competence) may be the more significant determiner of attention. Second is the retention phase, which involves the storage and retrieval of what was observed. Third is the reproduction phase, where the learner copies the observed behavior. Mental rehearsal, immediate enactment, and corrective feedback strengthen the reproduction of behavior. Fourth is the motivational phase, involving whether the learner is motivated to perform a certain type of behavior. Reinforcement or punishment for a role model's behavior, the learning situation, and the appropriateness of subsequent situations where the behavior is to be displayed all affect a learner's performance (Bandura, 1977; Gage & Berliner, 1998).

More recently, Bandura (2001) shifted his focus to sociocultural influences, viewing the learner as the agent through which learning experiences are filtered. As he argued, the human mind is not just reactive; it is "generative, creative, and reflective." Essentially, the individual engages in a transactional relationship between the social environment and the self, where sociocultural factors are mediated by "psychological mechanisms of the self-system to produce behavioral effects" (p. 4). In his model, he stressed the internal dynamics of personal selection, intentionality, self-regulation, self-efficacy, and self-evaluation in the learning process. This perspective applies particularly well to health behaviors and partially explains why some people select positive role models and effectively regulate their attitudes, emotions, and actions, whereas other people choose negative role models and engage in unhealthy and destructive behaviors. One of Bandura's (2001) principal research findings is that self-efficacy contributes to productive human functioning. The implication is that healthcare professionals need to find ways to encourage patients' feelings of competency and to promote wellness rather than fostering dependency, helplessness, and feelings of low self-worth.

The social learning theory extends the learning process beyond the teacher–learner relationship and directs experiences to the larger social world. The theory helps explain the socialization process as well as the breakdown of behavior in society. Responsibility is placed on the teacher or leader to be an exemplary role model and to choose socially healthy experiences for individuals to observe and repeat (requiring the careful evaluation of learning materials for stereotypes, mixed or hidden messages, and negative impacts). However, simple exposure to competent role models correctly performing a behavior that is rewarded (or performing some undesirable behavior that is punished) does not ensure learning. Attention to the learner's "self-system" and the dynamics of self-regulation may help sort out the varying effects of the social learning experience.

This organized approach to learning requires attention to the social environment, the behavior to be performed, and the individual learner. In health care, social learning theory has been applied to staff training and to interventions that address health problems such as alcoholism and teenage smoking. The major difficulty is that social learning theory is complex and not easily measured and assessed. The basic principles of social learning theory are as follows:

- Focus on role models, the reinforcement that a model has received, the social environment, and the four self-regulating processes within the learner.
- The role of the teacher is to act as a stellar role model, to use effective role models in teaching that are rewarded for their behavior, to assess the internal self-regulation of the learner, and to provide feedback for a learner's performance.

The final two theories to be reviewed in this chapter focus on the importance of emotions and feelings in the learning process.

Psychodynamic Learning Theory

Although not usually treated as a learning theory, some of the concepts from *psychodynamic theory* (based on the work of Sigmund Freud and his followers) have significant implications for learning and changing behavior (Notterman & Drewry, 1993). Largely a theory of motivation, the emphasis is on emotions rather than on responses to the environment or on perceptions and thoughts. A central principle of the theory is that behavior may be conscious or unconscious—in other words, people may or may not be aware of their motivations and why they feel, think, and act as they do.

According to the psychodynamic view of personality development, the most primitive source of motivation comes from the id, which involves our most basic instincts, impulses, and desires, such as aggression and the desire for pleasure and to live a full life or perhaps a wish for death and destruction. Patients who survive or die, despite all predictions to the contrary, provide an illustration of such motivations in action. The id, according to Freud, operates on the basis of the pleasure principle—to seek pleasure and avoid pain. For example, dry, dull lectures given by health professionals who go through the motions of instruction without much enthusiasm or emotion inspire few patients to listen, remember, or follow the advice. This does not mean, however, that only pleasurable presentations will be acceptable.

The id, with its primitive drives, is held in check by the superego, which involves the social values and standards children are taught. The superego forms the basis for a conscience. According to Freud, if a conscience is not formed by adolescence, it is unlikely to develop later in life. Because the id and the superego are in such conflict, they need to be mediated by the ego, which operates on the basis of the reality principle. Thus, rather than insisting on immediate gratification, people learn to take the long road to pleasure and to weigh the choices in the conflict between the id and superego.

Healthy ego (self) development is an important consideration in the health fields. For example, patients with ego strength can cope with painful medical treatments because they recognize the long-term value of enduring discomfort and pain to achieve a positive outcome. Patients with weak ego development, however, may miss their appointments, not comply with their treatments, or engage in short-term pleasurable activities that work against their healing and recovery. A significant aspect of the learning and healing process involves helping patients develop ego strength and adjust realistically to a changed body image or lifestyle brought about by disease and medical treatment. Health professionals, too, require personal ego strength to cope with the numerous predicaments in the everyday practice of medicine, as they face conflicting values, ethical responsibilities, and medical demands. Professional burnout, for example, often occurs among health professionals who have an overly idealistic notion of the healthcare role and unrealistic expectations for themselves in performing the role.

A particularly useful psychodynamic concept for health professionals to know involves the use of ego defense mechanisms. When the ego is threatened, as can easily occur in a stressful healthcare setting, defense mechanisms may be employed to protect the self. The short-term use of defense mechanisms is a way of coming to grips with reality. The danger comes in the overuse or long-term reliance on defense mechanisms, which allows individuals to avoid reality and may act as a barrier to learning. In Table 3-1, some of the more commonly used defense mechanisms are outlined.

TABLE 3-1   Ego Defense Mechanisms: Ways of Protecting the Self from Perceived Threat

Denial: Ignoring or refusing to acknowledge the reality of a threat

Rationalization: Excusing or explaining away a threat

Displacement: Taking out hostility and aggression on other individuals rather than directing anger at the source of the threat

Repression: Keeping unacceptable thoughts, feelings, or actions from conscious awareness

Regression: Returning to an earlier (less mature, more primitive) stage of behavior as a way of coping with a threat

Intellectualization: Minimizing anxiety by responding to a threat in a detached, abstract manner without feeling or emotion

Projection: Seeing one's own unacceptable characteristics or desires in other people

Reaction formation: Expressing or behaving the opposite of what is really felt

Sublimation: Converting repressed feelings into socially acceptable action

Compensation: Making up for weaknesses by excelling in other areas

As an example of defense mechanisms in health care, Elizabeth Kübler-Ross (1969) pointed out that many terminally ill patients' initial reaction to being told they have a serious illness is to employ the defense mechanism of denial. It is too overwhelming for patients to process the information that they are likely to die. Although most patients gradually accept the reality of their illness over time, the dangers are that if they remain in a state of denial, they may not seek treatment and care, and if their illness is contagious, they may not protect others against infection. A common defense mechanism employed by health professionals is to intellectualize rather than deal realistically at an emotional level with the significance of a patient as a person. Other defense mechanisms related to health care are identified in Table 3-1.

Another central assumption of the psychodynamic theory is that personality development occurs in stages, with much of adult behavior based on earlier childhood experiences and conflicts. For example, people's behavior when they are sick may reflect their emotional feelings and conflicts from childhood. One of the most widely used models of personality development is Erik Erikson's (1968) eight stages of life, organized around a psychosocial "crisis" to be resolved at each stage. For example, during infancy, the psychosocial crisis to be resolved is trust versus mistrust. The early childhood years involve issues of autonomy versus doubt, followed by initiative versus guilt. The school-aged child comes to terms with industry versus inferiority. Adolescence involves the crisis of identity versus role confusion. Young adults attempt to resolve the crisis of intimacy versus isolation. Middle-aged adults focus on generativity versus stagnation. Older adults struggle with integrity versus despair. Erikson noted that the two most significant periods of personality growth occur during adolescence and older adulthood—an important observation for health professionals to consider when working with members of these two age groups (see Chapter 5 for more on developmental stages).

Treatment plans, communication, and health education efforts need to include considerations of the patient's stage of personality development. For example, in working with 4- and 5-year-old patients, where the psychosocial crisis is "initiative versus guilt," health professionals should encourage these children to share their ideas and to make and do things themselves. Adults also must be careful not to make these children feel guilty for their illness or misfortune. As a second example, the adolescent's desire to have friends and to define their identity requires special attention in health care. Adolescent patients may need help and support adjusting to a changed body image and addressing their fears of weakness, lack of activity, and social isolation. One danger is that teenagers may treat their illness or injury as a significant dimension of their identity and self-concept.

The psychodynamic approach reminds teachers to pay attention to emotions, unconscious motivations, and the psychological development of all those involved in health care and learning. The teacher's role is to listen and ask questions. Teachers need to recognize how conscious and unconscious motivations affect learning and to work with id-ego-superego conflicts. The goal is to promote ego strength in learners. Forgetting information may be due to a desire not to remember it or as a result of emotional barriers to learning. This theory is well suited to understanding and working with patient and family noncompliance, trauma and loss, as well as the stresses of working with long-term care residents, palliative care, and the deeply emotional issues of terminal illness and death.

One problem with the psychodynamic approach is that much of the analysis of learners is open to different interpretations. Health professionals' biases, emotional conflicts, and motivations may distort their evaluation of other persons and situations. Another caution is that the psychodynamic theory may be used inappropriately; it is not the job of health professionals with little clinical psychology or psychiatric training to probe into the private lives and feelings of patients and speculate about their deep, unconscious motivations. A third danger is that health professionals may use the many psychodynamic principles as reasons to explain away, rather than deal with, people as individuals who need emotional care. As an illustration, researchers found that rather than using Kübler-Ross's (1969) model of death and dying to help terminally ill patients and their families discuss their fears and emotions, some health professionals used it to categorize, label, and dismiss the concerns of dying patients (Dunkel-Schetter & Wortman, 1982). When applied to learning, the basic principles of the psychodynamic theory are as follows:

- Focus on the learner's personality development, significant childhood experiences, conscious and unconscious motivations, id-ego-superego conflicts, and defensive behaviors.
- The teacher's role is to listen, ask probing questions about motivations and wishes, assess emotional barriers to learning, and make learning pleasurable while working to promote ego strength in learners.

Humanistic Learning Theory

Underlying the *humanistic theory* of learning are the assumptions that each individual is unique and that all individuals have a desire to grow in a positive way. Unfortunately, say the humanists, the natural inclination toward positive psychological growth may be undermined by some of society's values and expectations (beliefs such as males are less emotional than females, some ethnic groups are "inferior" to others, making money is more important than caring for people) and by adults' mistreatment of their children and each other (e.g., inconsistent or harsh discipline, humiliation and belittling, abuse and neglect). The cornerstones of a humanistic approach to learning include being open and spontaneous, recognizing the significance of emotions and feelings, respecting the right of individuals to make their own choices, and appreciating the potential for human creativity within each person.

Like the psychodynamic theory, the humanistic theory is largely a motivational theory. From a humanistic perspective, the motivation to act stems largely from each person's needs, feelings about the self, and the desire to grow in positive ways. Remembering information and transferring learning to other situations are helped by encouraging curiosity and a positive self-concept, and having open situations where people respect individuality and value freedom of choice. Under such conditions, flexibility in problem solving and creativity is enhanced.

According to humanistic principles, feelings and emotions are the keys to learning, communication, and understanding. Humanists worry that in today's stressful society people can easily lose touch with their feelings, which sets the stage for emotional problems and difficulties in learning. "Tell me how you feel" is a much more important statement than "tell me what you think," since thoughts and "the shoulds" may be at odds with true feelings (Rogers, 1961). Consider the implications of a young person who says, "I know I should go to nursing school and become a nurse because I am smart and that is what my parents want, but I don't feel comfortable with sick people—I don't even like them!" Or, consider the dying patient who says, "I realize that I am going to die and should be brave, but I feel so sad that I am losing my family, my friends, and my self; frankly, I am afraid of dying—all the pain and suffering, being a burden—I'm scared!" In both cases, humanists would argue, the overriding factor that will affect the behavior of the young person and the dying patient is their feelings, not their cognitions.

One of the best-known humanistic theorists is Abraham Maslow (1954, 1987), who identified a hierarchy of needs to explain motivation (Figure 3-4). At the bottom of the hierarchy are physiological needs (food, water, warmth, sleep); next come safety needs; then the need for belonging and love; followed by self-esteem. At the top of the hierarchy is the need for self-actualization (maximizing one's potential). An assumption is that basic-level needs must be met before individuals can

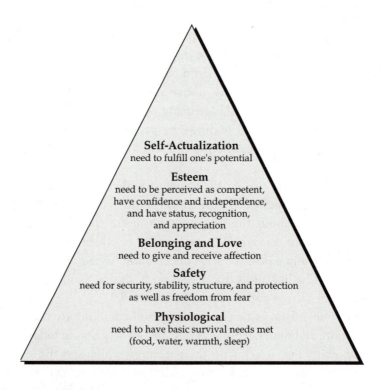

Self-Actualization
need to fulfill one's potential

Esteem
need to be perceived as competent,
have confidence and independence,
and have status, recognition,
and appreciation

Belonging and Love
need to give and receive affection

Safety
need for security, stability, structure, and protection
as well as freedom from fear

Physiological
need to have basic survival needs met
(food, water, warmth, sleep)

FIGURE 3-4   Maslow's Hierarchy of Needs
Source: Adapted from Maslow (1987).

be concerned with learning and self-actualizing. Thus, clients who are hungry, tired, and in pain will be motivated to have these biological needs met before being interested in learning about their medications, rules for self-care, and other health information. Although Maslow's theory is intuitively appealing, research has not been able to support the hierarchy of needs with much consistency. For example, although some people's basic needs may not be met, they may nonetheless engage in creative activities, extend themselves to other people, and enjoy learning (Pfeffer, 1985).

Besides personal needs, humanists contend that self-concept and self-esteem are necessary considerations in any learning situation. The therapist Carl Rogers (1961, 1994) argued that what people want most is unconditional positive self-regard (the feeling of being loved without strings attached). Experiences that are threatening, coercive, and judgmental undermine the ability and enthusiasm of individuals to learn. Thus, it is essential that those in positions of authority convey a fundamental respect for the people with whom they work. If a health professional is prejudiced against AIDS patients, then little will be healing or therapeutic in her relationship with them until she is genuinely able to feel respect for these patients as individuals.

Rather than acting as an authority, say humanists, the role of any teacher or leader is to be a facilitator (Rogers, 1994). Listening—rather than talking—is the skill that is needed. Because the uniqueness of each individual is fundamental to the humanistic perspective, much of the learning experience is based on a direct relationship between the teacher and the learner. Instruction is tailored to the needs, self-esteem, and positive growth of each learner. Learners, not teachers, choose what is to be learned. Teachers are to serve as resource persons whose job is to help guide learners to make wise choices. Mastering information and facts is not the central purpose of learning. Encouraging curiosity, enthusiasm, initiative, and responsibility is much more important and should be the primary goal of any educational effort. As an illustration, rather than inserting health education videos into television sets for hospital patients to view or routinely distributing lots of pamphlets and pages of small-print instructions, the humanist perspective indicates that efforts should be devoted to establishing rapport and becoming emotionally attuned to patients and their family members.

Humanistic principles are the foundation of self-help groups, wellness programs, and palliative care and are well suited to working with children and young patients undergoing separation anxiety due to illness, surgery, and recovery (Holyoake, 1998). Within this perspective, a principal emphasis is on client-centered care and the need for health professionals to learn and grow from their practice experiences. However, the theory has its weaknesses. Research has not been able to substantiate some of its strongest claims, and the theory has been criticized for promoting self-centered learners who cannot compromise or take criticism. The "touchy-feely" approach of humanists makes some people feel truly uncomfortable. Moreover, information, facts, memorization, drill, practice, and tedious work are often required to master knowledge. To summarize, humanistic theory suggests the following principles of learning:

- Focus on the learner's desire for positive growth, subjective feelings, needs, self-concept, choices in life, and interpersonal relationships.
- The teacher's role is to assess and encourage changes in learners' needs, self-concept, and feelings by providing support, freedom to choose, and opportunities for spontaneity and creativity.

APPLYING LEARNING THEORIES TO HEALTH CARE

A logical question is which of these theories "best" explains learning and would be the most useful to health professionals interested in increasing knowledge or in changing the behavior of patients, oneself, or others? The answer to this question is that each theory contributes to understanding certain aspects of the learning process. For example, behaviorist and social learning theories emphasize external factors in the environment that promote learning, whereas cognitive, psychodynamic, and humanistic theories as well as certain features of social learning theory focus on internal psychological factors in the learning process.

In practice, these learning theories can be used singly and in combination to help nurses and other health professionals teach patients or themselves to acquire new information and alter behavior. As an illustration, patients undergoing painful procedures are first taught relaxation exercises (behaviorist) and while experiencing pain or discomfort are encouraged to employ imagery, such as thinking about a favorite, beautiful place or imagining the healthy cells "gobbling up" the unhealthy cells (cognitive). Health professionals are respectful and emotionally supportive of each patient (humanistic), and they take the time to listen to patients discuss their fears and concerns (psychodynamic). Waiting rooms and lounge areas for patients and their families are designed to be comfortable, friendly, and pleasant in order to facilitate conversation and interaction (social learning).

At the same time, research indicates that some learning theories are better suited to certain kinds of individuals than to others. For example, patients who are not particularly verbal may learn more effectively when behaviorist techniques are used, and although some patients respond well to reinforcement and incentives, other patients do not seem to need—and may even resent—attempts to manipulate and reinforce them. Moreover, some clients learn by responding and taking action (behaviorist), whereas the route to learning for others may be through perceptions and thoughts (cognitive) or through feelings and emotions (humanistic and psychodynamic). Most patients and staff benefit from demonstration and example (social learning).

Taken together, the theories discussed in this chapter indicate that learning is a more complex process than any one theory implies. Besides the distinct considerations for learning suggested by each theory, the similarities in these perspectives point to some common features of learning. The issues raised at the beginning of the chapter can be addressed by considering how the learning theories might be applied to patients in the healthcare setting. Readers can also think about how the theories might apply to their own needs to acquire new knowledge or change behaviors and break bad habits.

How Does Learning Occur in the Healthcare Setting?

Learning takes place as patients interact with their environment and incorporate new information or experiences with what they already know or have learned. Environmental factors that affect their learning include the society's norms and values, the culture of the healthcare facility, and the particular structure of the learning situation. Role models need to be effective, patients may need reinforcement, feedback is required for the patients' correct and incorrect responses, and patients need to have opportunities to apply what they learned to different settings and new situations. However, the patient ultimately controls the learning process, often involving considerations of his or her developmental stage, past history (habits, cultural learning, socialization, childhood experiences, and conflicts), cognitive style, conscious and unconscious motivations, personality (stage of development, conflicts, self-concept), and emotions. Most patients have a preferred way of taking in information (visual, motor, auditory, or symbolic) and, although some patients learn best on their own, others will benefit from expert guidance, social interaction, and cooperative learning.

A critical influence on whether learning occurs is the patient's motivational level (see Chapter 6 for more on motivation). The learning theories reviewed here suggest that in order to learn, patients must want to gain something (receive rewards and pleasure, meet goals and needs, confirm expectations, grow in positive ways, resolve conflicts), which in turn creates tension (drives to be reduced, imbalance) and the motivation to acquire information or change behavior. The success or failure of a patient's actions may affect future learning experiences and their reactions to health care. In some cases, patients' previously learned information or habits may need to be replaced with more accurate information and more appropriate responses. It is, of course, easier to instill new learning than to correct faulty learning.

What Kinds of Experiences Help or Hinder Learning?

When health professionals are attempting to teach patients information or work with them to change their attitudes and behavior, the selection of learning principles and the structure of the learning experience strongly influence the course of learning. Teaching requires imagination, flexibility, and the ability to use a variety of educational methods. Teachers must know their material well and need good communication skills and the ability to motivate themselves and others. All the learning perspectives discussed in this chapter recognize the need to make learning a positive experience and the necessity of relating new information to patients' past experiences—their habits, culture, memories, and feelings about the self.

Ignoring these considerations, of course, may hinder learning. Some obstacles to learning may involve a lack of clarity and meaningfulness in what is to be learned, neglect or punishment, fear, negative or ineffective role models, and such factors as rewards for unhealthy behavior and confusing reinforcement. Other considerations include the appropriateness of educational materials for the patient's ability and needs, patients' readiness to learn, and their stage of cognitive and personality development. Moreover, patients are unlikely to want to learn if they have had damaging socialization experiences, are deprived of stimulating environments, and do not have reasonable goals and expectations for themselves.

What Helps Learning Become Relatively Permanent?

First, the likelihood of learning is enhanced by organizing the learning experience, making it meaningful and pleasurable, and pacing the presentation in keeping with a patient's ability to process information. This is especially crucial when teaching children and older adults. Second, practicing (mentally and physically) new knowledge or skills under varied conditions strengthens learning. The third issue concerns reinforcement. Although reinforcement may or may not be necessary, some psychologists have argued that it may be helpful because it serves as a signal that learning has occurred. Another consideration involves trying to assure that learning will transfer beyond the immediate healthcare setting to other environments. And finally, learning cannot be assumed to be relatively lasting or permanent; it must be assessed and evaluated soon after the learning experience as well as by follow-up measurements at later times. What is learned from evaluating the teaching situation can then be used to improve future learning experiences for patients.

SUMMARY

This chapter demonstrates that learning is complex, multifaceted, and challenging. Readers may feel overwhelmed by the different perspectives, various principles of learning, and cautions. Yet, like the blind men exploring the elephant, each theory highlights an important dimension that affects the overall learning process. Taken together the approaches to learning provide a wealth of useful options and tools to encourage learning and changing behavior in the healthcare setting. There is, of course, no single best way to approach learning, although all the theories indicate the need to be sensitive to the unique characteristics and motivations of each patient. Health professionals cannot be expected to know everything about the learning process. More important, perhaps, is that they can determine what needs to be known, where to find the necessary information, and how to help others benefit directly from a learning experience.

REVIEW QUESTIONS

1. What are the basic principles of learning for each of the five psychological theories discussed in this chapter?
2. What is the role of the teacher in each of the five learning theories?
3. What contribution does each of the following cognitive approaches make to help us understand the learning process: gestalt, developmental, information processing, and social cognition?
4. How does motivation act as the critical influence on whether learning occurs?
5. What are the ways that teachers can motivate learners?
6. Based on the various learning theories, what techniques are useful in helping patients remember information?
7. Using the theories of learning, what approaches can help patients break bad habits, such as smoking or a sedentary lifestyle?

REFERENCES

Bandura, A. (1977). *Social learning theory*. Englewood Cliffs, NJ: Prentice-Hall.

Bandura, A. (2001). Social cognitive theory: An agentic perspective. *Annual Review of Psychology, 52*, 1–26.

Berliner, D. C. & Calfee, R. C. (Eds.). (1996). *Handbook of educational psychology*. New York: Simon & Schuster Macmillan.

Bigge, M. L. & Shermis, S. S. (1992). *Learning theories for teachers* (5th ed.). New York: HarperCollins.

Brien, R. & Eastmond, N. (1994). *Cognitive science and instruction*. Englewood Cliffs, NJ: Educational Technology Publications.

Dunkel-Schetter, C. & Wortman, C. B. (1982). The interpersonal dynamics of career: Problems in social relationships and their impact on the patient. In H. Freeman (ed.), *Interpersonal issues* (pp. 69–100). New York: Academic Press.

Erikson, E. (1968). *Identity: Youth and crisis*. New York: Norton.

Fiske, S. T. & Taylor, S. E. (1991). *Social cognition*. New York: McGraw-Hill.

Gage, N. L. & Berliner, D. C. (1998). *Educational psychology* (6th ed.). Boston: Houghton Mifflin.

Gardner, H. (1978). *Developmental psychology: An introduction*. Boston: Little, Brown.

Hilgard, E. R. & Bower, G. H. (1966). *Theories of learning* (3rd ed.). New York: Appleton-Century Crofts.

Holyoake, D. D. (1998). A little lady called Pandora: An exploration of philosophical traditions of humanism and existentialism in nursing ill children. *Child Care, Health and Development, 24*, 325–336.

Klein, S. B. & Mowrer, R. R. (Eds.). (1989). *Contemporary learning theories: Pavlovian conditioning and the status of traditional learning theory*. Hillsdale, NJ: Lawrence Erlbaum.

Kohler, W. (1969). *The task of gestalt psychology*. Princeton, NJ: Princeton University Press.

Kübler-Ross, E. (1969). *On death and dying*. New York: Macmillan.

Marshall, H. H. (1998). Teaching educational psychology: Learner-centered constructivist perspectives. In N. M. Lambert & B. L. McCombs (Eds.), *How students learn: Reforming schools through learner-centered education* (pp. 449–473). Washington, DC: American Psychological Association.

Maslow, A. (1954). *Motivation and personality*. New York: Harper & Row.

Maslow, A. (1987). *Motivation and personality* (3rd ed.). New York: Harper & Row.

Miller, N. E. & Dollard, J. (1941). *Social learning and imitation*. New Haven, CT: Yale University Press.

Notterman, J. M. & Drewry, H. N. (1993). *Psychology and education*. New York: Plenum.

Pfeffer, J. (1985). Organizations and organizational theory. In G. Lindzey & E. Aronson (Eds.), *Handbook of social psychology* (3rd ed., vol. 1, pp. 379–440). New York: Random House.

Piaget, J. & Inhelder, B. (1969). *The psychology of the child* (H. Weaver, trans.). New York: Basic Books.

Redman, B. L. (2001). *The practice of patient education* (9th ed.). St. Louis: Mosby.

Rogers, C. (1961). *On becoming a person*. Boston: Houghton Mifflin.

Rogers, C. (1994). *Freedom to learn* (3rd ed.). New York: Merrill.

Skinner, B. F. (1974). *About behaviorism*. New York: Vintage Books.

Sternberg, R. J. (1996). Styles of thinking. In P. B. Baltes & U. M. Staudinger (Eds.), *Interactive minds: Life-span perspectives on the social foundation of cognition* (pp. 347–365). New York: Cambridge University Press.

PART II

Characteristics of the Learner

Determinants of Learning

Sharon Kitchie

KEY TERMS

determinants of learning
learning needs

learning styles
readiness to learn

OBJECTIVES

After completing this chapter, the reader will be able to
1. State the nurse's role as teacher in the learning process.
2. Identify the three elements included in the "determinants of learning."
3. Describe the steps involved in assessing learning needs.
4. Explain methods that are used in assessing learner needs.
5. Identify the four types of readiness to learn.
6. Describe what is meant by learning styles.
7. Identify the similarities and differences between the major learning style types.
8. Discuss ways to assess learning styles.

In a variety of settings, nurses have always provided education for patients and their families to learn the many different aspects of their health care. This learning includes such things as self-care activities, preparations for diagnostic tests, disease management, and health promotion. Several factors have made teaching of this vital knowledge and skills challenging for the nurse in today's healthcare environment. Often nurses have difficulty meeting patients' needs because of time constraints in clinical practice. For example, same-day surgery has shortened the time that the nurse has available to be with patients. The "teachable moment" is hard to capture because of decreased lengths of stay in hospitals and other healthcare settings.

To meet these challenges, the nurse must know what determines how well a person learns. These determinants of learning include:

- learning needs
- readiness to learn
- learning styles

This chapter will address the determinants of learning in relation to patient teaching in the practice of nursing.

THE NURSE'S ROLE AS TEACHER

Teaching can be one of the most challenging and essential interventions a nurse has to perform. To teach well, the nurse must identify the information each patient and family needs to know, as well as consider their readiness to learn and their styles of learning. Learning can actually occur without a teacher, but the nurse can enhance learning by serving as a facilitator. However, just providing information alone does not guarantee that learning will occur. The nurse plays a crucial role in the learning process by:

- Assessing problems or deficits
- Providing meaningful information and presenting the information in unique ways
- Identifying progress being made
- Giving feedback and follow-up
- Reinforcing learning in the attainment of new knowledge, the performance of a skill, or a change in attitude
- Evaluating the client's abilities

When learning new knowledge about an illness, a new skill, or a behavior it is vital that the nurse give the client the needed support, encouragement, and direction.

For example, the nurse can make the needed changes in the home environment, such as minimizing distractions by having family members turn the television off. A quiet environment will help the patient concentrate on the learning activity. Patients can always make self-care choices without the help of the nurse, but these choices may not be sufficient or may be inappropriate. The nurse can identify the best learning approaches and help the patient and family members choose the learning activities based on their individual needs, readiness to learn, and learning styles.

ASSESSMENT OF THE LEARNER

For years nurses have been taught that any direct physical and psychosocial care to meet the needs of patients should not be initiated unless the interventions are based on an assessment. Few would deny that this is the correct approach even when the intervention is teaching about aspects of self-care. Nursing assessment of needs, readiness, and styles of learning is the first and most important step in preparing to teach—but it is also the step most often neglected. Frequently, the nurse delves into teaching before assessing all of the determinants of learning. As a result, patients with the same condition often are taught with the same materials in the same way (Haggard, 1989). Thus, information given to patients is neither individualized nor based on sound educational principles.

The effectiveness of nursing care depends on the scope, accuracy, and comprehensiveness of assessment prior to interventions. What is it about assessment that is so important to patient education, and why is it often overlooked or only partially carried out? This initial step in the educational process confirms the need for teaching and the approaches to use in providing the patient with appropriate learning experiences. Individuals who desire or require information to maintain optimal health deserve a thorough assessment by the nurse so that the needs of every learner are correctly addressed.

Many factors must be considered with respect to the three determinants of learning. First, assessments of all three should be based on theories, concepts, and principles. Second, assessments assist in identifying and prioritizing behavioral goals and objectives that provide the background for selecting correct instructional interventions, and in evaluating if learning has occurred. Third, good assessments ensure that the best possible learning takes place with the least amount of stress and anxiety for the patient. Finally, assessments prevent unneeded repetition of known material, save time and energy of the patient and the nurse (Haggard, 1989), and increase the motivation to learn by addressing what the patient feels is most important to know or to be able to do. Lack of time, as a result of such factors as shortened hospital stays and limited contact between the nurse and patients, has led nurses to sometimes short-change the assessment phase. The nurse, in the role of a teacher, must become familiar and comfortable with all the elements of teaching, but particularly with the assessment phase because it provides the foundation for the rest of the educational process. To deliver quality and meaningful education, nurses must become skilled in accurately carrying out assessments so as to have ample time for actual teaching.

The following three determinants of learning are defined:

1. Learning needs—**what** the learner needs to learn
2. Readiness to learn—**when** the learner is receptive to learning
3. Learning style—**how** the learner best learns

ASSESSING LEARNING NEEDS

Of the three determinants, learning needs must be examined first to discover what has to be taught and to determine the extent of teaching required. Once the needs and interests of the learner are identified and prioritized, this information is used to set objectives and plan appropriate and effective teaching. Education should begin at a point suitable to the learner. Significant differences have been found between the perception of needs identified by patients and the needs identified by nurses caring for them (Roberts, 1982).

Learning needs are defined as gaps in knowledge that exist between a desired level of performance and the actual level of performance (Healthcare Education Association, 1985). A learning need is the gap between what someone knows and what someone needs to know. Such gaps exist because of a lack of knowledge, attitude, or skill.

Most learners, 90% to 95% of them, can master a subject with a high degree of success if given sufficient time and assistance (Bloom, 1968; Bruner, 1966; Carroll, 1963; Skinner, 1954). It is the task of the nurse to first discover what the needs of the learner are and then to find the best means of presenting the information so the patient and family members can master what is required of them to function independently. The following are important steps in the assessment of learning needs:

1. *Identify the learner.* Who is the audience? Are you teaching a group of patients or an individual and his or her significant others? Are their needs the same or different? Teaching opportunities, formal or informal, must be based on accurate identification of the learners. For example, a nurse may believe that all postpartum mothers need a class on safety issues for the newborn. This perception may be based on the nurse's interaction with one patient and may not be true of all postpartum mothers.

2. *Choose the right setting.* Establish an environment in which learners feel a sense of security in confiding information and believe their concerns are respected and taken seriously. Maintaining privacy and confidentiality is essential to establishing a trusting relationship (Rankin & Stallings, 2001).

3. *Collect important information about the learner.* Explore the health problems or issues that are of interest to your audience to determine the type and extent of content to be included in teaching as well as the teaching methods and instructional tools best suited to meet their needs. Patients and/or family members are usually the most important source of needs assessment information. Be sure to ask what is important to them, what types of social support systems are available, and how their social support system can help. Actively engaging learners in defining their own problems and needs motivates most patients because they have an investment in planning for their learning and allows the nurse to tailor teaching specifically to their unique circumstances.

4. *Involve members of the healthcare team.* Consult with other professionals to gain insight into the needs of patients and their families. Nurses must remember to collaborate with their colleagues, who can serve as excellent sources of information. In addition, representatives of health-related organizations, such as the American Cancer Society, American Diabetes Association, or American Heart Association, often can provide insight into the learning needs of people with specific health problems or concerns.

5. *Prioritize needs.* Setting priorities for teaching is often difficult when many learning needs have been identified in several areas. However, if basic needs are not attended to first and foremost, as indicated in Figure 4-1 of Maslow's hierarchy of needs (1970), learning of other information may either be delayed or be impossible to achieve. For example, learning about a low-sodium diet will likely not occur if a patient faces problems with basic physiological needs such as pain or discomfort. Prioritizing these needs helps the nurse in partnership with the patient set realistic and achievable learning goals. Another way to prioritize learning needs is based on the criteria of the Healthcare Education Association (1985), as outlined in Table 4-1.

Not all learners need to know everything, and assessment can help to discriminate the "need to know" from the "nice to know" information. If patients want to know the pathophysiology of their disease, then their curiosity should be satisfied, but it is not fundamental to them in learning how to carry out self-care activities essential for discharge from the hospital. It is always important to remember that patients "do not have to know how an engine works to be able

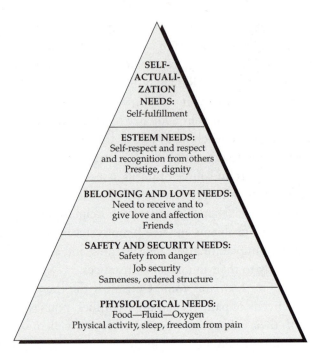

FIGURE 4-1   Maslow's Hierarchy of Needs
Source: Reprinted from M. LaFleur-Brooks, *Health Unit Coordinating*. Philadelphia: W.B. Saunders, 1979, p. 48.

TABLE 4-1	Criteria for Prioritizing Learning Needs
Criteria	**Learning Needs**
Mandatory	Needs that must be learned for survival or situations in which the learner's life or safety is threatened. Learning needs in this category must be met immediately. For example, a patient who has experienced a recent heart attack needs to know the signs and symptoms and when to get immediate help.
Desirable	Needs that are not life-dependent but are related to well-being or the ability to provide self-care. For example, it is important for patients who have cardiovascular disease to understand the effects of a high-fat diet on their condition.
Possible	Needs for information that is "nice to know" but not essential or required or situations in which the learning need is not directly related to daily activities. The patient who is newly diagnosed as having diabetes mellitus most likely does not need to know about traveling across time zones or staying in a foreign country because this information does not relate to the patient's everyday activities.

to drive a car." Often, highly technical information will serve only to confuse and distract patients from learning what they need to know to comply with their prescribed treatment (Hansen & Fisher, 1998; Ruzicki, 1989).

6. *Take time-management issues into account.* Because lack of time is a major barrier to carrying out a proper assessment, Rankin and Stallings (2001) suggest the nurse consider the following tips that, in the long term, are time-savers:

- Although close observation and active listening take time, it is much more efficient and effective to do a good initial assessment than to have to waste time going back to discover the obstacles to learning that prevented progress in the first place.
- Learners must be given time to offer their own thoughts about their learning needs if the nurse expects them to take charge and become actively involved in learning.
- Assessment can be made anytime and anywhere the nurse has contact with patients and families. There are many potential opportunities, such as when giving a bath, serving a meal, making rounds, distributing medications, and so forth.
- Informing patients ahead of time that the nurse wishes to spend time discussing problems or needs gives them advance notice to sort out their thoughts and feelings.
- Minimizing interruptions and distractions during planned assessment interviews allows the nurse to accomplish in 5 minutes what otherwise might have taken 15 minutes or more during an interview session that is frequently interrupted.

METHODS TO ASSESS LEARNING NEEDS

The nurse, as a teacher, must obtain information about the learning needs from the patient as well as information from others who are in contact with the patient. The following are various methods that can be used to assess client needs and should be used in combination with one another to yield the most reliable information (Haggard, 1989).

Casual Conversations

Often learning needs are discovered during conversations that take place when the nurse is performing patient care. The nurse must rely on active listening. Open-ended questions will encourage patients and family to reveal information about what they believe are gaps in their knowledge or skills.

Structured Interviews

The structured interview is perhaps the most common form of needs assessment to solicit the learner's point of view. As with the gathering of any information from a patient during assessment, the nurse should strive to establish a trusting environment, use direct and open-ended questions, choose a setting that is free of distractions, and allow the patient to state what is believed to be the needs for learning. It is important to remain nonjudgmental when collecting information about the learner's strengths, beliefs, and motivations. The telephone is a good tool to use for an interview if it is impossible to ask questions in person. The major drawback of a telephone interview, however, is the inability for the nurse to see the nonverbal cues from the respondent.

Interviews produce answers that may reveal uncertainties, conflicts, inconsistencies, unexpected problems, anxieties, and fears, as well as current knowledge base. Examples of questions that could be asked of a patient as learner are as follows:

- What do you think caused your problem?
- How severe is your illness?
- What does your illness/health mean to you?
- What do you do to stay healthy?
- What results do you hope to obtain from treatments?

Questionnaires

The patient's written responses to questions about learning needs can be obtained by this method. Checklists, one of the most common forms of questionnaires, are easy to administer, provide more privacy than interviews, and make it easy to tabulate data. Because checklists usually reflect what the nurse perceives as needs, there should also be a space for the patients and their family members to add any other items of interest or concern.

Observations

Observing health behaviors in several different time periods can help to determine established patterns of behavior. Actually watching the learner perform a task is an excellent way of assessing a skill. Are all steps performed correctly? Is there any difficulty with using the equipment? Does the learner require prompting? Learners may believe they can accurately perform a task (e.g., walking with crutches, changing a dressing, giving an injection), but the nurse can best determine what additional learning may be needed by directly observing the skill performance.

Patient Charts

Often documentation in patient charts will provide patterns that reveal learning needs. Physicians' progress notes, nursing care plans, nurses' notes, discharge planning forms, and documentation by other team members, such as physical therapists, social workers, respiratory therapists, and nutritionists, are important sources of information on learning needs.

READINESS TO LEARN

Once the learning needs have been identified, the next step is to determine the learner's readiness to receive information. *Readiness to learn* is defined as the time when the learner expresses or shows interest in learning the information necessary to maintain optimal health. Often, nurses have noted that when a patient asks a question, the "time is prime for learning." Readiness to learn occurs when the learner is receptive, willing, and able to participate in the learning process. The nurse must never overuse the expression "the patient is not ready to learn." It is the responsibility of the nurse to adapt the content to be learned to fit with what the learner wants and needs to learn to move the patient toward independence in self-care.

Assessing readiness to learn requires the nurse to understand what needs to be taught and to be skilled in collecting and verifying information. The same methods to assess learning needs can also be used for assessing readiness to learn, such as making observations, conducting interviews, gathering information from the learner as well as other healthcare team members, and reviewing written data in charts.

No matter how important the information is or how much the nurse feels the patient needs the information, if the patient is not ready to learn, the information will not be absorbed. If educational objectives are set by the nurse before assessing readiness to learn, then both the nurse's and the patient's time could very well be wasted, because the established objectives may be beyond the readiness of the patient.

Timing—that is, the point at which teaching should take place—is very important, because anything that affects physical or psychological comfort can influence a learner's ability and willingness to learn. A learner who is not receptive to information at one time may be more receptive to the same information at another time. Within the healthcare system, the nurse often has limited contact with pa-tients and family members due to short hospital stays or outpatient visits. Therefore, teaching must be brief and basic. Adults, whether patient or family members, are eager to learn when the subject of teaching is relevant to their every-day concerns.

Before teaching can begin, the nurse must take the time to first take a PEEK (Lichtenthal, 1990) at the four types of readiness to learn, which are determined by the learner's characteristics as follows: **P**hysical readiness, **E**motional readiness, **E**xperiential readiness, and **K**nowledge readiness (see Table 4-2).

TABLE 4-2   Take Time to Take a PEEK at the Four Types of Readiness to Learn

P = Physical readiness
- Measures of ability
- Complexity of task
- Environmental effects
- Health status
- Gender

E = Emotional readiness
- Anxiety level
- Support system
- Motivation
- Risk-taking behavior
- Frame of mind
- Developmental stage

E = Experiential readiness
- Level of aspiration
- Past coping mechanisms
- Cultural background
- Locus of control
- Orientation

K = Knowledge readiness
- Present knowledge base
- Cognitive ability
- Learning disabilities
- Learning styles

Source: From C. Lichtenthal, *A Self-Study Model on Readiness to Learn,* August 1990. Reprinted with permis-sion from Cheryl Lichtenthal Hardy.

Physical Readiness

Physical readiness factors need to be considered by the nurse because they may have an adverse impact on the degree to which learning will occur (Singer, 1972). There are five major components to physical readiness: measures of ability, complexity of task, environmental effects, health status, and gender.

Measures of Ability   Ability to perform a task may require fine and/or gross movements using the large and small muscles of the body. Walking on crutches is a good example of a task for which a patient must have the physical ability to be ready to learn. The nurse must assess that adequate strength, flexibility, and endurance are present. In addition, for information to be accurately processed, the sense organs of seeing and hearing, in particular, must be adequately functioning. For example, if a person has a visual deficit, are eyeglasses available to allow the patient to see the lines on an insulin syringe? If not, then the individual is not physically ready to learn. The nurse can help the patient by providing a clip-on magnifier that will help to overcome visual problems. By using instructional tools to match learners' sensory abilities or providing equipment to overcome their sensory deficits the nurse will help increase interest in learning.

Complexity of Task   The nurse must take into account the difficulty level of the subject or task to be mastered by the learner. The more complex the task, the more changes in behavior are necessary to acquire a skill. For example, some skills require a high degree of dexterity and physical energy output. Once acquired, however, these behaviors are usually retained better and longer than cognitive learning that requires knowledge of facts (Greer, Hitt, Sitterly, & Slebodnick, 1972). Once a skill becomes routine in nature, it is more difficult for the patient to alter it, if necessary to do so, because it has become a habit. For instance, if a procedure or equipment changes, the learner will need to unlearn the tasks and relearn them in a new way. This may increase the difficulty to perform the task, put additional physical demands on the learner, and lengthen the amount of time needed to adjust to doing something in a different way. In particular, older adults or those with low literacy skills will likely be confused or overwhelmed and may even refuse to make a change.

Environmental Effects   An environment favorable to learning will help to keep the learner's attention and stimulate interest in learning. On the other hand, unfavorable conditions, such as extremely high levels of noise, can interfere with the accuracy and precision of performance. Use of a jackhammer in the street outside the patient's home, for example, is more disruptive to the patient's ability to learn a new skill the nurse is teaching than a constant roar of traffic coming from the same street.

The older adult, in particular, needs more time to react and respond to stimuli because of a decreased ability to receive and transmit information that occurs with aging. Thus, tasks requiring large amounts of strength, endurance, speed, or flexibility can prove difficult. Complex motor tasks, with too much information given during demonstration by the nurse, may result in older adults becoming overwhelmed. Instead, they may focus on irrelevant information rather than on cues critical to accomplishing the task at hand. When an activity is self-paced, the older adult will respond more favorably. For all learners, increasing their physical readiness to learn can be accomplished by breaking down complex learning material into more simplified steps. This technique is helpful for improving retention of information, reducing inattention and confusion, and decreasing energy demands.

Health Status   Assessment of the patient's health status is important to determine the amount of energy available for learning. For example, the pain or discomfort associated with acute illness requires the learner to expend large amounts of physical and psychic energy, with little reserve left for actual learning. Any learning that does occur is usually related to treatments, tests, and symptom control. As these patients stabilize or improve, they can then focus on learning how to manage their disease and avoid complications. However, medicines that can induce side effects, such as drowsiness, mental depression, or decreased ability to concentrate, will impact on the patient's ability to learn. Giving a patient a sedative prior to a learning experience will result in less apprehension, but mental functioning and manual dexterity will be impaired, thus requiring more time, more physical output, and more frustration for the learner to master a skill (Greer, Hitt, Sitterly, & Slebodnick, 1972).

Chronic illness, on the other hand, is by definition long-term in duration. The physiological and psychological demands vary and are not always predictable. Patients go through different stages in adjusting to their illness. Boyd, Gleit, Graham, and Whitman (1998) suggested that these stages are similar to what a person who has experienced a loss goes through. Corbin and Strauss (1999) propose that chronic illness occurs in phases. Burton (2000) describes the continuous adaptation required to cope with a chronic condition, and Patterson (2001) suggests that living with chronic illness is an ongoing and continually shifting process. Understanding these cycles is important when assessing a chronically ill person's readiness to learn. The nurse should never assume that an approach to teaching and learning that worked before will be just as effective again. There may be periods of time when learners are more receptive to learning.

In contrast, healthy learners have energy available for learning, but their readiness to learn about health-promoting behaviors is based on their perception of self-responsibility. If they believe there is a threat to their quality of life, more information will be sought in an attempt to avoid the negative impact of an illness (Bubela & Galloway, 1990). This type of response behavior can be best understood by examining the Health Belief Model and the Health Promotion Model described in Chapter 6.

Gender   Research has indicated that women are generally more receptive to medical care and take less risks regarding their health than men (Ashton, 1999; Bertakis, Rahman, Helms, Callahan, & Robbins, 2000; Stein & Nyamathi, 2000). This may be because women traditionally have been in the role of caregivers and therefore are more open to health promotion teaching. In addition, they have more frequent contacts with health providers while bearing and raising children. Men, on the other hand, tend to be less receptive to healthcare interventions and are more likely to be risk takers. Because a good deal of this behavior is thought to be socially induced, changes are beginning to be seen in the health-seeking behavior of men and women. More than ever before men are focusing increased attention on practicing healthier lifestyles, and both men and women are being affected by a blending of gender roles in the home and workplace.

Emotional Readiness

Like physical readiness, emotional readiness also includes several components that need to be assessed. These components influence how emotionally ready someone is to learn.

Anxiety Level   Anxiety influences the ability to perform mental or physical tasks. Depending on the level of anxiety, patients may be better or less able to learn new skills. Fear, a major contributor to anxiety, often negatively impacts on readiness to learn. For example, a patient having to learn self-administration of a medicine by injection may be afraid to inflict pain on oneself. Or, a family member may have real difficulty mastering a skill because of the fear of harming a loved one who is ill or of failing to do a procedure correctly.

Also, fear may lead patients to deny their illness, which interferes with their ability to learn. In addition, if a situation is life-threatening or overwhelming, anxiety will be very high, and learning usually can take place only if instructions are repeated over and over again by the nurse. In such circumstances, families or other support persons should be taught instead. In later stages of adaptation individuals will be more receptive to learning because anxiety levels will be less acute.

Some degree of anxiety is a motivator to learn, but low or high anxiety will interfere with readiness to learn. On either end of the continuum, mild or severe anxiety
may lead to an inability to learn, whereas moderate anxiety will drive someone to take
action. As the level of anxiety begins to increase, emotional readiness peaks and then
begins to decrease (see Figure 4-2). A moderate level of anxiety is best for success in
learning and is considered the optimal time for learning. Discovering what stressful
events or major life changes the learner is experiencing will give the nurse clues as to
that person's emotional readiness to learn.

Support System   The availability and strength of a support system also influence
emotional readiness and are closely tied to how anxious someone might feel. If people in the patient's support system are available to assist with self-care activities at
home, then they should be present during at least some of the teaching sessions to
learn how to help the patient if the need arises. A strong support system decreases
anxiety, whereas the lack of one may increase anxiety levels. Beddoe (1999) describes
the unique opportunity that nurses have to provide emotional support to patients.
She labels this opportunity as the "reachable moment"—the time when a nurse truly
connects with clients without prejudice or bias. When the client feels emotionally
supported, it sets the stage for the "teachable moment," when the client will be most
receptive to learning.

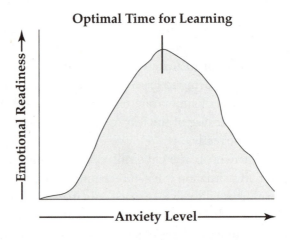

FIGURE 4-2   Effect of Anxiety on Emotional Readiness to Learn

Motivation   Assessment of emotional readiness involves determining the level of motivation, not necessarily the reasons for the motivation. A learner may have many reasons why he or she is motivated to learn, and almost any reason to learn is valid. The level of motivation is related to what learners perceive as an expectation of themselves or others. Patients who are ready to learn show an interest and willingness to participate or to ask questions. Prior learning experiences, whether they are past accomplishments or failures, usually influence the extent to which someone is motivated for learning (see Chapter 6 for more on motivation).

Risk-Taking Behavior   Taking risks, at least to some extent, is part of everyday living. Many activities are done without thinking about the outcome. According to Joseph (1993), some patients, by the very nature of their personality, will take more risks than others. Wolfe (1994) stated that taking risks can be threatening when the outcomes are not guaranteed. Nurses can, however, help these patients develop strategies to reduce the risk of their choices. If patients prefer to participate in activities that may shorten their life spans, rather than expecting them to comply with a rigid treatment plan, the nurse must be willing to teach patients how to recognize what to do if something goes wrong.

Frame of Mind   This factor involves concern about the here and now. If survival is of primary concern, then readiness to learn will be focused on meeting basic human needs. Physical needs such as food, warmth, comfort, and safety as well as psychosocial needs of feeling accepted and secure must be met before someone can focus on other learning. People from lower socioeconomic levels tend to pay immediate attention to present-day concerns because they are trying to satisfy everyday needs. Children also regard life in the here and now because they are developmentally focused on what makes them happy and satisfied. In addition, their thinking is concrete rather than abstract. Adults who have reached self-actualization (see Figure 4-1) and whose basic needs are met tend to plan for their future and are more ready to learn health promotion tasks.

Developmental Stage   Each stage associated with human development produces a peak time for readiness to learn certain tasks, known as a "teachable moment" (Tanner, 1989). Unlike children, adults can build on meaningful past experiences and are strongly driven to learn information that will help them to cope better with real-life tasks. They see learning as relevant when they can apply new knowledge to help them solve immediate problems. Children, on the other hand, desire to learn for learning's sake. They actively seek out experiences that give them pleasure and comfort (see Chapter 5 for more on developmental stages) and involve themselves in activities that stimulate their physical and psychosocial development.

Experiential Readiness

Before starting to teach, the nurse should assess whether previous learning experiences have been positive or negative in overcoming problems or accomplishing new tasks. Someone who has had negative experiences with learning is not likely to be motivated or willing to take a risk in trying to change behavior or acquire new behaviors. Five components of this type of readiness must be assessed.

Level of Aspiration   Previous failures and past successes influence what goals learners set for themselves. Early successes in accomplishing skills are important motivators for learning. Satisfaction, once achieved, elevates the level of desire, and this in turn increases the probability of continued efforts to change or acquire new behavior.

Past Coping Mechanisms   The coping mechanisms someone has been using must be explored to understand how the learner has dealt with previous problems. Once these mechanisms are identified, the nurse must determine if past coping strategies have been effective and, if so, whether these will work well under the present learning situation.

Cultural Background   Knowledge by nurses about other cultures and their ability to be sensitive to behavioral differences between cultures are important to avoid teaching in opposition to cultural beliefs (see Chapter 8 for more on cultural attributes). Assessment of what an illness means from the patient's cultural perspective is important in determining readiness to learn. Remaining sensitive to cultural influences allows nurses to bridge the gap, when necessary, between the medical healthcare culture and the patient's culture. Building on the learner's knowledge base or belief system (unless it is dangerous to well-being), rather than attempting to change it or claiming it is wrong, will encourage rather than dampen readiness to learn.

Language is also a part of culture and may prove to be a significant obstacle to learning if the nurse and the learner do not fluently speak the same language. A qualified interpreter will be necessary to help the nurse and the patient to communicate with one another. Enlisting the help of someone else, such as a relative or a friend who is not a trained interpreter, to bridge the language differences may have a negative impact on learning. There may be instances when a patient does not want to have family members or friends know about a health concern or be present when a sensitive topic is discussed.

Also, medical terminology in and of itself may be a foreign language to many patients, whether or not they are from another culture or their primary language is not English. In addition, sometimes a native language does not have an equivalent word to describe the terms that are being used in the teaching situation. Differences in language compound the cultural barrier. Teaching should not be started unless you have determined that the learner understands you and that you have an understanding of the learner's culture (see Chapter 8 for more on cultural attributes).

Locus of Control　When patients are internally motivated to learn, they have what is known as an internal locus of control. They are ready to learn when they feel a need to know about something. Patients with an external locus of control depend on the expectations and initiatives of others to get them motivated to learn. How assertive and responsible a person tends to be indicates their locus of control type.

Orientation　The tendency to adhere to a parochial or cosmopolitan point of view is known as orientation. Patients with a parochial orientation tend to be more conservative in their thinking and their approach to situations. They are not as willing to accept change and tend to place their trust in traditional authority figures, such as the physician. This type of orientation is seen most often in people who have been raised in a small-town atmosphere or who come from cohesive neighborhoods or sheltered family environments. Conversely, people who exhibit a cosmopolitan orientation are more likely to have a worldly perspective on life due to broader experiences outside their immediate spheres of influence. These individuals tend to be more receptive to new ideas and to opportunities to learn new ways of doing things. One must be careful not to unfairly stereotype individuals, but when asked, learners will label themselves as being liberal, moderate, or conservative. Also their lifestyle, attitudes, and behaviors will often indicate their predominant orientation.

Knowledge Readiness

This refers to the learner's present knowledge base, the level of learning capability, and the preferred style of learning. These components must be assessed to determine readiness to learn, and teaching should be planned accordingly.

Present Knowledge Base　How much someone already knows about a particular subject is an important component that needs to be assessed before implementing teaching. If the nurse makes the mistake of teaching some topic that the patient already knows then he or she risks insulting the learner. This could produce resistance to further learning. Always find out what the patient already knows prior to teaching, and build on this knowledge base to encourage readiness to learn.

Cognitive Ability　The nurse must match behavioral objectives to the ability of the learner, or failure to achieve will result. The learner who demonstrates problem solving or who can apply information to everyday situations is functioning at a higher level than the learner who can memorize or recall information but can't apply this information to everyday situations. The level at which the learner is able to learn is of major importance when planning to teach.

Individuals with limited cognitive abilities present a special challenge to the nurse and will require simple explanations and step-by-step instruction with frequent repetition. Teaching members of the patient's support system the necessary skills for self-care will allow them to positively contribute to the reinforcement of information or assume responsibility for activities of daily living when the patient is at home.

Learning Disabilities   People with learning disabilities and low-level reading skills will require special approaches to teaching. It is easy for those who struggle with learning in traditional ways to become discouraged unless the nurse recognizes their special needs and seeks ways to help them adapt or overcome their problems with processing information (see Chapters 7 on literacy and 9 on special populations).

Learning Styles   A variety of preferred styles of learning exist. Assessing how someone learns best will help the nurse to vary teaching approaches accordingly. Knowing what teaching methods and materials a learner is most comfortable with or, conversely, does not tolerate well will help the nurse to tailor teaching according to how someone learns best. Meeting the needs of individuals with different styles of learning increases their readiness to learn. The following discussion on learning styles provides further information on the uniqueness of individuals' preferences for learning.

LEARNING STYLES

Learning styles refer to the way individuals process information (Guild & Garger, 1998). Each learner is unique and complex, with distinct learning style preferences that distinguish one learner from another. Certain characteristics of learning style are biological in origin, whereas others are developed as a result of sociological and environmental influences. Accepting diversity of style can help nurses create an atmosphere for learning that offers experiences that encourage each individual to reach his or her full potential. No learning style is either better or worse than another. The more flexible the nurse is in using different approaches to teaching, the greater the likelihood that learning will occur.

Six Learning Style Principles

Six principles have emerged from research about learning styles based on the work of Friedman and Alley (1984). The six principles provide a basic foundation for the nurse to understand learning styles and are as follows:

1. *Both the style by which the nurse prefers to teach and the style by which the patient prefers to learn can often be identified.* Identification of different styles offers clues as to the way a person learns.

2. *Nurses need to guard against teaching exclusively by their own preferred learning styles.* Nurses should realize that just because they like to learn a certain way does not mean that everyone else can or wants to learn this way. It is much easier for the nurse to change the teaching approach than for the learner to adapt to the teacher's style.

3. *Nurses should assist patients to identify their own style preferences.* Awareness of individual style preferences will help patients to understand what teaching and learning approaches work best for them.

4. *Patients should have the opportunity to learn through their preferred style.* Visual learners, for example, should be given videos, computer simulations, illustrations, and models for learning rather than written materials alone to get the information they need.

5. *Nurses should encourage patients to diversify their style preferences.* Once patients have a good understanding of the content and are comfortable in the learning situations the nurse should try other approaches to teaching that will help patients to learn to their fullest potential. The more frequently learners are exposed to different ways of learning, the more likely their comfort level will increase.

6. *Nurses must become aware of various methods and materials available to address and augment the different learning styles.* To be effective, teaching should be geared to different learning styles because using only a limited number of approaches will exclude many learners.

To determine a person's learning style, three mechanisms can be used—observation, interviews, and learning style instruments. For example, by observing the learner in action, the nurse can discover how a patient approaches information and solves problems. During an interview, the nurse can ask questions to get responses about what type of environment and which methods of teaching are most preferred. Does the temperature of the room or the noise level in the surroundings affect concentration? Is group discussion more preferable than one-to-one instruction? Once data are gathered through interview and observations the nurse can validate learning style and choose methods and materials for instruction to match the preferences of the learner. By administering learning style instruments, learning style preferences can be measured. However, because it is not always practical in a clinical setting to actually administer these instruments to every patient, the following discussion will focus on the popular theories on learning styles rather than on the instruments used to measure styles of learning.

Adapting educational experiences to coincide with how someone best processes information increases the likelihood that learning will take place. Recognizing that various styles exist is useful when making decisions about choosing the most effective approaches to teaching patients and their families.

Theorists define learning styles differently, but many of the concepts are overlapping. The remainder of this chapter will look at some of the well-known theories on learning styles. These do not offer any single framework for teaching but do provide the nurse with a better understanding of how learners perceive and process information (Villejo & Meyers, 1991).

Right-Brain/Left-Brain and Whole-Brain Thinking

Twenty-five years ago Dr. Roger Sperry and his research team established that in many ways the brain functions as two brains (Herrman, 1988; Sperry, 1977). The brain is composed of two hemispheres that have separate and complementary functions. Studies were conducted on people whose hemispheres were separated to observe how each hemisphere functions. The left hemisphere of the brain was found to be the vocal and analytical side, which is used for verbalization and for reality-based and logical thinking. The right hemisphere was found to be the emotional, visual-spatial, nonverbal hemisphere. Thinking processes using the right brain are intuitive, subjective, relational, holistic, and time-free. Sperry and his colleagues also discovered that learners are able to use both sides of the brain because of a connector between the two hemispheres called the corpus callosum.

There is no correct or wrong side of the brain. Each hemisphere gathers the same sensory information but handles the information in different ways. Nurses need to know that each side of the brain is better equipped for certain kinds of tasks and, thus, what is the most effective and efficient way to present information to learners who may have a dominant brain hemisphere (see Table 4-3). Also, knowledge of one's own brain hemispherical performance can aid nurses in identifying their strengths and weaknesses as teachers.

Recent advances in brain research, mainly due to neuroimaging techniques such as positron emission tomography (PET) and magnetic resonance imaging (MRI) provide new knowledge about how the brain works. Such technology has contributed to better understanding of brain hemispherical performance and has confirmed the importance of right–left brain functioning on individual differences in learning

TABLE 4-3 Examples of Hemisphere Functions	
Left-Hemisphere Functions	**Right-Hemisphere Functions**
Thinking is critical and logical	Thinking is creative and intuitive
Prefers talking	Prefers drawing and manipulating objects
Responds to verbal instructions and explanations	Responds to written instructions
Recognizes and remembers names	Recognizes and remembers pictures and faces
Solves problems by logically breaking them into parts	Solves problems by looking at the whole, sees patterns and uses hunches
Good organizational skills	Loose organizational skills
Likes stability, willing to adhere to rules	Likes change, uncertainty
Conscious of time and schedules	Frequently loses contact with time and schedules
Controls emotions	Free with emotions

(Caulfield, Kidd, & Kocher, 2000; Iaccino, 1993; McIntosh, 1998; Stover, 2001; Sylvester, 1995).

Statistics show that most Americans have left-brain dominance and that only approximately 30% have right-brain dominance (Gondringer, 1989). This may be because our educational system at the primary and secondary grade levels is geared toward rewarding left-brain skills of structural, logical, and concrete thinking to the extent that right-brain skills go undeveloped. Teaching strategies aimed at helping learners to use the less dominant side of their brain will facilitate more effective and efficient learning. For example, teachers might choose to play soft music in the background at a slow, even rhythm, to stimulate right-brain functioning in those who are left-brain dominant. Whole-brain thinking allows the learner to get the best of both worlds. Duality of thinking should be encouraged to help learners reach their fullest learning potentials.

Because the brain does more than just mental processing, other variables such as a person's feelings and desires must be taken into account (Gardner, 1999). For example, the culture in which one lives is important in the development and expression of one's learning style.

Dunn and Dunn Learning Style

Dunn and Dunn (1978) identified five basic stimuli (see Figure 4-3) that affect a person's ability to learn:

1. Environmental elements (such as sound, light, temperature, design), which are biological in nature.
2. Emotional elements (such as motivation, persistence, responsibility, and structure), which are developmental and emerge over time as a result of experiences that have happened at home, school, and play or work.
3. Sociological patterns, which indicate the desire to work alone or in groups.
4. Physical elements (such as perceptual strength, intake, time of day, and mobility), which are also biological in nature and relate to the way learners function physically.
5. Psychological elements, which indicate the way learners process and react to information.

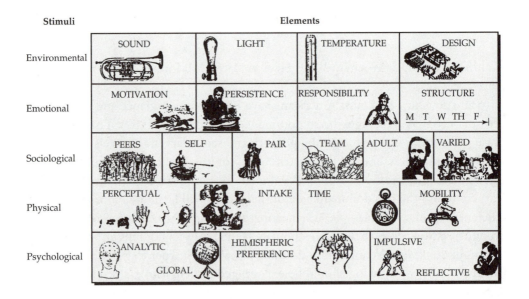

FIGURE 4-3   Dunn and Dunn's Learning Style Elements
Source: R. Dunn, "Can Students Identify Their Own Learning Styles?" *Educational Leadership, 40,* 5:61. Reprinted by permission of the Association for Supervision and Curriculum Development.
Copyright © 1983 by ASCD. All rights reserved.

Certain characteristics of Dunn and Dunn's identified stimuli are very relevant to the role of the nurse as teacher. The nurse needs to consider the following selected characteristics when assessing a patient's or a family member's learning style.

The Environmental Elements

Sound   Individuals react to sound in different ways. Some need complete silence, others are able to block out sounds around them, and others require sound in their environment for learning.

Light   Some learners work best under bright lights and others need dim or low lighting.

Temperature   Some learners have difficulty thinking or concentrating if a room is too hot or, conversely, if it is too cold.

The Emotional Elements

Motivation   Motivation, or the desire to achieve, increases when learning success increases. Unmotivated learners need short learning assignments that enhance their strengths. Motivated learners, by comparison, are eager to learn and should be told exactly what they are required to do, with resources available so they can self-pace their learning.

Responsibility   Responsibility involves the desire to do what learners think is expected of them. Individuals with low responsibility scores usually are nonconforming and will do something according to their own time frame and in their own way. Conversely, those who demonstrate high levels of responsibility will usually undertake to complete a task immediately and as directed.

The Sociological Elements

Learning Alone   Some people learn on their own and, therefore, self-instruction or one-to-one interaction is the best approach for learning. For those who prefer to learn with family members or friends, group discussion and role playing are effective to facilitate learning.

Presence of an Authority Figure   Some learners feel more comfortable when someone with authority or recognized expertise is present during learning. Others become timid, are embarrassed to demonstrate their skills, and often become too tense to concentrate. Depending on the style of the learner, either one-to-one interaction or self-study, for example, may be the appropriate approach.

The Physical Elements

Perceptual Strengths   Four types of learners are distinguished in this category: those with auditory preferences, who learn best while listening to verbal instruction; those with visual preferences, who learn best by reading or observing; those with tactile preferences, who learn best when they can underline as they read, take notes when they listen, and otherwise keep their hands busy; and those with kinesthetic preferences, who absorb and retain information best when allowed to participate in simulated or real-life experiences.

Auditory learners should be introduced to new information first by hearing about it, followed by verbal feedback for reinforcement of the information. Group discussion is a teaching method best suited to their style. Visual learners should be allowed to view, watch, and observe; therefore, videotapes and demonstration approaches are most beneficial to their learning. Tactile learners should be given the opportunity to touch, manipulate, and handle objects. The use of models and computer-assisted instruction is most suitable for their learning style. Kinesthetic learners, who like learning by doing and experiencing things, profit from opportunities for role playing and participating in return demonstration.

Time of Day   Some learners perform better at one time of day than another. The nurse needs to identify these preferences with an effort toward structuring teaching and learning to occur during the times that are most suitable for the learner. Dunn (1995) contends that among adults, 55% are "morning people" and 28% work best in the evening. Many adults experience energy lows in the afternoon. School-age children, on the other hand, tend to have high energy levels in the late morning and early afternoon. About 13% of high school students work best in the evening. This means that it may be more difficult for a person to learn a new skill or behavior at certain times of the day than at other times.

Dunn and Dunn stress that these characteristics yield information regarding the patterns through which learning occurs but do not assess the finer aspects of an individual's skills. These learning style elements indicate how people prefer to learn, not the abilities they possess.

The Psychological Elements

Global versus Analytic   Some learners are global in their thinking and learn best by first understanding an issue, problem, or concept from a broad, overall perspective before focusing on the specific parts. Other learners are analytic in their thinking, like details, and process information best by using a step-by-step approach to learning.

Impulsive versus Reflective Impulsive learners tend to prefer opportunities to participate in groups and answer questions spontaneously. Reflective learners are not as likely to volunteer information unless they are asked to do so, prefer to contemplate information, and tend to be less comfortable in groups (Dunn, 1984).

Jung and Myers-Briggs Typology

C. G. Jung (1921, 1971), a Swiss psychiatrist, developed a theory that explains personality similarities and differences by identifying the ways people prefer to take in and make use of data from the world around them. Jung proposed that each individual will tend to develop comfortable patterns, which dictate behavior in certain predictable ways. Jung used the word "types" to identify these styles of personality.

According to Jung's typology all people can be classified using three criteria called dimensions or preferences:

1. *Extraversion-Introversion (EI)* reflects an orientation to either the outside world of people and things or to the inner world of concepts and ideas. This dimension describes the extent to which our behavior is determined by our attitudes toward the world. Jung invented the terms from Latin words meaning outward turning (extraversion) or inward turning (introversion). Jung said extraverts operate comfortably and successfully by interacting with things external to themselves, such as other people, experiences, and situations. Extraverts like to clarify thoughts and ideas through talking and doing. Those who operate more comfortably in an extraverted way think aloud. Introverts, on the other hand, are more interested in the internal world of their minds, hearts, and souls. They like to brew over thoughts and actions, reflecting on them until they become more personally meaningful. Those who operate more comfortably in an introverted way are often thoughtful, reflective, and slow to act because they need time to translate internal thoughts to the external world. Introverts have their thoughts well formulated before they are willing to share them with others.

2. *Sensing-Intuition (SN)* describes perception as coming directly through the five senses or indirectly by way of the unconscious. This dimension explains how people understand what is experienced. People who fall into the sensing category view the world through their senses—vision, hearing, touch, taste, and smell. They observe what is real, what is factual, and what is actually happening. Seeing (or other sensory experiences) is believing. These sensing functions allow the individual to observe carefully, gather facts, and focus on practical actions. Conversely, those people who are associated with the intuition category tend to

read between the lines, focus on meaning, and attend to what is and what might be. Intuitives view the world through possibilities and relationships and are tuned into subtleties of body language and tones of voice. This kind of perception leads them to examine problems and issues in creative and original ways.

3. *Thinking-Feeling (TF)* is the approach used by individuals to arrive at judgments through impersonal, logical, or subjective processes. Thinkers analyze information, data, situations, and people and make decisions based on logic. They are careful and slow in the analysis of the data because accuracy and thoroughness are important to them. They trust objectivity and put faith in logical predictions and rational arguments. Thinkers explore and weigh all alternatives, and the final decision is reached unemotionally and carefully. In the feeling dimension, on the other hand, the approach to decision making is through a subjective, perceptive, empathetic, and emotional perspective. Feeling people search for the effect of a decision on themselves and others. They consider alternatives and examine evidence to develop a personal reaction and commitment. They believe the decision-making process is complex and not totally objective. Circumstantial evidence is extremely important, and they see the world as gray rather than black and white.

Jung said that everyone uses these opposing perceptions to some degree in each of the three dimensions (EI, SN, TF) when dealing with people and situations, but each person has a preference for one way of looking at the world. Individuals become more skilled in arriving at a decision in either a thinking or feeling way and can function as extraverts at one time and as introverts at another time, but they tend to develop patterns that are most typical and comfortable.

Katherine Briggs and her daughter Isabel Briggs Myers became convinced that Jung's theories had an application for increasing human understanding (Myers, 1980). In addition to Jung's dimensions, Myers and Briggs discovered another dimension, Judgment-Perception (JP), whereby an individual comes to a conclusion about something or becomes aware of something (see Figure 4-4). Each individual has a preference for either the judging function or the perceptive function. The desire to regulate and bring closure to circumstances in life is called judgment, and the desire to be open-minded and understanding is known as perception.

The different combinations of the dimensions can be useful for the nurse to understand the many different ways in which learners process information when learning (see Table 4-4). These preferences can be reflected in how the nurse teaches and how the learner learns. It is the responsibility of the nurse to strive to adapt teaching to meet the style of the learner.

Extraversion (E) ←——————→ Introversion (I)

Sensing (S) ←——————→ Intuition (N)

Thinking (T) ←——————→ Feeling (F)

Judgment (J) ←——————→ Perception (P)

FIGURE 4-4   Myers-Briggs Dichotomous Dimensions or Preferences

TABLE 4-4   Jung and Myers-Briggs Types: Examples of Learning

EXTRAVERT	**INTROVERT**
Likes group work	Likes quiet space
Dislikes slow-paced learning	Dislikes interruptions
Likes action and to experience things so as to learn	Likes learning that deals with thoughts and ideas
Offers opinions without being asked	Offers opinions only when asked
Asks questions to check on the expectations of nurse	Asks questions to allow understanding of learning activity
SENSING	**INTUITION**
Practical	Always likes something new
Realistic	Imaginative
Observation	Sees possibilities
Learns from orderly sequence of details	Prefers the whole concept versus details
THINKING	**FEELING**
Low need for harmony	Values harmony
Finds ideas and things more interesting than people	More interested in people than things or ideas
Analytical	Sympathetic
Fair	Accepting
JUDGMENT	**PERCEPTION**
Organized	Open-ended
Methodical	Flexible
Work-oriented	Play-oriented
Controls the environment	Adapts to the environment

Kolb's Cycle of Learning

In Kolb's model (Kolb, 1984), known as the Cycle of Learning, learning is a continuous process. He acknowledges that the learner is not a blank slate and that every learner approaches a topic to be learned based on past experiences, heredity, and the demands of the present environment. These factors combine to produce different orientations (modes) to learning. By understanding Kolb's theory, the nurse is better equipped to provide teaching to meet the needs of each individual's preferred style of learning.

The Cycle of Learning, which includes four modes of learning, reflects two major dimensions: perception and processing. Kolb believes that learning results from the way learners perceive information as well as how they process information.

The *dimension of perception* includes two opposing viewpoints—learners either perceive through concrete experience (CE mode) or they perceive through abstract conceptualization (AC mode). Those oriented to CE learning tend to rely more on feelings than on thinking when dealing with problems and situations. Learners who fall into this category like relating with people, benefit from group experiences, and are sensitive to others. They learn best by getting in touch with their feelings. Those with an AC orientation to learning, on the other hand, rely on logic and ideas rather than on feelings to handle problems or situations. They learn best by thinking and analyzing.

The *process dimension* also includes two opposing orientations. Learners either process information through active experimentation (AE mode) or through reflective observation (RO mode). Those with an AE orientation to learning tend to like to be actively involved and prefer to experiment with things to influence or change situations. They are risk takers and learn best by doing. Those with an RO orientation to learning rely on objectivity, careful judgment, personal thoughts, and feelings to form opinions. People who fall into this category look for the meaning of things by viewing them from different perspectives. They learn best by watching and listening.

Kolb labeled learning styles as "types" by combining the modes (CE, AC, AE, and RO) to define the strengths and weaknesses of a learner. The learner predominantly demonstrates characteristics of one of the following style types (see Figure 4-5).

1. The *diverger* combines the modes of CE and RO. People with this learning style are good at viewing concrete situations from many points of view. They like to observe, gather information, and gain insights rather than take action. Working in groups to generate ideas appeals to them. They place a high value on understanding for knowledge's sake and like to personalize learning by connecting information with something familiar in their experiences. They have active imaginations, enjoy being involved, and are sensitive to feelings. Divergent thinkers

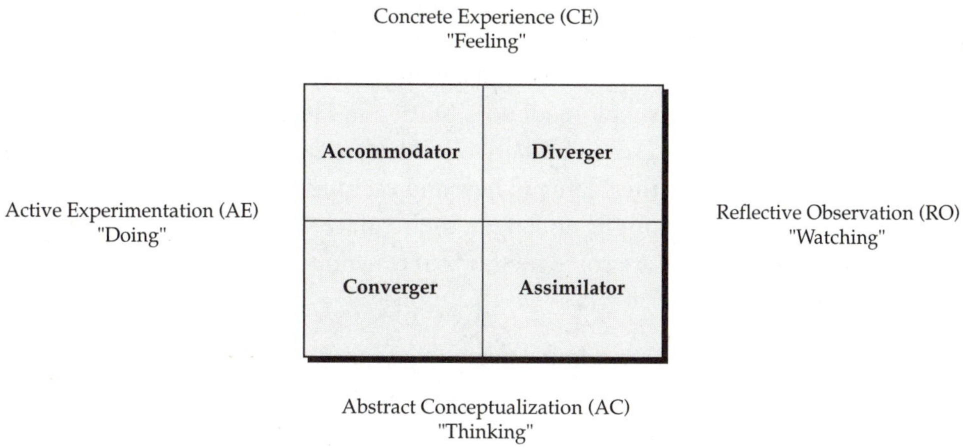

Concrete Experience (CE)
"Feeling"

Accommodator	Diverger
Converger	Assimilator

Active Experimentation (AE)
"Doing"

Reflective Observation (RO)
"Watching"

Abstract Conceptualization (AC)
"Thinking"

FIGURE 4-5   Kolb's Cycle of Learning

Source: Kolb, D. *Experiential Learning: Experience as Source of Learning and Development.* © 1984, Figure 4.2.

learn best, for example, through group discussions and participating in brainstorming sessions.

2. The *assimilator* combines the modes of AC and RO. People with this learning style demonstrate the ability to understand large amounts of information by putting it into concise and logical form. They are less interested in people and more focused on abstract ideas and concepts. They are good at inductive reasoning, value theory over practical application of ideas, and need time to reflect on what has been learned and how new information is related to their past experiences. They rely on knowledge from experts. Assimilative thinkers learn best, for example, through lecture, one-to-one instruction, and self-instruction methods with ample reading materials to support their learning.

3. The *converger* combines the modes of AC and AE. People with this learning style find practical application for ideas and theories and have the ability to use deductive reasoning to solve problems. They like structure and factual information, look for specific solutions to problems, and prefer technical tasks rather than dealing with social and interpersonal issues. Convergent thinkers learn best, for example, through demonstration–return demonstration methods of teaching accompanied by handouts and diagrams.

4. The *accommodator* combines the modes of CE and AE. People with this learning style learn best by hands-on experience and enjoy new and challenging situations. They act on intuitive and "gut feelings" rather than on logic. They are risk takers who like to explore all possibilities and learn by experimenting with materials and objects. Accommodative thinkers are perhaps the most challenging to nurses because they demand new and exciting experiences and are willing to take chances that might endanger their safety. Role playing, gaming, and computer simulations are some methods of teaching most preferred by this style of learner.

Kolb believes that understanding a person's learning style, including its strengths and weaknesses, represents a major step toward increasing learning power and helping learners to get the most from their learning experiences. The nurse, by using different teaching strategies to address these four learning styles, can match particular modes of learning, at least some of the time, with appropriate methods of teaching. For most groups of learners, about 25% will fall into each of the four categories. If the educator predominantly uses only one method of teaching, such as the lecture, then 75% of all learners will be excluded from the opportunity to be presented with information in the way they learn best.

Therefore, when teaching groups of learners who have different orientations to learning, instruction should begin with activities best suited to the divergent thinker and progress sequentially to include activities for the assimilator, converger, and accommodator, respectively (Arndt & Underwood, 1990). This pattern works because learners must first have foundational knowledge of a subject before they can test out information. Otherwise, they will be operating from a level of ignorance. It is important that they have familiarity with facts and ideas before they can explore and test concepts.

Gardner's Seven Types of Intelligence

Children also have their own way of learning. Learning styles of children can be assessed from the standpoint of growth and each individual's unique pattern of neurological functioning. Psychologist Howard Gardner (1983) developed a theory of seven different kinds of intelligence, and this theory is useful in looking at styles of learning in children. He identified seven kinds of intelligence located in different parts of the brain: linguistic, logical-mathematical, spatial, musical, bodily-kinesthetic, interpersonal, and intrapersonal. All learners have each of the seven kinds of intelligence but in different proportions.

1. *Linguistic intelligence:* Children who have a preference for this type of intelligence have highly developed auditory skills and think in words. They like to write, tell stories, spell words accurately, and read, and can recall names, places, and dates. These children learn best by verbalizing, hearing, or seeing words. Word games or crossword puzzles are excellent methods for helping these children learn new material.

2. *Logical-mathematical intelligence:* The children who are strong in this intelligence explore patterns, categories, and relationships. In the adolescent years, they can think logically with a high degree of abstraction. As learners, they question a lot and ask where, what, and when. A question this learner could ask is, "If people are always supposed to be good to each other, then why do people always say they are sorry?" They can do arithmetic problems quickly in their heads, like to learn by computers, and do experiments to test concepts they do not understand. They enjoy strategy board games such as chess or checkers.

3. *Spatial intelligence:* These children learn by images and pictures. They enjoy such things as building blocks, jigsaw puzzles, and daydreaming. They like to draw or do other art activities, can read charts and diagrams, and learn with visual methods such as videos or photographs.

4. *Musical intelligence:* These children can be found singing a tune, telling you when a note is off-key, playing musical instruments with ease, dancing to music, and keeping time rhythmically. They are also sensitive to sounds in the environment such as the sound of walking on snow on a cold winter morning. Often musically intelligent children learn best with music playing in the background.

5. *Bodily-kinesthetic intelligence:* These children learn by processing knowledge through bodily sensations. They need to learn by moving or acting things out. It is difficult for these learners to sit still for long periods of time. They are good at sports and have highly developed fine-motor coordination. Use of body language to communicate and copying people's behaviors or movements come easily for this group of learners.

6. *Interpersonal intelligence:* These children understand people, are able to notice others' feelings, tend to have many friends, and are gifted in the social skills. They learn best in groups and gravitate toward activities that involve others.

7. *Intrapersonal intelligence:* These children have strong personalities and prefer the inner world of feeling and ideas and like being alone. They are very private individuals, like a quiet area to learn, and many times need to be by themselves in order to learn. They tend to be self-directed and self-confident. They learn well with independent, self-paced instruction.

Educators should approach a child's learning using concepts from the seven intelligences (Armstrong, 1987). Often it can be difficult to assess the preferred learning style of a child when the child is facing an illness or surgery. Asking some key questions of the child or parents may give the educator some clues as to the preferred style of learning:

- What does the child already know how to do?
- What subjects does the child excel in or like best?
- What kinds of hobbies does the child have?
- What excites this child?
- What kinds of toys does the child play with?
- What inner qualities does the child possess, such as courage, playfulness, curiosity, friendliness, or creativity?
- What talents does the child have?
- Does the child like to take things apart and put them back together?

By using the theory of the seven intelligences, the educator can assess each child's style of learning and tailor teaching accordingly. For example, if the nurse wants to assist a child in learning about a kidney disorder, then one of seven different approaches can be used, depending on the child's style of learning:

1. *Linguistic:* Practice verbally quizzing the child on the different parts of the kidney, the disease itself, and how to take care of oneself.
2. *Spatial:* Have a diagram or chart that allows the child to associate different colors or shapes with concepts. Storytelling can be used illustrating a child with the same chronic illness.
3. *Bodily-kinesthetic:* Have a kidney model available that can be felt, taken apart, and manipulated. Have the child identify tactile features of the kidney or "act out" appropriate behavior.
4. *Logical-mathematical:* Group concepts into categories, starting with simple generalizations or health behaviors. Reasoning works well in showing the child the consequences of actions.
5. *Musical:* Teach self-care or the material to be learned by putting information into a song. Soft music also serves as a relaxing influence on the child.
6. *Interpersonal:* Have a group of children play a card game that matches information with medical pictures or pictures of healthcare activities and procedures. Use group work for problem-solving activities.
7. *Intrapersonal:* Suggest that the child get active in writing to friends, family, or local and state government officials to advocate for kidney disease. They need to

research the facts and then convey these findings to others. These children learn best by one-to-one teaching and through use of self-learning modules.

INTERPRETATION OF LEARNING STYLES

Learning style is an important consideration in the teaching–learning process. However, caution must be used in assessing styles in order not to ignore other factors that are equally important in learning such as readiness to learn, educational and cultural backgrounds, and gender differences in learning. Styles, which vary from person to person, also differ from capabilities in that the style by which someone learns describes how that individual processes stimuli as opposed to defining how much and how well the information is processed (Thompson & Crutchlow, 1993). Many learning theorists advocate that learning style be matched with a similar teaching style for learners to attain an optimum level of achievement. However, it may be that learning occurs not so much as a result of matching teacher and learner styles, but that learners feel less stressed when the nurse uses a variety of different teaching approaches rather than relying on just one. As a result, learners will be more satisfied overall with the learning experience and, hence, will be more motivated to learn. Nevertheless, using teaching methods that coincide with the dominant learning style of individuals usually has the greatest influence on learning achievement (de Tornay & Thompson, 1987). Application of learning style theory allows the nurse to approach learners holistically, recognizing they do not all process information in the same way (Arndt & Underwood, 1990).

Although individuals have a certain dominant learning style that prevails over time, they may temporarily gravitate to using other styles depending on the circumstances at any given moment. The following general guidelines should be followed when assessing individual learning styles:

- Become familiar with the ways in which styles are classified so that it becomes easier to recognize various approaches to learning.
- Identify key elements of an individual's learning style by observing and asking questions to verify observations and then matching instructional methods and materials to those unique qualities. For example, such questions could include the following: "Do you prefer to attend group classes or one-on-one teaching with the nurse?" "Which do you like to do better, reading or viewing a video?" "Would you like me to demonstrate this skill first, or would you rather learn by doing while I talk you through the procedure?"

- Always give learners the opportunity to say when the teaching method is not working for them.
- Place emphasis on assessing learning styles as a way to increase understanding both from the nurse's and the learner's perspectives. No one style is better than another, and everyone should realize that there are a variety of learning modalities.
- Be cautious about saying that certain instructional methods are always more effective for certain styles. Remember that everyone is unique, and there are many different ways to influence learning.
- Provide learning choices that enable learners to recognize and choose the style in which they prefer to learn.

Caution must be exercised to avoid stereotyping learners as to their style. The goal should be to identify preferred styles of learning to ensure that each individual is given an equal opportunity to learn the best or most comfortable way. Understanding learning styles helps the nurse choose diverse teaching methods and materials to meet the needs of all learners.

SUMMARY

Learning is a complex concept that depends on many factors influencing a learner to change or learn new behavior. This chapter stressed the importance of assessing each individual's learning needs, readiness to learn, and learning styles prior to planning and implementing any teaching intervention. Assessment of these three determinants provides the information necessary for decision making about who and what needs to be taught, when teaching should take place, and where and how teaching should be carried out.

Identifying and prioritizing learning needs is the first step and requires the nurse to find out what information the learner feels is important or wants to know. Once these needs are established, the nurse must assess the learner's readiness to learn based on the physical, emotional, experiential, and knowledge components particular to each learner. The last determinant of learning examines individual learning styles. Assessment of learning style by way of interviewing and observing can reveal how people best learn as well as how they prefer to learn. By accepting the diversity of style among learners, the nurse can provide optimal experiences that encourage all learners to reach their fullest potentials. Effective and efficient patient and family education demands that the nurse in the role of a teacher attend to determinants of learning. Whoever the audience may be, the nurse must be able to identify and select the most appropriate teaching methods and instructional materials that facilitate learning.

REVIEW QUESTIONS

1. What are the three determinants of learning?
2. How are the terms *learning needs, readiness to learn,* and *learning styles* defined?
3. What are six important steps to assess learning needs?
4. What are the four types of readiness to learn and the components of each type?
5. What are the six learning style principles that should guide the nurse in teaching any audience of learners?
6. Why is it important to assess learning style?
7. What are similarities and differences between the learning style types?

REFERENCES

Armstrong, T. (1987). *In their own way.* New York: St. Martin's Press.

Arndt, M. J. & Underwood, B. (1990). Learning style theory and patient understanding. *Journal of Continuing Education in Nursing, 21*(1), 28–31.

Ashton, K. C. (1999). How men and women with heart disease seek care: The delay experience. *Progress in Cardiovascular Nursing, 14*(2), 53–60.

Beddoe, S. S. (1999). Reachable moment. *Image: Journal of Nursing Scholarship, 31*(3), 248.

Bertakis, K. D., Rahman, A., Helms, L. J., Callahan, E. J., & Robbins, J. A. (2000). Gender differences in the utilization of health care services. *Journal of Family Practice, 49*(2), 147–152.

Bloom, B. (1968). *Learning for mastery.* Instruction and Curriculum, Topical Papers and Reprints No. 1 (Durham, NC: National Laboratory for Higher Education).

Boyd, M. D., Gleit, C. J., Graham, B. A., & Whitman, N. I. (1998). *Health teaching in nursing practice: A professional model* (3rd ed.). Stamford, CT: Appleton & Lange.

Bruner, J. (1966). *Toward a theory of instruction.* Cambridge, MA: Harvard University Press.

Bubela, N. & Galloway, S. (1990). Factors influencing patients' informational needs at time of hospital discharge. *Patient Education and Counseling, 16,* 21–28.

Burton, C. (2000). Re-thinking stroke rehabilitation: The Corbin and Strauss chronic illness trajectory framework. *Journal of Advanced Nursing, 32*(3), 595–602.

Carroll, I. (1963). A model of school learning. *Teachers College Record, 64,* 723–733.

Caulfield, J., Kidd, S., & Kocher, T. (2000). Brain-based instruction in action. *Educational Leadership, 58*(3), 62–66.

Corbin, J. M. & Strauss, A. (1999). A nursing model for chronic illness management based upon the trajectory framework. *Scholarly Inquiry for Nursing Practice: An International Journal, 5*(3), 155–174.

deTornay, R. & Thompson, M. A. (1987). *Strategies for teaching nursing* (3rd ed.). Albany, NY: Delmar.

Dunn, R. (1984). Learning style: State of the science. *Theory into Practice, 23*(1), 10–19.

Dunn, R. (1995). *Strategies for educating diverse learners.* Bloomington, IN: Phi Delta Kappa Educational Foundation.

Dunn, R. & Dunn, K. (1978). *Teaching students through their individual learning styles: A practical approach.* Reston, VA: National Association of Secondary School Principals.

Friedman, P. & Alley, R. (1984). Learning/teaching styles: Applying the principles. *Theory into Practice, 23*(1), 77–81.

Gardner, H. (1983). *Frames of mind.* New York: Basic Books.

Gardner, H. (1999). *The disciplined mind: What all students should understand.* New York: Simon and Schuster.

Gondringer, N. (1989). Whole brain thinking: A potential link to successful learning. *Journal of the American Association of Nurse Anesthetists, 57*(3), 217–219.

Greer, G., Hitt, J. D., Sitterly, T. E., & Slebodnick, E. B. (1972). An examination of four factors impacting on psychomotor performance effectiveness. In D. P. Ely (ed.), *Psychomotor domain: A resource book for media specialists.* Washington, DC: Gryphon House.

Guild, P. B. & Garger, S. (1998). *Marching to different drummers* (2nd ed.). Alexandria, VA: Association for Supervision and Curriculum Development.

Haggard, A. (1989). *Handbook of patient education.* Rockland, MD: Aspen.

Hansen, M. & Fisher, J. C. (1998). Patient-centered teaching: From theory to practice. *American Journal of Nursing, 98*(1), 56–60.

Healthcare Education Association. (1985). *Managing hospital education.* Laquana Niquel, CA: Healthcare Education Associates.

Herrman, N. (1988). *The creative brain.* Lake Lure, NC: Brain Books.

Iaccino, J. F. (1993). *Left-brain right-brain differences: Inquiries, evidence and new approaches.* Hillsdale, NJ: Lawrence Erlbaum.

Joseph, D. H. (1993). Risk: A concept worthy of attention. *Nursing Forum, 28*(1), 12–16.

Jung, C. G. (1971). Psychological types. In *Collected works* (Vol. 6, R. F. C. Hull, Trans.). Princeton, NJ: Princeton University Press. (Originally published in German as *Psychologische Typen,* Zurich: Rasher Verlag, 1921.)

Kolb, D. A. (1984). *Experiential learning: Experience as the source of learning and development.* Englewood Cliffs, NJ: Prentice-Hall.

Lichtenthal, C. (1990). *A self-study model on readiness to learn.* Unpublished.

Maslow, A. (1970). *Motivation and personality.* New York: Harper & Row.

McIntosh, A. R. (1998). Understanding neural interactions in learning and memory using functional neuroimaging. *Annals of the New York Academy of Sciences. Olfaction and Taste XII: An International Symposium, 855,* 556–571.

Myers, I. B. (1980). *Gifts differing.* Palo Alto, CA: Consulting Psychologists Press.

Patterson, B. L. (2001). The shifting perspectives model of chronic illness. *Journal of Nursing Scholarship, 33*(1), 21–26.

Rankin, S. H. & Stallings, L. D. (2001). *Patient education: Issues, principles and practices* (4th ed.). Philadelphia: Lippincott.

Roberts, C. (1982). Identifying the real patient problems. *Nursing Clinics of North America, 17*(3), 484–485.

Ruzicki, D. A. (1989). Realistically meeting the educational needs of hospitalized acute and short-stay patients. *Nursing Clinics of North America, 24*(3), 629–636.

Singer, R. N. (1972). The psychomotor domain: General considerations. In D. P. Ely (ed.), *Psychomotor domain: A resource book for media specialists.* Washington, DC: Gryphon House.

Skinner, B. F. (1954). The science of learning and the art of teaching. *Harvard Educational Review, 24,* 86–97.

Sperry, R. W. (1977). Bridging science and values: A unifying view of mind and brain. *American Psychologist, 32*(4), 237–245.

Stein, J. A. & Nyamathi, A. (2000). Gender differences in behavioural and psychosocial predictors of HIV testing and return for test results in a high-risk population. *AIDS Care, 12*(3), 343–356.

Stover, D. (2001). Applying brain research in the classroom is not a no-brainer. *Education Digest, 66*(8), 26–29.

Sylvester, R. (1995). *A celebration of neurons: An educator's guide to the human brain.* Alexandria, VA: Association for Supervision and Curriculum Development.

Tanner, G. (1989). A need to know. *Nursing Times, 85*(31), 54–56.

Thompson, C. & Crutchlow, E. (1993). Learning style research: A critical review of the literature and implications for nursing education. *Journal of Professional Nursing, 9*(1), 34–40.

Villejo, L. and Myers, C. (1991). Brain function, learning styles, and cancer patient education. *Seminars in Oncology Nursing, 7*(2), 97–104.

Wagner, P. S. & Ash, K. L. (1998). Creating the teachable moment. *Journal of Nursing Education, 37*(6), 278–280.

Wolfe, P. (1994). Risk taking: Nursing's comfort zone. *Holistic Nurse Practice, 8*(2), 43–52.

CHAPTER 5

Developmental Stages of the Learner

Susan B. Bastable and Michelle A. Dart

CHAPTER HIGHLIGHTS

Developmental Characteristics
The Developmental Stages of Childhood
    Infancy (0–12 Months of Age) and
       Toddlerhood (1–3 Years of Age)
    Preschooler (3–6 Years of Age)
    School-Aged Childhood (6–12 Years
      of Age)
    Adolescence (12–18 Years of Age)

The Developmental Stages of Adulthood
    Young Adulthood (18–40 Years of Age)
    Middle-Aged Adulthood (40–65 Years
      of Age)
    Older Adulthood (65 Years of Age
      and Older)
The Role of the Family in Patient Education

KEY TERMS

ageism
andragogy
cognitive development
crystallized intelligence
developmental stage
fluid intelligence

gerogogy
imaginary audience
pedagogy
personal fable
physical maturation
psychosocial development

OBJECTIVES

After completing this chapter, the reader will be able to

1. Identify the physical, cognitive, and psychosocial characteristics of learners that influence learning at various stages of growth and development.
2. Recognize the role of the nurse as teacher in assessing stage-specific learner needs according to maturational levels.
3. Discuss appropriate teaching strategies effective for learners at different developmental stages.
4. Determine the role of the family in patient education.

When planning, designing, and implementing patient education, the nurse must carefully consider the characteristics of learners with respect to their developmental stage in life. The more diverse the audience, the more complex teaching will be to meet the needs of patients and their family members. Conversely, teaching a group of learners with the same characteristics will be more straightforward.

An individual's developmental stage significantly influences his or her ability to learn. Three major factors associated with learner readiness—physical, cognitive, and psychosocial maturation—must be taken into account at each developmental period throughout the life cycle. It is well recognized that the willingness and ability of individuals to make use of instruction depends to a large extent on their stage of growth and development.

A deliberate attempt has been made to minimize reference to age as the criterion for categorizing learners. Chronological age per se is not a good predictor of learning ability (Whitener, Cox, & Maglich, 1998). At any given age, there can be a wide variation in abilities related to physical, cognitive, and psychosocial maturation. Age ranges, included after each developmental stage heading in this chapter, are intended to be used only as general guidelines. They do not imply that chronological ages necessarily correspond to the various stages of development. Thus, the term *developmental stage* will be used based on the fact that human growth and development are sequential but not always specifically age-related.

This chapter has specific implications for staff nurses because of the recent mandates by the Joint Commission on Accreditation of Healthcare Organizations (JCAHO). For healthcare agencies to meet JCAHO accreditation requirements, teaching plans developed by nurses must address stage-specific competencies of the learner. Therefore, this chapter emphasizes the role of the nurse in assessing stage-specific learner needs, the role of the family in the teaching-learning process, and the teaching strategies specific to meeting the needs of learners at various developmental stages of life. Middle-aged and older adults account for the largest percentage of the patient population, so emphasis is placed on the learning needs of the adult learner.

DEVELOPMENTAL CHARACTERISTICS

As stated earlier, actual chronological age is only a relative indicator of someone's physical, cognitive, and psychosocial stage of development. Unique as each individual is, however, some typical developmental trends have been identified as standard milestones of normal progression through the life cycle. When dealing with the teaching-learning process, it is important to look at which developmental stage each learner is at to understand the cognitive, affective, and psychomotor behavioral changes that are occurring. However, other important factors such as past experiences, physical and emotional health, personal motivation, stress, environmental conditions, and available support systems also affect a person's ability and readiness to learn.

The major question underlying the planning for patient education is: When is the most appropriate or best time to teach the learner? The answer is when the learner is ready—the "teachable moment" as defined by Havighurst (1976)—that point in time when a person is most receptive to learning. It is important to remember that the nurse does not always have to wait for teachable moments to occur. Instead, the teacher can create these opportunities by taking an interest in and paying attention to the needs of the learner (Hussey & Hirsh, 1983).

THE DEVELOPMENTAL STAGES OF CHILDHOOD

Pedagogy is the art and science of helping children to learn. The different stages of childhood are divided according to specific patterns of behavior seen in particular phases of growth and development. The following is a review of the teaching strategies to be used in the four stages of childhood in relation to physical, cognitive, and psychosocial maturational levels (Table 5-1).

Infancy (0–12 Months of Age) and Toddlerhood (1–3 Years of Age)

At no other time is physical, cognitive, and psychosocial maturation so changeable as during the very early years of childhood. Because of the dependency of this age group, the main focus of instruction is geared toward the parents, who are considered to be the primary learners rather than the very young child.

Physical, Cognitive, and Psychosocial Development

Physical maturation is never so rapid as during the period of development from infancy to toddlerhood. The environment is an important factor in a child's physical development. Patient education must focus on teaching the parents of very young children the need for stimulation, good nutrition, and the practice of safety measures to prevent illness and injury.

Piaget (1951, 1952, 1976), the noted expert in defining the key milestones in the cognitive development of children, labeled the stage of infancy to toddlerhood as the *sensorimotor* period. During this stage, children learn through their senses. Motor activities help them understand their world and develop an awareness of themselves as well as how others respond to their actions.

TABLE 5-1   Stage-Appropriate Teaching Strategies

Learner	General Characteristics	Teaching Strategies	Nursing Interventions
Infancy-Toddlerhood			
Approximate age: Birth–3 yr Cognitive stage: Sensorimotor Psychosocial stage: Trust vs. mistrust (Birth–12 mo) Autonomy vs. shame and doubt (1–3 yr)	Dependent on environment Needs security Explores self and environment Natural curiosity	Orient teaching to caregiver Use repetition and imitation of information Stimulate all senses Provide physical safety and emotional security Allow play and manipulation of objects	Welcome active involvement Forge alliances Encourage physical closeness Provide detailed information Answer questions and concerns Ask for information on child's strengths/limitations and likes/dislikes
Preschooler			
Approximate age: 3–6 yr Cognitive stage: Preoperational Psychosocial stage: Initiative vs. guilt	Egocentric Thinking precausal, concrete, literal Believes illness self-caused and punitive Limited sense of time Fears bodily injury Cannot generalize Animistic thinking (objects possess life or human characteristics) Centration (focus is on one characteristic of an object) Separation anxiety Motivated by curiosity Active imagination, prone to fears Play is his/her work	Use warm, calm approach Build trust Use repetition of information Allow manipulation of objects and equipment Give care with explanation Reassure not to blame self Explain procedures simply and briefly Provide safe, secure environment Use positive reinforcement Encourage questions to reveal perceptions/feelings Use simple drawings and stories Use play therapy, with dolls and puppets Stimulate senses: visual, auditory, tactile, motor	Welcome active involvement Forge alliances Encourage physical closeness Provide detailed information Answer questions and concerns Ask for information on child's strengths/limitations and likes/dislikes

TABLE 5-1   Stage-Appropriate Teaching Strategies (continued)

Learner	General Characteristics	Teaching Strategies	Nursing Interventions
School-Aged Childhood Approximate age: 6–12 yr Cognitive stage: Concrete operations Psychosocial stage: Industry vs. inferiority	More realistic and objective Understands cause and effect Deductive/inductive reasoning Wants concrete information Able to compare objects and events Variable rates of physical growth Reasons syllogistically Understands seriousness and consequences of actions Subject-centered focus Immediate orientation	Encourage independence and active participation Be honest, allay fears Use logical explanation Allow time to ask questions Use analogies to make invisible processes real Establish role models Relate care to other children's experiences; compare procedures Use subject-centered focus Use play therapy Provide group activities Use drawings, models, dolls, painting, audio- and videotapes	Welcome active involvement Forge alliances Encourage physical closeness Provide detailed information Answer questions and concerns Ask for information on child's strengths/limitations and likes/dislikes
Adolescence Approximate age: 12–18 yr Cognitive stage: Formal operations Psychosocial stage: Identify vs. role confusion	Abstract, hypothetical thinking Can build on past learning Reasons by logic and understands scientific principles Future orientation Motivated by desire for social acceptance Peer group important Intense personal preoccupation, appearance extremely important (imaginary audience) Feels invulnerable, invincible/immune to natural laws (personal fable)	Establish trust, authenticity Know their agenda Address fears/concerns about outcomes of illness Identify control focus Include in plan of care Use peers for support and influence Negotiate changes Focus on details Make information meaningful to life Ensure confidentiality and privacy Arrange group sessions Use audiovisuals, role-play, contracts, reading materials Provide for experimentation and flexibility	Explore emotional and financial support Determine goals and expectations Assess stress levels Respect values and norms Determine role responsibilities and relationships Allow for 1:1 teaching without parents present, but with adolescent's permission, inform family of content covered

(continues)

TABLE 5-1 Stage-Appropriate Teaching Strategies (continued)

Learner	General Characteristics	Teaching Strategies	Nursing Interventions
Young Adulthood Approximate age: 18–40 yr Cognitive stage: Formal operations Psychosocial stage: Intimacy vs. isolation	Autonomous Self-directed Uses personal experiences to enhance or interfere with learning Intrinsic motivation Able to analyze critically Makes decisions about personal, occupational, and social roles Competency-based learner	Use problem-centered focus Draw on meaningful experiences Focus on immediacy of application Encourage active participation Allow to set own pace, be self-directed Organize material Recognize social role Apply new knowledge through role-playing and hands-on practice	Explore emotional, financial, and physical support system Assess motivational level for involvement Identify potential obstacles and stressors
Middle-Aged Adulthood Approximate age: 40–65 yr Cognitive stage: Formal operations Psychosocial stage: Generativity vs. self-absorption and stagnation	Sense of sense well-developed Concerned with physical changes At peak in career Explores alternative lifestyles Reflects on contributions to family and society Reexamines goals and values Questions achievements and successes Has confidence in abilities Desires to modify unsatisfactory aspects of life	Focus on maintaining independence and reestablishing normal life patterns Assess positive and negative past experiences with learning Assess potential sources of stress due to midlife crisis issues Provide information to coincide with life concerns and problems	Explore emotional, financial, and physical support system Assess motivational level for involvement Identify potential obstacles and stressors

TABLE 5-1   Stage-Appropriate Teaching Strategies (continued)

Learner	General Characteristics	Teaching Strategies	Nursing Interventions
Older Adulthood			
Approximate age: 65 yr and over Cognitive stage: Formal operations Psychosocial stage: Ego integrity vs. despair	Cognitive changes Decreased ability to think abstractly, process information Decreased short-term memory Increased reaction time Increased test anxiety Stimulus persistence (afterimage) Focuses on past life experiences	Use concrete examples Build on past life experiences Make information relevant and meaningful Present one concept at a time Allow time for processing/response (slow pace) Use repetition and reinforcement of information Avoid written exams Use verbal exchange and coaching Establish retrieval plan (use one or several clues) Encourage active involvement Keep explanations brief Use analogies to illustrate abstract information	Involve principal caregivers Encourage participation Provide resources for support (respite care) Assess coping mechanisms Provide written instructions for reinforcement Provide anticipatory problem solving (what happens if . . .)
	Sensory/motor deficits Auditory changes Hearing loss, especially high-pitched tones, consonants (S, Z, T, F, and G), and rapid speech Visual changes Farsighted (needs glasses to read) Lenses become opaque (glare problem)	Speak slowly, distinctly Use low-pitched tones Face client when speaking Minimize distractions Avoid shouting Use visual aids to supplement verbal instruction Avoid glares, use soft white light Provide sufficient light Use white backgrounds and black print	

(continues)

TABLE 5-1   Stage-Appropriate Teaching Strategies (*continued*)

Learner	General Characteristics	Teaching Strategies	Nursing Interventions
Older Adulthood (*continued*)	Smaller pupil size (decreased visual adaptation to darkness) Decreased peripheral perception	Avoid color coding with blues, greens, purples, and yellows Increase safety precautions/ provide safe environment	
	Yellowing of lenses (distorts low-tone colors: blue, green, violet) Distorted depth perception Fatigue/decreased energy levels Pathophysiology (chronic illness)	Ensure accessibility and fit of prostheses (i.e., glasses, hearing aid) Keep sessions short Provide for frequent rest periods Allow for extra time to perform Establish realistic short-term goals	
	Psychosocial changes Decreased risk taking Selective learning Intimidated by formal learning	Give time to reminisce Identify and present pertinent material Use informal teaching sessions Demonstrate relevance of information to daily life Assess resources Make learning positive Identify past positive experiences Integrate new behaviors with formerly established ones	

The toddler has the capacity for basic reasoning, has the beginnings of memory, and begins to develop a simple understanding of the concept of causality (what causes something to happen). With limited ability to recall past happenings or anticipate future events, the toddler is oriented primarily to the "here and now" and has little tolerance for delayed gratification. The child who has lived with strict routines and plenty of structure will have more of a grasp of time than the child who lives in an unstructured environment. Children at this stage have short attention spans, are easily distracted, are egocentric in their thinking, and are not easily swayed from their own ideas. Unquestionably, they believe their own perceptions to be reality. Asking questions is the hallmark of this age group, and they are undoubtedly curious. They can respond to simple, step-by-step commands and obey such directives as "kiss Daddy goodnight" or "put your hat on" (Levine, 1983; Petrillo & Sanger, 1980). Language skills increase rapidly during this period, and parents should be encouraged to talk with and listen to their child. As they progress through this phase, children begin to engage in fantasizing and "make-believe" play. Because they are unable to distinguish fact from fiction and have limited understanding of cause and effect, a child may feel that illness and hospitalization are a punishment for something done wrong.

According to Erikson (1963), the noted authority on psychosocial development, the period of infancy is one of *trust versus mistrust*. During this time, children must work through their first major challenge of developing a sense of trust with their primary caretaker (see Table 5-2). As the infant matures into toddlerhood, *autonomy versus shame and doubt* emerges as the central issue. During this period of psychosocial growth, toddlers must learn to balance feelings of love and hate and learn to cooperate and control willful desires (Table 5-2). Children progress sequentially through accomplishing the tasks of developing basic trust in their environment to reaching increasing levels of independence. Children may have difficulty in making up their minds, and their level of frustration and feelings of ambivalence may be expressed in negative words and behaviors, such as in exhibiting temper tantrums to release tensions (Falvo, 1994). With peers, play is a parallel activity, and it is not unusual for them to end up in tears because they have not yet learned about fairness or the rules of sharing (Babcock & Miller, 1994).

Toddlers like routine because it gives them a sense of security when carrying out activities of daily living. Separation anxiety is also characteristic of this stage of development. It is particularly apparent when children are hospitalized because they feel insecure in an unfamiliar environment and with people who are strangers to them.

TABLE 5-2   Erikson's Eight Stages of Psychosocial Development

Developmental Stages	Psychosocial Crises	Strengths
Infancy	Trust vs. mistrust	Hope
Toddlerhood	Autonomy vs. shame and doubt	Will
Preschooler	Initiative vs. guilt	Purpose
School-aged childhood	Industry vs. inferiority	Competence
Adolescence	Identity vs. role confusion	Fidelity
Young adulthood	Intimacy vs. isolation	Love
Middle-aged adulthood	Generativity vs. self-absorption and stagnation	Care
Older adulthood	Ego integrity vs. despair	Wisdom

Source: Adapted from Ahroni, J. H. (1996). Strategies for teaching elders from a human development perspective. *Diabetes Educator, 22*(1), 48.

Teaching Strategies

Patient education for this stage of development usually centers on wellness care. Time is mostly spent with parents on teaching them the aspects of normal development, safety, health promotion, and disease prevention. When the child is ill, the first priority before teaching is to assess the parent's and child's anxiety levels and help them cope with their feelings of stress related to uncertainty and guilt. Anxiety on the part of the child and parent can interfere with their readiness to learn.

Although teaching activities primarily are directed to the main caregiver(s), toddlers are capable of some degree of understanding procedures that they may experience. It is important that a primary nurse be assigned to establish a relationship with the child and parents to provide consistency in the teaching-learning process, which will help reduce the child's fear of strangers. Parents should be present whenever possible during learning activities to decrease stress caused by separation anxiety.

Ideally, health teaching should take place in an environment familiar to the child, such as the home or day-care center. When the child is hospitalized, the environment selected for teaching and learning sessions should be as safe and secure as possible, such as the child's bed or the playroom, to increase the child's sense of feeling protected.

Movement is an important mechanism by which toddlers communicate. Immobility tends to increase children's anxiety by restricting activity. Nursing interventions should be chosen that promote children's use of their motor abilities and that stimulate their visual, auditory, and tactile senses. The approach to children should be warm, honest, calm, accepting, and matter-of-fact. A smile, a warm tone of voice, a gesture of encouragement, or a word of praise goes a long way in attracting their attention and helping children adjust to new circumstances. Fundamental to the child's response is how the parents respond to healthcare personnel and medical interventions.

The following teaching strategies are suggested to promote the child's need for play, active participation, and sensory stimulation.

For Short-Term Learning

- Read simple stories from books with lots of pictures or use simple audiotapes with music and videotapes with cartoon characters to help them understand what is happening.
- Use dolls and puppets for children to act out their feelings.
- Role play to bring the child's imagination closer to reality.
- Perform procedures on a teddy bear or doll first to help the child understand what an experience will be like.
- Give the child something to do—squeeze your hand, hold a Band-Aid, cry if it hurts.
- Keep teaching sessions brief (no longer than about 5 minutes each) because of the child's short attention span.
- Cluster teaching sessions close together so that children can remember what they learned.
- Explain things in simple, straightforward, and nonthreatening terms because children take their world literally and concretely.
- Pace teaching according to the child's responses and level of attention.

For Long-Term Learning

- Focus on rituals, imitation, and repetition of information to hold the child's attention.
- Use reinforcement as an opportunity for children to learn through practice.
- Use games as a means by which children can learn about the world and test their ideas.
- Encourage parents to act as role models because they influence the child's development of attitudes and behaviors.

Preschooler (3–6 Years of Age)

Preschool children's sense of identity becomes clearer, and their world expands to involve others outside the family unit. Children in this developmental category acquire new behaviors that allow them to care for themselves more independently. Learning during this time period occurs through interactions with others and through mimicking or modeling the behaviors of playmates and adults (Whitener et al., 1998).

Physical, Cognitive, and Psychosocial Development

Fine and gross motor skills become increasingly more developed so that they are able to carry out activities of daily living with greater physical independence. Although their efforts are more coordinated, supervision of activities is still required because they lack judgment in carrying out the skills they have developed.

The preschooler's stage of cognitive development is labeled by Piaget (1951, 1952, 1976) as the *preoperational* period. The young child continues to be egocentric and is essentially unaware of others' thoughts or the existence of others' points of view. Preschoolers can recall past experiences and anticipate future events. They can classify objects into groups and categories, but have only a vague understanding of their relationships. Thinking remains literal and concrete—they believe what is seen and heard.

Preschoolers are very curious and pose questions about almost anything. They want to know the why, but because their thinking is precausal they don't understand the how. Children in this cognitive stage mix fact and fiction, tend to generalize, think magically, develop imaginary playmates, and believe they can control events with their thoughts.

The preschooler also continues to have a limited sense of time. For children of this age, being made to wait 15 minutes before they can do something can feel like an eternity. They do, however, understand the timing of familiar events in their daily lives, such as when breakfast or dinner is eaten and when they can play or watch their favorite television program. Their attention span begins to lengthen such that they can usually remain quiet long enough to listen to a song or hear a short story read.

Children at this stage begin to have an understanding of their bodies. They can name external body parts but do not know the function of internal organs (Kotchabhakdi, 1985). Preschoolers see illness as a punishment for something they did wrong. Health, on the other hand, may be identified with doing things right. Health allows them to play with friends and participate in desired activities; illness prevents them from doing so (Hussey & Hirsh, 1983).

Erikson (1963) has labeled the preschooler's psychosocial maturation level as the period of *initiative versus guilt*. Children take on tasks for the sake of being involved and on the move (Table 5-2). Excess energy and a desire to dominate may lead them to frustration and anger. They are impulsive in their actions, and their growing imagination can lead to many fears—of separation, disapproval, pain, punishment, and aggression from others, which significantly affects their willingness to interact with healthcare personnel (Poster, 1983; Vulcan, 1984).

In this stage of development, children begin interacting with playmates rather than just playing alongside one another. Appropriate social behaviors demand that they learn to wait for others, give others a turn, and recognize the needs of others. Play is their work and the way in which they learn about the physical and social world (Whitener et al., 1998). It helps the child act out feelings and experiences to master fears, develop role skills, and express joys, sorrows, and hostilities. Through play, the preschooler also begins to share ideas and imitate parents of the same sex. Role playing is typical of this age as the child attempts to learn the responsibilities of family members and others in society.

Teaching Strategies

The nurse's interactions with preschool children and their parents are often sporadic, usually occurring during occasional well-child visits to the pediatrician's office or when minor medical problems arise. During these visits, teaching should include health promotion and disease prevention, guidance regarding normal growth and development, and medical recommendations when illnesses do arise. Parents can help the nurse in working with children in this developmental phase, and they should be included in all aspects of the teaching plan (Ryberg & Merrifield, 1984; Woodring, 2000). Parents can provide insight into the child's disabilities, likes and dislikes, and favorite activities—all of which may affect the child's ability to learn (Hussey & Hirsh, 1983).

Children's fear of pain and bodily harm is uppermost in their minds, whether they are well or ill. Because of preschoolers' fantasies and active imaginations, it is most important for the nurse to reassure them and allow them to express themselves openly about their fears (Heiney, 1991). Choose your words carefully when describing procedures. Preschoolers are familiar with many words, but using terms like "cut" or "knife" is frightening to them. Instead, use less threatening words like "fix," "sew," or "cover up the hole." "Band-Aids" rather than "dressings" is a much more understandable term, and bandages are often thought by children to have magical healing powers (Babcock & Miller, 1994).

Although the preschooler has begun to have increasing contact with the outside world and is usually able to interact more comfortably with others, teaching should be directed to the significant adults in a child's life. Family members can provide support to the child, substitute as the teacher if the child is reluctant to interact with the nurse, and reinforce teaching. They are the learners who will assist the child in achieving desired health outcomes (Hussey & Hirsh, 1983; Kennedy & Riddle, 1989; Whitener et al., 1998). The following specific teaching strategies are recommended.

For Short-Term Learning

- Provide physical and visual stimuli because language ability is still limited.
- Keep teaching sessions short (no more than 15 minutes) and scheduled at close intervals so that information is not forgotten.
- Relate information needs to activities and experiences familiar to the child.
- Encourage the child to participate by choosing the instructional methods and tools, such as playing with dolls or reading a story, which promote active involvement and help to establish nurse–client rapport.
- Arrange small group sessions with peers to make teaching less threatening and more fun.
- Give praise and approval through both verbal expressions and nonverbal gestures, which are real motivators for learning.
- Give tangible rewards, such as badges or small toys, to reinforce learned skills.
- Allow the child to manipulate equipment and play with replicas or dolls to learn about body parts. Special kidney dolls, ostomy dolls with stomas, or orthopedic dolls with splints and tractions provide opportunity for hands-on experience.
- Use storybooks to help the child identify with particular people and situations.

For Long-Term Learning

- Have the parents help by being role models of healthy habits, such as practicing safety measures and eating a balanced diet.
- Reinforce positive health behaviors and new skills learned.

School-Aged Childhood (6–12 Years of Age)

School-aged children have progressed in their physical, cognitive, and psychosocial skills to the point where most begin formal training in structured school systems. They approach learning with enthusiastic anticipation, and their minds are open to new and varied ideas. They are motivated to learn because of their natural curiosity and their desire to understand more about themselves, their environment, society, and the world (Hussey & Hirsh, 1983; Whitener et al., 1998). This stage is a period of great change for them, when attitudes, values, and perceptions are shaped and expanded.

Physical, Cognitive, and Psychosocial Development

The gross- and fine-motor abilities of school-aged children are increasingly more coordinated so that they are much better able to control their movements. Involvement in activities helps them to fine-tune their psychomotor skills. Physical growth during this phase is highly variable, with the rate of development differing from child to child.

Piaget (1951, 1952, 1976) has labeled the cognitive development in the school-aged child as the period of *concrete operations*. During this time, logical thought processes and the ability to think inductively and deductively develop. Also, they begin to reason syllogistically—that is, they can consider two premises and draw a logical conclusion from them (Elkind, 1984). In addition, concepts are beginning to be mastered, such as conservation—a piece of clay weighs the same no matter whether it changes shape (Babcock & Miller, 1994). They are able to classify objects and systems, use sarcasm, and express concrete ideas about relationships and people (Lambert, 1984).

Although they can separate fiction and fantasy from fact and reality, nevertheless, their thinking remains quite literal, with only a vague understanding of abstractions. Early on in this phase, children are reluctant to do away with magical thinking in exchange for reality thinking. Cherished beliefs, such as the existence of Santa Claus or the tooth fairy, are clung to for the fun and excitement that the fantasy provides them, even when they have information that proves contrary to their beliefs.

School-aged children have developed the ability to concentrate for extended periods, can tolerate delayed gratification, and can generalize from experience. They understand time, are oriented to the past and present, and have some grasp and interest in the future. However, they understand only to a limited extent the seriousness or consequences of their choices.

In the shift from precausal to causal thinking, the child at this stage of cognitive development begins to incorporate the idea that illness is related to cause and effect and can recognize that germs create disease. Illness is thought of in terms of social consequences and role alterations, such as the realization that they will miss school and outside activities, people will feel sorry for them, and they will be unable to maintain their independence and usual routines (Banks, 1990). However, differences exist in children's reasoning skills based on their experiences with illness. Children suffering from chronic diseases have been found to have more sophisticated understanding of illness causality and body functioning than do their healthy peers, but the stress and anxiety resulting from having to live with a chronic illness can interfere with a child's general cognitive performance (Perrin, Sayer, & Willett, 1991).

Erikson (1963) characterizes school-aged children's psychosocial stage of life as *industry versus inferiority*. During this period, children begin to gain an awareness of their unique talents and special qualities that distinguish them from one another (Table 5-2). Also, they begin to establish their self-concept as members of a social group larger than their own nuclear family and start to compare family values with those of the outside world. With less dependency on family, they extend their intimacy to include special friends and social groups. Relationships with peers and adults outside the home environment become important influences in their development of self-esteem and their susceptibility to social forces outside the family unit. School-aged children fear failure and being left out of groups. They worry about their inabilities and become self-critical as they compare their own accomplishments to those of their peers.

Teaching Strategies

School-aged children and their families must be taught how to maintain health and manage illness. Woodring (2000) emphasizes the importance of following sound teaching principles with the child and family, such as identifying individual learning styles, determining readiness to learn, and accommodating particular learning needs and abilities to achieve positive health outcomes.

With their increased ability to understand information and their desire for active involvement and control of their lives, it is very important to include school-aged children in patient education efforts. The nurse should explain illness, treatment plans, and procedures in simple, logical terms in accordance with the child's level of understanding and reasoning. Although school-aged children are able to think logically, their ability for abstract thought remains limited. Therefore, teaching should be presented in concrete terms with step-by-step instructions (Pidgeon, 1985). Observe children's reactions and listen to their verbal feedback to confirm that information shared has not been misinterpreted or confused.

Parents should be informed of what their child is being taught. Teaching parents directly is encouraged so that they may be involved in fostering their child's independence, providing emotional support and physical assistance, and giving guidance regarding the correct techniques or regimens in self-care management. Siblings and peers should also be considered as sources of support (Hussey & Hirsh, 1983).

Education for health promotion and health maintenance is most likely to occur in the school system. The school nurse, in particular, is in an excellent position to coordinate the efforts of all other providers. The parents as well as nurses outside the school setting should be told what content is being addressed so that information then can be reinforced and expanded on when with the child in other care settings.

The specific conditions that may come to the attention of the nurse when caring for children at this phase of development include problems such as behavioral disorders, hyperactivity, learning disorders, diabetes, asthma, and enuresis. Extensive teaching may be needed to help children and parents understand a particular condition and learn how to overcome or deal with it. The need to sustain or bolster their self-image and self-esteem requires that children be invited to participate, to the extent possible, in planning for and carrying out learning activities. Because of children's fears of falling behind in school, being separated from peer groups, and being left out of social activities, teaching must be geared toward fostering normal development despite any limitations that may be imposed by illness or disability (Falvo, 1994).

Lifelong health attitudes and behaviors begin in early childhood and remain consistent throughout the stage of middle childhood. The development of understanding health and illness follows a systematic progression parallel to the stage of general cognitive development. As the child matures, beliefs about health and illness become less concrete and more abstract, less egocentric, and increasingly differentiated. Motivation, self-esteem, and self-perception are personal characteristics that influence health behavior (Farrand & Cox, 1993; Whitener et al., 1998). Teaching should be directed at assisting them to incorporate positive health actions into their daily lives. Because of the importance of peer influence, group activities are an effective method of teaching health behaviors, attitudes, and values.

Because school-aged children are used to the structured, direct, and formal learning in the school environment, they are receptive to a similar teaching-learning approach when hospitalized or confined at home. The following teaching strategies are suggested when caring for children in this developmental stage of life.

For Short-Term Learning

- Allow school-aged children to take responsibility for their own health care because they are not only willing, but also capable of manipulating equipment with accuracy.

- Teaching sessions can be extended to last as long as 30 minutes each because the increased attention span and cognitive abilities of school-aged children aids in the retention of information. However, lessons should be spread apart to allow for comprehension of large amounts of content and to provide opportunity for the practice of newly acquired skills between sessions.
- Use diagrams, models, pictures, videotapes, and printed materials as adjuncts to various teaching methods.
- Choose audiovisual and printed materials that show peers undergoing similar procedures or facing similar situations.
- Clarify any scientific terminology and medical jargon used.
- Use analogies as an effective means of providing information in meaningful terms, such as "A chest x-ray is like having your picture taken" or "White blood cells are like police cells that can attack and destroy infection."
- Use one-to-one teaching sessions as a method to individualize learning relevant to the child's own experiences.
- Provide time for clarification, validation, and reinforcement of what is being learned.
- Select individual instructional techniques that provide an opportunity for privacy, because this group of learners often feels quite self-conscious and modest when learning about bodily functions.
- Use group teaching sessions with others of similar age and with similar problems or needs to help children avoid feelings of isolation and to assist them in identifying with their own peers.
- Prepare children for a procedure well in advance to allow them time to cope with their feelings and fears, to anticipate events, and to understand what the purpose of a procedure is, how it relates to their condition, and how much time it will take.
- Encourage participation in planning for procedures and events because active involvement will help the child to learn information more readily.
- Provide nurturance and support, always keeping in mind that young children are not just small adults.

For Long-Term Learning

- Help school-aged children acquire skills that they can use to assume self-care responsibility for carrying out therapeutic treatment regimens on an ongoing basis with minimal assistance.

- Assist them in learning to maintain their own well-being and prevent illnesses from occurring.

Adolescence (12–18 Years of Age)

The stage of adolescence marks the transition from childhood to adulthood. How adolescents think about themselves and the world significantly influences many healthcare issues facing them, from anorexia to diabetes. Teenage thought and behavior give insight into the etiology of some of the major health problems of this group of learners (Elkind, 1984). Adolescents are known to be among the nation's most at-risk populations (American Association of Colleges of Nursing, 1994). For patient education to be effective, an understanding of the characteristics of the adolescent phase of development is crucial.

Physical, Cognitive, and Psychosocial Development

Adolescents vary greatly in their biological, psychological, social, and cognitive development. From a physical maturation standpoint, they must adapt to rapid and significant bodily changes, which can temporarily result in clumsiness and poor coordination. Alterations in physical size, shape, and function of their bodies, along with the appearance and development of secondary sex characteristics, bring about a significant preoccupation with their appearance (Falvo, 1994).

Piaget (1951, 1952, 1976) termed this stage of cognitive development as the period of *formal operations*. Adolescents are capable of abstract thought and logical reasoning that is both inductive and deductive. Adolescents can debate various points of view, understand cause and effect, comprehend complex concepts, and respond appropriately to multiple-step directions (Day, 1981; Heiney, 1991).

With the capacity for formal operational thought, teenagers can become obsessed with what others are thinking and begin to believe that everyone is focusing on the same things they are—namely, themselves and their activities. Elkind (1984) labeled this belief as the *imaginary audience*, which has considerable influence over an adolescent's behavior. The imaginary audience explains why adolescents are self-conscious. On the one hand, they may feel embarrassed because they believe everyone is looking at them yet, on the other hand, they desire to be looked at and thought about because this attention confirms their sense of specialness and uniqueness.

Adolescents are able to understand the concept of health and illness, the multiple causes of diseases, and the influence of variables on health status. They can also identify healthy behaviors and understand the benefits of health promotion and disease prevention activities; however, they may reject practicing them or begin to engage in risk-taking behaviors because of the social pressures they receive from peers as well as their belief that they are invincible. Elkind (1984) has called this belief the *personal fable*. The personal fable leads the adolescent to think that other people get hurt and die if they don't wear their seat belts, but that won't happen to them. It leads teenagers to believe they are protected from bodily harm despite any risks to which they may subject themselves. They can understand implications of future outcomes, but their immediate concern is with the present. Although children in the mid-to-late adolescent period appear to be aware of the risks they take and the consequences of these risks, it is important, nevertheless, to recognize that this population continues to need support and guidance (Cauffman & Steinberg, 2000).

Erikson (1968) has labeled the psychosocial dilemma adolescents face as one of *identity versus role confusion*. These children indulge in comparing their self-image with an ideal image (Table 5-2). Adolescents find themselves in a struggle to establish their own identity. They work to separate themselves from their parents, so that they can emerge as more distinct and independent. Teenagers have a strong need for peer acceptance and peer support. Their concern over personal appearance and their need to look and act like their peers drive them to conform to the dress and behavior of this age group. This usually contradicts values of their parents' generation. Conflict, toleration, or alienation often characterizes the relationship between adolescents and their parents and other authority figures.

Adolescents demand personal space, control, privacy, and confidentiality. To them, illness or injury means dependency, loss of identity, a change in body image and functioning, bodily embarrassment, confinement, and separation from peers. Knowledge about how to protect their health and prevent disease and injury is not enough. They need coping skills to successfully complete this stage of development (Grey, Kanner, & Lacey, 1999).

Teaching Strategies

Challenges adolescents may face include chronic illness, a range of disabilities as a result of injury, or psychological problems as a result of depression or physical and/or emotional maltreatment. In addition, adolescents are considered at high risk for teen pregnancy, the effects of poverty, drug or alcohol abuse, suicide, and sexually trans-mitted diseases. Despite all of these potential threats to their well-being, adolescents use medical services the least frequently of all age groups. Unfortunately, adolescent health has not been a national priority and their health issues have been largely ignored by the healthcare system (American Association of Colleges of Nursing, 1994). Thus, the educational needs of adolescents are broad and varied.

Healthy teens have difficulty imagining themselves as sick or injured. Those with an illness or disability often comply poorly with medical regimens and continue to indulge in risk-taking behaviors. They view health recommendations as a threat to their autonomy and sense of control. Probably the greatest challenge to the nurse responsible for teaching the adolescent, whether healthy or ill, is to be able to develop a mutually respectful, trusting relationship. Adolescents are able to participate fully in all aspects of learning, but they need privacy, understanding, an honest and straightforward approach, and unqualified acceptance in the face of their fears of losing independence, identity, and self-control.

Patient education should be done directly with adolescents to respect their right to individuality, privacy, and confidentiality. The nurse should give guidance and support to families to help them to better understand adolescent behavior. Parents may need to be taught how to set realistic limits while at the same time foster the adolescent's sense of independence. Look for potential sources of stress. Because of the ambivalence the adolescent feels while in this transition stage from childhood to adulthood, healthcare teaching, to be effective, must consider the learning needs of both the adolescents and their parents (Falvo, 1994).

The following teaching strategies are suggested when caring for adolescents.

For Short-Term Learning

- Use one-to-one instruction to ensure confidentiality.
- Choose peer group discussion sessions as an effective approach to deal with health topics such as smoking, alcohol and drug use, safety measures, and teenage sexuality.
- Use group discussion, role playing, and gaming as methods to clarify values and problem solve. Getting groups of peers together can be very effective in helping teens confront health challenges and learn how to significantly change behavior (Fey & Deyes, 1989).
- Use instructional tools; models, diagrams, audiotapes, videotapes, simulated games, and computers are attractive and comfortable approaches to learning.
- Clarify any scientific terminology and medical jargon used. Do not assume they understand.
- Allow them to participate in decision making.
- Include them in formulating teaching plans related to teaching strategies and expected outcomes to meet their needs for autonomy.

- Offer options so that they feel they have a choice about courses of action.
- Give a rationale for all that is said and done to help adolescents feel a sense of control.
- Approach them with respect, tact, openness, and flexibility to elicit their attention and encourage their involvement.
- Expect negative responses, which are common when their self-image and self-integrity are threatened.
- Avoid confrontation and acting like an authority figure. Acknowledge their thoughts and then casually suggest an alternative viewpoint, such as "Yes, I can see your point, but what about the possibility of . . . ?"

For Long-Term Learning

- Accept adolescents' personal fable and imaginary audience as valid.
- Acknowledge that their feelings are very real.
- Allow them the opportunity to test their own convictions. When safe and appropriate, let them try out some of their ideas.

THE DEVELOPMENTAL STAGES OF ADULTHOOD

Andragogy, the term coined by Knowles (1990) to describe his theory of adult learning, is the art and science of helping adults learn. Education within this framework is more learner-centered and less teacher-centered; that is, instead of one party imparting knowledge to another, the power relationship between the educator and the adult learner is much more equal (Milligan, 1997).

The following basic assumptions about adult learning have major implications for teaching this population of learners (Knowles, Holton, & Swanson, 1998):

1. Adults' self-concept moves from one of being a dependent personality to being an independent, self-directed human being.
2. Adults accumulate a growing reservoir of previous experiences that serve as a rich resource for learning.
3. Readiness to learn becomes increasingly oriented to the developmental tasks of social roles in adulthood.
4. Adults desire knowledge for immediate application in solving life's problems.

The period of adulthood consists of three major developmental stages—that of the young adult, the middle-aged adult, and the older adult (see Table 5-1). Because adults have essentially reached the peak of their cognitive development, Piaget's

(1951, 1952, and 1976) cognitive stage of formal operations, which begins in adolescence, carries through all three periods of adulthood. Erikson (1963), on the other hand, continues to identify distinct psychosocial characteristics of the different stages of adulthood.

The emphasis for adult learning revolves around differentiation of life tasks and social roles with respect to employment, family, and other activities beyond the responsibilities of home and career (Boyd, Gleit, Graham, & Whitman, 1998). In contrast to childhood learning, which is subject centered, adult learning is problem centered. The prime motivator to learn in adulthood is to be able to apply knowledge and skills for the solution of immediate problems. Unlike children, who enjoy learning for the sake of learning, most adults need to see the relevance of acquiring new behaviors or changing old ones for them to be willing and eager to learn. In the beginning of any teaching encounter, therefore, adults want to know the benefit they will derive from their efforts at learning.

As compared with the characteristics of the child as learner, adults are much more self-directed and independent in seeking information, their past experiences form the basis for further learning, they already have a rich resource of stored information from which to draw upon, they grasp relationships quickly, and they usually do not tolerate learning isolated facts (Table 5-3). Because adults already have established ideas, values, and attitudes, they tend to be more resistant to change. In addition, adults must overcome obstacles to learning, such as the burdens of family, work, and social responsibilities, which can diminish their time, energy, and concentration for learning. In addition, they may feel too old or too out of touch with the formal learning of the school years, and if past experiences with learning were not positive, they may shy away from assuming the role of learner for fear of the risk of failure (Boyd et al., 1998). Although we accept the adult learner as autonomous, self-directed, and independent, these individuals often really want and need structure, clear and concise specifics, and direct guidance. As such, Taylor, Marienau, and Fiddler (2000) label adults as paradoxical learners.

Only recently has it been recognized that learning is a lifelong process that begins at birth and does not cease until the end of life. Growth and development are a process of "becoming." As a person matures, learning is a significant and continuous task to maintain and enhance oneself.

Obviously, there are many differences between child and adult learners (Table 5-1). As the following discussion will clearly reveal, there also are differences in the characteristics of adult learners within the three developmental stages of adulthood.

TABLE 5-3 Summary of Adult Learning Principles	
ADULTS LEARN BEST WHEN:	
Principle #1	Learning is related to an immediate need, problem, or deficit.
Principle #2	Learning is voluntary and self-initiated.
Principle #3	Learning is person centered and problem centered.
Principle #4	Learning is self-controlled and self-directed.
Principle #5	The role of the teacher is one of facilitator.
Principle #6	Information and assignments are pertinent.
Principle #7	New material draws on past experiences and is related to something the learner already knows.
Principle #8	The threat to self is reduced to a minimum in the educational situation.
Principle #9	The learner is able to participate actively in the learning process.
Principle #10	The learner is able to learn in a group.
Principle #11	The nature of the learning activity changes frequently.
Principle #12	Learning is reinforced by application and prompt feedback.

Source: Adapted from Burgireno, J. (1985). Maximizing learning in the adult with SCI. *Rehabilitation Nursing, 10*(5), 20–21.

Young Adulthood (18–40 Years of Age)

Early adulthood is a time for establishing long-term, intimate relationships with other people, choosing a lifestyle and adjusting to it, deciding on an occupation, and managing a home and family. All of these decisions lead to changes in the lives of young adults that can be a potential source of stress for them.

Physical, Cognitive, and Psychosocial Development

During this period, physical abilities for most young adults are at their peak, and the body is at its optimal functioning capacity. The vast majority of individuals at this stage can master, if they so desire, almost any psychomotor skill they undertake to accomplish.

Young adults continue in the formal operations stage of cognitive development that began in adolescence (Piaget, 1951, 1952, 1976). The cognitive capacity of young adults is fully developed, but with maturation, they continue to accumulate new knowledge and skills through formal and informal experiences. These experiences add to their perceptions, allow them to generalize to new situations, and improve their abilities to critically analyze, problem solve, and make decisions about their personal, occupational, and social roles. Their interests for learning are oriented toward those experiences that are relevant for immediate application to problems and tasks in their daily lives.

Erikson (1963) describes the young adult's stage of psychosocial development as the period of *intimacy versus isolation*. During this time, individuals work to establish a trusting, satisfying, and permanent relationship with others (Table 5-2). They strive to establish commitment to others in their personal, occupational, and social lives. The independence and self-sufficiency they worked to obtain in adolescence they are now working to maintain.

Young adults face many challenges as they take steps to control their lives. Many of the events they experience are happy and growth promoting from an emotional and social perspective, but they also can prove disappointing and psychologically draining. The new experiences and multiple decisions they must make regarding choices for a career, marriage, parenthood, and higher education can be quite stressful. Young adults realize that the avenues they pursue will affect their lives for years to come.

Teaching Strategies

Young adults are generally very healthy and tend to have limited exposure to health professionals. Their contact with the healthcare system is usually for pre-employment, college, or pre-sport physicals; for a minor episodic complaint; or for pregnancy and contraceptive care. At the same time, young adulthood is a crucial period for the establishment of behaviors that help individuals to lead healthy lives, both physically and emotionally. Many of the choices young adults make, if not positive ones, will be difficult to modify later. As Havighurst pointed out, this stage is full of "teachable moment" opportunities, but it is the most neglected stage of life for teaching positive health behaviors (Johnson-Saylor, 1980).

The nurse must find a way of reaching and communicating with this audience about health promotion and disease prevention measures. Readiness to learn does not always require the nurse to wait for it to develop. Rather, such readiness can be fostered through experiences the nurse creates. Knowledge of the individual's lifestyle can provide cues to concentrate on when determining specific aspects of education for the young adult. For example, if the individual is planning marriage, then family planning, contraception, and parenthood are potential topics to address. The motivation for adults to learn comes in response to internal drives, such as need for self-esteem, a better quality of life, or job satisfaction (Babcock & Miller, 1994).

When young adults are faced with acute or chronic illnesses, many of which may significantly alter their lifestyles, they are stimulated to learn so as to maintain their independence and return to normal life patterns. It is likely they will view an illness or disability as a serious setback to achieving their immediate or future life goals.

Because adults typically desire active participation when learning, it is important for the nurse to include them in health education decision making. They should be encouraged to select what to learn (objectives), how they want material to be presented (instructional methods and tools), and which indicators will be used to determine the achievement of learning goals (evaluation) (Gessner, 1989). Also, it must be remembered that adults bring to the teaching-learning situation a variety of experiences that can serve as a foundation on which to build new learning. Consequently, it is important to draw on their experiences to make learning relevant, useful, and motivating. Young adults tend to be reluctant to expend the resources of time, money, and energy to learn new information, skills, and attitudes if they do not see these efforts as relevant to their current lives or anticipated problems (Babcock & Miller, 1994).

Teaching strategies must be directed at encouraging young adults to seek information that expands their knowledge base, helps them control their lives, and bolsters their self-esteem. Whether they are well or ill, young adults need to know about the opportunities available for learning. These opportunities must be convenient and accessible to them in terms of their lifestyle with respect to work and family responsibilities.

Because they tend to be very self-directed, young adults do well with written teaching materials and audiovisual tools that allow them to independently self-pace their learning. Group discussion is an attractive method for teaching and learning because it provides young adults with the opportunity to interact with others of similar age and situation, such as parenting groups, prenatal classes, or marital adjustment sessions.

Middle-Aged Adulthood (40–65 Years of Age)

Just as adolescence is the link between childhood and adulthood, midlife is the transition period between young adulthood and older adulthood. During middle age, many individuals have reached the peak in their careers, their sense of who they are is well developed, their children are grown, and they have time to pursue other interests. It is a time for them to reflect on the contributions they have made to family and society and to reexamine their goals and values.

Physical, Cognitive, and Psychosocial Development

At this stage of maturation, a number of physiological changes begin to take place. Skin and muscle tone decreases, metabolism slows down, body weight tends to increase, endurance and energy levels lessen, hormonal changes bring about a variety of symptoms, and hearing and visual acuity begin to diminish. All these physical changes and others affect middle-aged adults' self-image, ability to learn, and motivation for learning about health promotion, disease prevention, and maintenance of health.

The ability to learn from a cognitive standpoint remains at a steady state throughout middle age as the adults continue in the formal operations stage of cognitive development (Piaget, 1951, 1952, 1976). For many, the accumulation of life experiences and their proven record of accomplishments allow them to come to the teaching-learning situation with confidence in their abilities as learners. However, if their past experiences with learning were minimal or not positive, their motivation likely will not be at a high enough level to facilitate learning. Physical changes, especially with respect to hearing and vision, may impede learning as well.

Erikson (1963) labeled this psychosocial stage of adulthood as *generativity versus self-absorption and stagnation*. Midlife marks a point at which adults realize that half of their life has been spent. This realization may cause them to question their level of achievement and success. Middle-aged adults, in fact, may choose to modify aspects of their lives that they perceive as unsatisfactory or adopt a new lifestyle as a solution to dissatisfaction. Developing concern for the lives of their grown children, recognizing the physical changes in themselves, dealing with the new role of being a grandparent, and taking responsibility for their own parents whose health may be failing—all are factors that may cause them to become aware of their own mortality (Table 5-2). At this time, middle-aged adults may either feel greater motivation to follow health recommendations more closely or, just the opposite, may deny illnesses or abandon healthy practices altogether (Falvo, 1994).

The later years of middle adulthood are the phase in which productivity and contributions to society are valued. They offer an opportunity to feel a real sense of accomplishment from having cared for others—children, spouse, friends, parents, and colleagues for whom they have served as mentor. During this time, individuals often become oriented away from self and family to the larger community. New social interests and leisure activities are pursued as they find more free time from family responsibilities and career demands. As they move toward their retirement years, individuals begin to plan for what they want to do after culminating their career. This transition sparks their interest in learning about financial planning, alternative lifestyles, and ways to remain healthy as they approach the later years.

Teaching Strategies

When teaching members of this age group, the nurse must be aware of their potential sources of stress, the health risk factors associated with this stage of life, and the concerns typical of midlife. Misconceptions regarding physical changes such as menopause are common. Stress may interfere with their ability to learn or may stimulate them to seek the help of healthcare providers. Those who have lived healthy and productive lives are often motivated to make contact with health professionals to ensure maintenance of their healthy status. It is an opportune time on the part of the nurse to reach out to assist these middle-aged adults in coping with stress and maintaining optimal health status. Many need and want information related to chronic illnesses that can arise at this phase of life.

Adult learners need to be reassured or complimented on their learning competencies. Reinforcement for learning is internalized and serves to reward them for their efforts. Teaching strategies for learning are similar to those instructional methods and tools used for the young adult learner, but the content is different to coincide with the concerns and problems specific to this group of learners.

Older Adulthood (65 Years of Age and Older)

Older persons constitute approximately 12% of the U.S. population, and those aged 85 and older make up the fastest-growing segment of the population in our country today. By 2020, 16.5% (or 52 million) of the population is expected to be aged 65 years and older (Gollop, 1997). Most older persons suffer from at least one chronic condition, and many have multiple conditions. On the average, they are hospitalized longer than persons in other age categories. Also, because many older persons did not have the formal educational opportunities that are available to the young today, one-third of older adults have completed only 8 years or less of schooling, and 45% of them have less than a high school education (Pearson & Wessman, 1996). Low educational levels in the older adult population contribute to difficulty reading and comprehending written health materials (Jackson, Davis, Murphy, Bairnsfather, & George, 1994). Of the total amount of healthcare expenditures, 36% are incurred by those older than 65 years of age (Pearson & Wessman, 1996). Given the high cost of health care and the fact that the educational needs of older adults are generally greater and more complex than those of individuals in any of the other developmental stages, teaching efforts to improve their health status would be a cost-effective measure (Pearson & Wessman, 1996; Weinrich et al., 1989).

Ageism describes prejudice against the older adult that perpetuates the negative stereotype of aging as a period of decline. Ahroni (1996) suggests that ageism, in many respects, is similar to the discriminatory attitudes of racism and sexism. Because our society values physical strength, beauty, social networking, productivity, and integrity of body and mind, we fear the natural losses that accompany the aging process. However, many older persons respond to these changes as challenges rather than defeats. Many aspects of older adulthood can be pleasurable, such as becoming a grandparent and experiencing retirement, which give older adults time to pursue life-long interests, as well as freedom to explore new avenues of endeavor. Ageism, which interferes with interactions between the older adult and younger age groups, must be counteracted because it "prevents older people from living lives as actively and happily as they might" (Ahroni, 1996, p. 48). Given that the aging process is universal, eventually everyone is potentially subjected to this type of prejudice. New research that focuses on healthy development and positive lifestyle adaptations, rather than on illnesses and impairments, in the older adult can serve to reverse the stereotypical images of aging. Teaching to inform people of the significant variations that occur in the way that individuals age and teaching to help the older adult learn to cope with irreversible losses can combat the prejudice of ageism as well.

The teaching of older persons, known as *gerogogy*, is different from teaching young and middle-aged adults (andragogy) and children (pedagogy). To be effective, gerogogy must accommodate the normal physical, cognitive, and psychosocial changes that occur at this phase of growth and development (Weinrich & Boyd, 1992). Until recently, little has been written about the special needs of older adults as a result of these aging changes that affect their ability to learn. Nurses must understand these changes and adapt appropriate teaching interventions to meet the older person's needs (Ahroni, 1996; Alford, 1982; Culbert & Kos, 1971; Ellison, 1985; Palmore, 1977; Pearson & Wessman, 1996; Weinrich & Boyd, 1992; Weinrich et al., 1989).

Physical, Cognitive, and Psychosocial Development

With advancing age, so many physical changes occur that it becomes difficult to establish normal boundaries. The senses of sight, hearing, touch, taste, and smell are usually the first areas of decreased functioning noticed by older persons.

Visual and auditory changes relate most closely to learning capacity. Hearing loss, which is very common beginning in the late forties and fifties, includes diminished ability to discriminate high-pitched sounds. Visual changes such as cataracts, reduced pupil size, and presbyopia prevent older persons from being able to see small print, read words printed on glossy paper, or drive a car. Yellowing of the ocular lens produces color distortions and diminished color perceptions.

Other physiological changes affect organ functioning, which results in decreased cardiac output, lung performance, and metabolic rate; these changes reduce energy levels and lessen the ability to cope with stress. Nerve conduction velocity also is thought to decline by as much as 15%, influencing reflex times and muscle response rates. The interrelatedness of each body system has a total negative cumulative effect on individuals as they grow older.

Aging affects the mind as well as the body. According to Piaget (1951, 1952, 1976), this population remains in the stage of formal operations. Cognitive ability changes as a result of loss of neurons in the brain. People have two kinds of intellectual ability—crystallized and fluid intelligence. *Crystallized intelligence* is the intelligence absorbed over a lifetime, such as vocabulary, understanding social interactions, and math reasoning. This kind of intelligence actually increases with experience as people age (Theis & Merritt, 1994) unless the brain is impaired by disease states, such as Alzheimer's dementia (Matsuda & Saito, 1998). *Fluid intelligence*, which is the capacity to perceive relationships, to reason, and to perform abstract thinking, declines as degenerative changes occur and results in the following:

1. **Slower processing time:** Older adults need more time to process and react to information. However, if the factor of speed is removed from task performance, older adults can usually do as well as those who are younger (Kray & Lindenberger, 2000).
2. **Persistence of stimulus (afterimage):** Older adults can confuse a previous symbol or word with a new word or symbol just introduced.
3. **Decreased short-term memory:** As people age, they sometimes have difficulty remembering events or conversations that occurred just hours or days before.
4. **Increased test anxiety:** Older people are especially anxious about making mistakes when performing. If they do make an error, they become easily frustrated. Because of their anxiety, they may require more time to respond to questions, particularly on tests that are written rather than verbal.
5. **Altered time perception:** For older persons, life becomes more finite; issues of the here and now are more important.

Despite the changes in cognition as a result of aging, older adults can learn and remember if special care is taken to slow the pace of presenting information, to ensure relevance of material, and to give appropriate feedback when teaching (Figure 5-1).

Erikson (1963) labeled the major psychosocial developmental task at this stage in life as *ego integrity versus despair*. Older adulthood includes dealing with the reality of aging and death, looking at past failures in the light of present and future concerns, and developing a sense of purpose for those years remaining (Table 5-2). The most common psychosocial tasks of aging involve changes in lifestyle and social status as a result of

- Retirement (often mandatory at 70 years in this country)
- Illness or death of spouse, relatives, and friends
- The moving away of children, grandchildren, and friends
- Relocation to an unfamiliar environment such as a nursing home or senior citizens center

Depression, grief, and loneliness are common among older persons experiencing multiple losses over a short period of time with respect to a previous support network of home, friends, family, and job. These losses result in isolation, financial insecurity, diminished coping mechanisms, and a decreased sense of identity, personal value, and societal worth. With aging, individuals begin to question their potential for a "meaningful life"—one that includes further enjoyment, pleasure, and satisfaction.

Separate from biological aging but closely related are the many sociocultural factors that affect how older adults see themselves as competent individuals. The following traits regarding personal goals in life and the values associated with them are significantly related to motivation and learning (Culbert & Kos, 1971; Ellison, 1985; Gessner, 1989):

1. **Independence:** The ability to provide for one's needs is the most important aim of the majority of older persons, regardless of their state of health. Health teaching is the tool to help them maintain or regain independence.
2. **Social acceptability:** Receiving approval from others is a common goal of most older adults. Despite declining physical attributes, the older adult often has residual fitness and functioning potentials. Health teaching can help to channel these potentials.
3. **Adequacy of personal resources:** Economic and social resources are important considerations when assessing the older adult's current ability to support their life patterns, as well as new requirements.

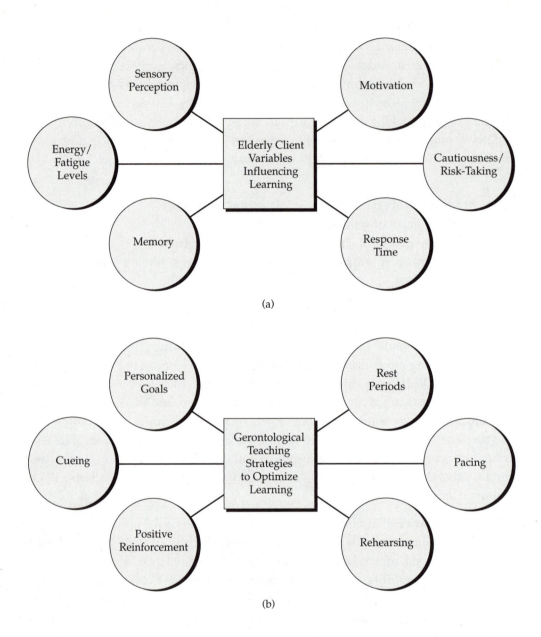

(a)

(b)

FIGURE 5-1 (a) Elderly Client Variables Influencing Learning; (b) Gerontological Teaching Strategies to Optimize Learning.
Source: Reprinted with permission from Rendon, D. C., Davis, D. K., Gioiella, E. C., & Tranzillo, M. J. (1986). The right to know, the right to be taught. *Journal of Gerontological Nursing, 12*(12), 36.

4. **Coping mechanisms:** The ability to cope with change during the aging process indicates a person's readiness for health teaching. Positive coping mechanisms allow for self-change. Negative coping mechanisms indicate their focus on losses. The emphasis in teaching is on exploring alternatives, determining realistic goals, and supporting large and small accomplishments.
5. **Meaning of life:** Health teaching must be directed at ways older adults can maintain optimal health so that they can derive pleasure from their leisure years.

Teaching Strategies

Understanding older persons' developmental tasks will allow nurses to alter how they approach both well and ill individuals in terms of counseling, teaching, and establishing a therapeutic relationship. Social isolation, loneliness, and sensory deprivation may lead to decreased cognitive functioning and often may prevent or delay early disease detection and intervention. A decline in psychomotor performance affects their reflex responses, energy levels, and ability to handle stress. These cognitive and psychomotor changes have implications with respect to how they care for themselves (food, dress, taking medications) as well as the extent to which they understand the nature of their illnesses.

In working with older adults, reminiscing is a beneficial approach to use to establish a therapeutic relationship. Memories can be quite powerful. Talking with older persons about their experiences can be very stimulating. Furthermore, their answers will give the nurse an insight into their successes, abilities, and concerns (Ellison, 1985).

It is easy to fall into the habit of believing the myths that older people are unteachable and unmotivated (Kick, 1989). Nurses may not even be aware of their stereotypical attitudes toward older adults. Think about the last time you gave instruction to an older patient, and ask yourself:

- Did I talk to the family and ignore the patient when I described some aspect of care or discharge planning?
- Did I tell the older person not to worry when he or she asked a question? Did I say, "Just leave everything up to the doctors and nurses"?
- Did I eliminate information that I normally would have given a younger patient?

Remember, older adults can learn, but their abilities and needs differ from those of younger persons. The process of teaching and learning is much more rewarding and successful for both the nurse and the patient if it is tailored to fit the older adult's physical, cognitive, motivational, and social differences.

Because changes as a result of aging vary considerably from one individual to another, it is essential to assess each learner's physical, cognitive, and psychosocial functioning level before developing and implementing any teaching plan. It is important to keep in mind that older adults have an overall lower educational level of formal schooling than the population as a whole. Also, they were raised in an era when consumerism and health education were practically nonexistent. As a result, older people may feel uncomfortable in the teaching-learning situation and may be reluctant to ask questions.

Health teaching for older persons should be directed at promoting their participation in activities and involvement in decision making (Ahroni, 1996; Morra, 1991; Weinrich et al., 1989). They need to feel important for what they once were as well as for what they are today. Interaction needs to be respectful and supportive, not judgmental. Interventions work best when they take place in a casual, informal atmosphere.

Some of the more common aging changes that affect learning and the teaching strategies specific to meeting the needs of the older adult are summarized in Table 5-1. The following are specific tips for creating an environment for learning that takes into account major changes in older adults' physical, cognitive, and psychosocial functioning (Ahroni, 1996; Alford, 1982; Hallburg, 1976; Picariello, 1986; Weinrich and Boyd, 1992).

Physical Needs

1. Compensate for visual changes by teaching in an environment that is brightly lit but without glare. Visual aids should include large print, well-spaced letters, and the use of primary rather than pastel colors. Bright colors and a visible name tag should be worn by the nurse. Tasks that require older adults to discriminate shades of color, such as test strips measuring the presence of sugar in the urine or taking medicines according to the color of their pills, can lead to error because light greens, blues, and yellows may all appear gray in color. Use white, flat matte paper and black print for posters, diagrams, and other written materials. For patients who wear glasses, be sure they are readily accessible, the lenses are clean, and the frames are properly fitted.

2. Compensate for hearing losses by eliminating extraneous noise, avoiding covering your mouth when speaking, directly facing the learner, and speaking slowly. The hearing impaired often watch people's faces for cues about what is being said. Low-pitched voices are heard best, but be careful not to drop the tone of your voice at the end of words or phrases. Avoid shouting, because the decibel level (loudness) is usually not the problem. Ask for feedback from the learner to deter-

mine whether you are speaking too softly, too fast, or not distinctly enough. Be alert to nonverbal cues from older adults who are having difficulty with hearing your message, such as them leaning forward, turning the "good" ear to the speaker, or cupping their hands to their ears. Ask older persons to repeat verbal instructions to be sure the entire message was heard and interpreted correctly.

3. Compensate for musculoskeletal problems, decreased efficiency of the cardio-vascular system, and reduced kidney function, by keeping sessions short, sched-uling frequent breaks to allow for use of bathroom facilities, and allowing time for stretching to relieve painful, stiff joints and to stimulate circulation.

4. Compensate for any decline in central nervous system functioning, metabolic rates, strength, and coordination by setting aside more time for the giving and receiving of information and for the practice of psychomotor skills. Be careful not to misinterpret the loss of energy and motor skills as a lack of motivation.

Cognitive Needs

1. Compensate for a decrease in fluid intelligence by providing older persons with more opportunities to process and react to information and to see relationships between concepts. Research has shown that older adults can learn anything if new information is tied to familiar concepts drawn from relevant past experi-ences. Avoid presenting long lists by dividing a series of directions for action into short, discrete, step-by-step messages and then waiting for a response after each one.

2. Compensate for decreased short-term memory by coaching and using repeti-tion to assist them with recall. Memory can also be enhanced by involving the client in devising ways to remember how or when to perform a procedure.

3. Reduce anxiety by explaining procedures simply and thoroughly, giving reassur-ance that you are not testing them.

4. Be aware of the effects of medications and energy levels on concentration, alert-ness, and coordination. Try to schedule teaching sessions before or well after medications are taken and when the person is rested.

5. Ask what an individual already knows about a healthcare issue or technique before explaining it to avoid repeating information already known.

6. Find out about older persons' health habits and beliefs before trying to change their ways or teach something new. Anything that is entirely strange or that upsets established habits is likely to be far more difficult for them to learn. As perception slows, the older person's mind has more trouble accommodating new routines.

7. Arrange for brief teaching sessions, due to shortened attention spans. In addition, if the material is relevant and focused on the here and now, older persons are more likely to be attentive to the information being presented.
8. Take into account that the ability to think abstractly becomes more difficult with aging. Conclude each teaching session with a summary of the information presented and allow for a question and answer period to correct any misconceptions (Figure 5-2).

Psychosocial Needs

1. Assess family relationships to determine how dependent the older person is on other members for financial and emotional support. In turn, explore the level of involvement by family members in reinforcing the lessons you are teaching and in giving assistance with self-care measures. Do they help the older person to function independently, or do they foster dependency? With permission of the patient, include family members in teaching sessions and enlist their support.
2. Determine availability of resources, because they may not be able to follow health care recommendations if they cannot afford transportation, buying or renting equipment, or purchasing medications or certain foods.
3. Encourage active involvement of older adults to improve their self-esteem and to stimulate them both mentally and socially. Teaching must be directed at helping them find meaningful ways to use their talents acquired over a lifetime.
4. Identify coping mechanisms. No other time in the life cycle carries with it the number of developmental tasks associated with adaptation to loss of roles, social and family contacts, and physical and cognitive capacities. Teaching must include offering constructive methods of coping.

The older person's ability to learn may be affected by the methods and tools chosen for teaching. One-to-one instruction provides a nonthreatening environment in which to meet their individual needs and promote their active participation in learning. Group teaching also can be a beneficial approach for fostering social skills and maintaining contact with others through shared experiences. Written materials may be very appropriate, but it is important to know the client's mental, visual, physical, and literacy abilities. Introducing newer teaching methods and tools, such as use of computers and videos, without adequate instructions on how to operate these technical devices may inhibit learning by increasing anxiety and frustration.

Games, role playing, demonstration, and return demonstration to rehearse problem solving and psychomotor skills require consideration of the energy levels

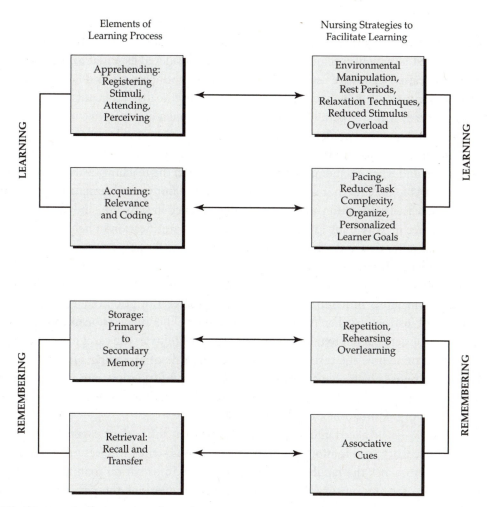

FIGURE 5-2 A Basic Gerontological Teaching-Learning Model for Nursing
Source: Reprinted with permission from Rendon, D. C., Davis, D. K., Gioiella, E. C., & Tranzillo, M. J. (1986). The right to know, the right to be taught. *Journal of Gerontological Nursing, 12*(12), 36.

and sensory abilities of the older adult before they are chosen to determine the effectiveness of these methods for teaching.

THE ROLE OF THE FAMILY IN PATIENT EDUCATION

The role of the family is considered one of the key variables influencing patient teaching outcomes. Family members provide critical emotional, physical, and social support to the patient (Gilroth, 1990; Reeber, 1992). Under recent JCAHO accreditation standards, healthcare organizations must show evidence that significant others are included in patient teaching efforts, which is considered essential to the provision of quality care. Nurses are responsible for assisting both patients and families to gain the knowledge and skills necessary to meet ongoing healthcare needs (Hartman & Kochar, 1994). Clinical pathways have become a popular and effective method of prioritizing and meeting predetermined goals and objectives for learning. Such guidelines provide patients and their families with a better understanding of what needs to be learned and when including the family members in the teaching-learning has positive benefits for the learner as well as the teacher. Family involvement helps clients derive increased satisfaction and greater independence in self-care, and allows nurses to experience increased job satisfaction and personal gratification in helping clients to reach their potentials and achieve successful outcomes (Barnes, 1995).

In patient education, the nurse may be tempted to teach as many family members as possible. In reality, it is difficult to coordinate the instruction of so many different people. The more individuals involved, the greater the potential for misunderstanding of instruction. The family must make the deliberate decision as to who is the most appropriate person to take the primary responsibility as the caregiver. The nurse must determine how the caregiver feels about the role of providing supportive care, how the caregiver feels about learning the necessary information, and what the caregiver's learning style preferences, cognitive abilities, fears and concerns, and current knowledge of the situation are (Phillips, 1989).

The caregiver needs information similar to what the patient is given to provide support, feedback, and reinforcement of self-care consistent with prescribed regimens of care. Sometimes the family members need more information than the patient to compensate for any sensory deficits or cognitive limitations the patient may have. Anticipatory teaching with family caregivers can reduce their anxiety, uncertainty, and lack of confidence. What the family is to do is important, but what the family is to expect also is essential information to be shared during the teaching-learning process. The greatest challenge for caregivers is to develop confidence in their ability to do what is right for the patient. Teaching is the means to help them confront this challenge.

The family can be the nurse's greatest ally in preparing the patient for discharge and in helping the patient to become independent in self-care. The patient's family is perhaps the single most significant determinant of the success or failure of the teaching plan (Haggard, 1989). The role of the family has been stressed in each developmental section in this chapter. Table 5-1 outlines the appropriate nursing interventions with the family at different stages in the life cycle.

SUMMARY

It is important to understand the specific and varied tasks associated with each developmental stage to individualize the approach to teaching in meeting the needs and desires of clients and their families. Assessment of physical, cognitive, and psychosocial maturation within each developmental period is crucial in determining the strategies to be used to facilitate the teaching-learning process. The younger learner is, in many ways, very different from the adult learner. Issues of dependency, extent of participation, rate of and capacity for learning, and situational and emotional obstacles to learning vary significantly according to phases of development.

Readiness to learn in children is very subject centered and highly influenced by their physical, cognitive, and psychosocial maturation. Motivation to learn in the adult is very problem centered and more oriented to psychosocial tasks related to roles and expectations of work, family, and community activities. For teaching to be effective, the nurse must create an environment conducive to learning by presenting information at the learner's level, inviting participation and feedback, and identifying whether parental and/or peer involvement is appropriate or necessary. Nurses, as the main resource for health education, must determine what needs to be taught, when to teach, how to teach, and who should be the focus of teaching in light of the developmental stage of the learner.

REVIEW QUESTIONS

1. What are the seven stages of development?
2. What are the definitions of pedagogy, andragogy, and gerogogy?
3. Who is the expert in cognitive development? What are the terms or labels used by this expert to identify the key cognitive milestones?
4. Who is the expert in psychosocial development? What are the terms or labels used by this expert to identify the key psychosocial milestones?
5. What are the salient characteristics at each stage of development that influence the ability to learn?
6. What are three main teaching strategies for each stage of development?
7. How does the role of the nurse vary when teaching individuals at different stages of development?
8. What is the role of the family in the teaching and learning process in each stage of development?

REFERENCES

Ahroni, J. H. (1996). Strategies for teaching elders from a human development perspective. *Diabetes Educator, 22*(1), 47–52.

Alford, D. M. (1982). Tips for teaching older adults. *Nursing Life, 2*(5), 60–63.

American Association of Colleges of Nursing. (1994). *AACN issue bulletin*. Washington, DC: Author.

Babcock, D. E. & Miller, M. A. (1994). *Client education: Theory & practice*. St. Louis: Mosby-Year Book.

Banks, E. (1990). Concepts of health and sickness of preschool- and school-aged children. *Children's Health, 19*(1), 43–48.

Barnes, L. P. (1995). Finding the "win/win" in patient/family teaching. *MCN: American Journal of Maternal Child Nursing, 20*(4), 229.

Boyd, M. D., Gleit, C. J., Graham, B. A., & Whitman, N. I. (1998). *Health teaching in nursing practice: A professional model* (3rd ed.). Norwalk, CT: Appleton & Lange.

Burgireno, J. (1985). Maximizing learning in the adult with SCI. *Rehabilitation Nursing, 10*(5), 20–21.

Cauffman, E. & Steinberg, L. (2000). (Im)maturity of judgment in adolescence: Why adolescents may be less culpable than adults. *Behavioral Science Law, 18*, 741–760.

Culbert, P. A. & Kos, B. A. (1971). Aging: Considerations for health teaching. *Nursing Clinics of North America, 6*(4), 605–614.

Day, M. C. (1981). Thinking at Piaget's stage of formal operations. *Educational Leadership, 39*, 44–47.

Elkind, D. (1984). Teenage thinking: Implications for health care. *Pediatric Nursing, 10*(6), 383–385.

Ellison, S. A. (1985). Geriatric oncology: A developmental approach. *Cancer Nursing, Supplement 1*, 28–32.

Erikson, E. H. (1963). *Childhood and society* (2nd ed.). New York: Norton.

Erikson, E. H. (1968). *Identity: Youth and crisis*. New York: Norton.

Falvo, D. R. (1994). *Effective patient education: A guide to increased compliance* (2nd ed.). Gaithersburg, MD: Aspen.

Farrand, L. L. & Cox, C. L. (1993). Determinants of positive health behavior in middle childhood. *Nursing Research, 42*(4), 208–213.

Fey, M. S. & Deyes, M. J. (1989). Health and illness self care in adolescents with IDDM: A test of Orem's theory. *Advances in Nursing Science, 12*(1), 67–75.

Gessner, B. A. (1989). Adult education: The cornerstone of patient teaching. *Nursing Clinics of North America, 24*(3), 589–595.

Gilroth, B. E. (1990). Promoting patient involvement: Educational, organizational, and environmental strategies. *Patient Education and Counseling, 15*, 29–38.

Gollop, C. J. (1997). Health information-seeking behavior and older African American women. *Bulletin of the Medical Library Association, 85*(2), 141–146.

Grey, M., Kanner, S., & Lacey, K. O. (1999). Characteristics of the learner: Children and adolescents. *Diabetes Educator, 25*(6), 25–33.

Haggard, A. (1989). *Handbook of patient education*. Rockville, MD: Aspen.

Hallburg, J. C. (1976). The teaching of aged adults. *Journal of Gerontological Nursing, 2*(3), 13–19.

Hartman, R. A. & Kochar, M. S. (1994). The provision of patient and family education. *Patient Education and Counseling, 24*, 101–108.

Havighurst, R. (1976). Human characteristics and school learning: Essay review. *Elementary School Journal*, 77, 101–109.

Heiney, S. P. (1991). Helping children through painful procedures. *American Journal of Nursing*, *91*(11), 20–24.

Hussey, C. G. & Hirsh, A. M. (1983). Health education for children. *Topics in Clinical Nursing*, *5*(1), 22–28.

Jackson, R. H., Davis, T. C., Murphy, P., Bairnsfather, L. E., & George, R. B. (1994). Reading deficiencies in older patients. *American Journal of the Medical Sciences, 308*(2), 79–82.

Johnson-Saylor, M. T. (1980). Seize the moment: Health promotion for the young adult. *Topics in Clinical Nursing, 2*(2), 9–19.

Kennedy, C. M. & Riddle, I. I. (1989). The influence of the timing of preparation on the anxiety of preschool children experiencing surgery. *Maternal-Child Nursing Journal, 18*(2), 117–132.

Kick, E. (1989). Patient teaching for elders. *Nursing Clinics of North America, 24*(3), 681–686.

Knowles, M. (1990). *The adult learner: A neglected species* (4th ed.). Houston: Gulf.

Knowles, M. S., Holton, E. F., & Swanson, R. A. (1998). *The adult learner: The definitive classic in adult education and human resource development* (5th ed.). Houston: Gulf.

Kotchabhakdi, P. (1985). School-age children's conceptions of the heart and its function. Monograph 15. *Maternal-Child Nursing Journal, 14*(4), 203–261.

Kray, J. & Lindenberger, U. (2000). Adult age differences in task switching. *Psychology and Aging, 15*(1), 126–147.

Lambert, S. A. (1984). Variables that affect the school-age child's reaction to hospitalization and surgery: A review of the literature. *Maternal-Child Nursing Journal, 13*(1), 1–18.

Levine, M. D. (1983). *Developmental-behavioral pediatrics*. Philadelphia: Lippincott.

Matsuda, O. & Saito, M. (1998). Crystallized and fluid intelligence in elderly patients with mild dementia of the Alzheimer type. *International Psychogeriatrics, 10*(2), 147–154.

Milligan, F. (1997). In defense of andragogy. Part 2: An educational process consistent with modern nursing's aims. *Nurse Education Today, 17*, 487–493.

Morra, M. E. (1991). Future trends in patient education. *Seminars in Oncology Nursing, 7*(2), 143–145.

Palmore, E. (1977). Facts on aging: A short quiz. *Gerontologist, 17*(4), 1–5.

Pearson, M. & Wessman, J. (1996). Gerogogy. *Home Healthcare Nurse, 14*(8), 631–636.

Perrin, E. C., Sayer, A. G., & Willett, J. B. (1991). Sticks and stones may break my bones . . . Reasoning about illness causality and body functioning in children who have a chronic illness. *Pediatrics, 88*(3), 608–619.

Petrillo, M. & Sanger, S. (1980). *Emotional care of hospitalized children* (2nd ed.). Philadelphia: Lippincott.

Phillips, L. R. (1989). Elder-family caregiver relationships: Determining appropriate nursing interventions. *Nursing Clinics of North America, 24*(3), 795–807.

Piaget, J. (1951). *Judgment and reasoning in the child*. London: Routledge and Kegan Paul.

Piaget, J. (1952). *The origins of intelligence in children*. New York: International Universities Press.

Piaget, J. (1976). *The grasp of consciousness: Action and concept in the young child*. Susan Wedgwood (translator). Cambridge, MA: Harvard University Press.

Picariello, G. (1986). A guide for teaching elders. *Geriatric Nursing, 7*(1), 38–39.

Pidgeon, V. (1985). Children's concepts of illness: Implications for health teaching. *Maternal-Child Nursing Journal, 14*(1), 23–35.

Poster, E. C. (1983). Stress immunization: Techniques to help children cope with hospitalization. *Maternal-Child Nursing Journal, 12*(2), 119–134.

Reeber, B. J. (1992). Evaluating the effects of a family education intervention. *Rehabilitation Nursing, 17*(6), 332–336.

Rendon, D. C., Davis, D. K., Gioiella, E. C., & Tranzillo, M. J. (1986). The right to know, the right to be taught. *Journal of Gerontological Nursing, 12*(12), 36.

Ryberg, J. W. & Merrifield, E. B. (1984). What parents want to know. *Nurse Practitioner, 9*(6), 24–32.

Taylor, K., Marienau, C., & Fiddler, M. (2000). *Developing adult learners: Strategies for teachers and trainers.* San Francisco: Jossey-Bass.

Theis, S. L. & Merritt, S. L. (1994). A learning model to guide research and practice for teaching of elder clients. *Nursing and Health Care, 15*(9), 464–468.

Vulcan, B. (1984). Major coping behaviors of a hospitalized 3-year-old boy. *Maternal-Child Nursing Journal, 13*(2), 113–123.

Weinrich, S. P. & Boyd, M. (1992). Education in the elderly. *Journal of Gerontological Nursing, 18*(1), 15–20.

Weinrich, S. P., Boyd, M., & Nussbaum, J. (1989). Continuing education: Adapting strategies to teach the elderly. *Journal of Gerontological Nursing, 15*(11), 19–21.

Whitener, L. M., Cox, K. R., & Maglich, S. A. (1998). Use of theory to guide nurses in the design of health messages for children. *Advances in Nursing Science, 20*(3), 21–35.

Woodring, B. C. (2000). If you have taught—have the child and family learned? *Pediatric Nursing, 26*(5), 505–509.

CHAPTER 6

Motivation, Compliance, and Health Behaviors of the Learner

Eleanor Richards and Wendy Sayward

CHAPTER HIGHLIGHTS

Motivation
    Motivational Factors
    Motivational Axioms
    Assessment of Motivation
    Motivational Strategies
Compliance
Compliance and Control

Health Behaviors of the Learner
    Health Belief Model
    Health Promotion Model (Revised)
    Self-Efficacy Theory
    Stages of Change Model
    Therapeutic Alliance Model

KEY TERMS

adherence
compliance
Health Belief Model
Health Promotion Model
hierarchy of needs
locus of control
motivation

motivational axioms
motivational incentives
noncompliance
readiness to learn
Self-Efficacy Theory
Stages of Change Model
Therapeutic Alliance Model

OBJECTIVES

After completing this chapter, the reader will be able to
1. Define the terms *motivation*, *compliance*, and *adherence* as related to behaviors of the learner.
2. Discuss motivation and compliance concepts and theories.
3. Identify incentives and obstacles that affect motivation to learn.
4. Discuss axioms of motivation relevant to learning.
5. Assess levels of learner motivation.
6. Outline strategies that facilitate motivation and compliance.
7. Compare and contrast selected health behavior frameworks and their influence on learning.

The nurse as teacher of patients needs to understand what drives the learner to learn and what factors promote or hinder the learning process. Motivation and compliance are concepts in many health behavior models.

The learner's level of motivation can indicate potential involvement in health education programs. Sands and Holman (1985) noted that compliance often has been used by researchers as a measure of outcomes of these programs. Becker, Drachman, and Kirscht (1974) found motivation to be significantly related to measures of compliance with a medical regimen.

Factors that determine health outcomes are complex. Ross and Rosser (1989) indicated that information alone does not account for changes in health behavior. Knowledge alone does not guarantee that the learner will engage in health-promoting behaviors or attain desired outcomes. The most well-thought-out educational program or plan of care will not achieve the desired goals if the learner is not understood in the context of factors associated with motivation and compliance. An understanding of the relationship between receiving information and the application of information, as well as those factors that impede or promote desired health outcomes, is essential for the nurse as patient teacher.

This chapter discusses the concepts of motivation and compliance as they relate to the learning situation with a focus on health behaviors. The discussion includes factors such as assessment of motivation, obstacles and facilitating factors for motivation and compliance, and motivational axioms. An overview and comparison of selected models of health behaviors is presented with an emphasis on the role of the nurse as a teacher of patients.

MOTIVATION

Motivation has been defined as a psychological force that moves a person toward some kind of action (Haggard, 1989) and as a willingness of the learner to embrace learning, with readiness as evidence of motivation (Redman, 2001). According to Kort (1987), it is the result of both internal and external factors and not the result of external manipulation alone. Motivation is movement in the direction of meeting a need or toward reaching a goal. Ideally, the nurse's role is to help the learner reach a desired goal and to prevent untimely delays.

Maslow (1943), a well-known early theorist, developed the theory of human motivation that is still widely used. The major premises of Maslow's motivation theory are integrated wholeness of the individual and a *hierarchy of needs*. These needs are organized by level of potency—physiological, safety, love/belonging, self-esteem, and self-actualization. Some individuals are highly motivated, whereas others are weakly motivated. When a need is fairly well satisfied, then the next potent need emerges. An example of the hierarchy of basic needs is the strong need to satisfy hunger. This need may be met by the nurse who assists the post-stroke patient with feeding. The nurse–patient interaction may also satisfy the next most potent needs, those of safety, love/belonging, and self-esteem.

There are relationships between motivation and learning; between motivation and behavior; and between motivation, learning, and behavior. Each theory presented in this chapter attempts to address the complex and somewhat elusive quality of motivation.

Motivational Factors

Factors that influence motivation can serve as incentives or obstacles to achieve desired behaviors. Both creating incentives and decreasing obstacles to motivation pose a challenge for the nurse as a teacher of patients. The cognitive (thinking processes), affective (emotions and feelings), social, and psychomotor (skill) domains of the learner can be influenced by the patient teacher, who can act as a motivational facilitator or blocker.

Motivational incentives need to be considered in the context of the individual. What may be a motivational incentive for one learner may be a motivational obstacle to another.

Facilitating or blocking factors that shape motivation to learn can be classified into three major categories, which are not mutually exclusive:

1. Personal attributes, which consist of physical, developmental, and psychological components of the individual learner
2. Environmental influences, which include the surroundings, and the attitudes of others
3. Learner relationship systems, such as those of significant other, family, community, and teacher-learner interaction

Personal Attributes
The factors that can shape an individual's motivation to learn include personal attributes such as:

- Developmental stage
- Age
- Gender

- Emotional readiness
- Values and beliefs
- Sensory functioning
- Cognitive ability
- Educational level
- Actual or perceived state of health
- Severity and/or chronicity of illness
- Level of natural curiosity
- Capacity for short-term and long-term memory

Ability to achieve behavioral outcomes is determined by an individual's physical, emotional, and cognitive status. One's perception of the difference between current and expected states of health can be a motivating factor in health behavior and can drive readiness to learn. Also, the learner's views about the complexity or extent of changes that are needed can shape motivation.

Environmental Influences

The environment can create, promote, or detract from learning. Environmental factors that influence the motivational level of the individual include:

- Physical characteristics of the learning environment
- Accessibility and availability of human and material resources
- Different types of behavioral rewards

Pleasant, comfortable, and adaptable individualized surroundings can promote a state of readiness to learn. Conversely, noise, confusion, interruptions, and lack of privacy can interfere with the capacity to concentrate and learn.

Accessibility and availability of resources include physical and psychological aspects. Can the client physically access a health facility, and once there, will the healthcare personnel be psychologically available to the client? Psychological availability refers to the healthcare system and whether it is flexible and sensitive to patients' needs. It includes factors such as promptness of services, sociocultural competence, emotional support, and communication skills. Attitude influences the client's engagement with the healthcare system.

The manner in which the healthcare system is perceived by the client affects the client's willingness to participate in health-promoting behaviors. Behavioral rewards support learner motivation. Rewards can be extrinsic, such as praise or acknowledgment. Alternatively, they can be intrinsically based, such as feelings of a personal sense of fulfillment, gratification, or self-satisfaction.

Relationship Systems

Family or significant others in the support system; cultural identity; work, school, and community roles; and teacher–learner interaction—all influence an individual's motivation. The learner exists in the context of relationship systems. Individuals are viewed in the context of family/community/cultural systems that have lifelong effects on the choices that individuals make, including healthcare seeking and healthcare decision making.

These significant other systems may have even more of an influence on health outcomes than commonly acknowledged. The health-promoting use of these systems needs to be taken into account. All of these factors are forces that affect motivation, and serve to facilitate or block the desire to learn.

Motivational Axioms

Axioms are premises on which an understanding of a phenomenon is based. The nurse as patient teacher needs to understand what is involved in promoting motivation of the learner. *Motivational axioms* are rules that set the stage for motivation. They include (1) the state of optimum anxiety, (2) learner readiness, (3) realistic goal setting, (4) learner satisfaction/success, and (5) dialogue about uncertainty.

State of Optimum Anxiety

Learning occurs best when a state of moderate anxiety exists. A moderate state of anxiety can be comfortably managed and is known to promote learning. In this optimum state for learning, one's ability to observe, focus attention, learn, and adapt is operative (Peplau, 1979). Above this optimum level, at high or severe levels of anxiety, the ability to perceive the environment, concentrate, and learn is reduced. For example, a patient who has been diagnosed recently with insulin-dependent diabetes and who has a high level of anxiety will not retain information at an optimum level when instructed about insulin injections. When the nurse is able to aid the client in reducing anxiety, through techniques such as guided imagery, use of humor, or relaxation tapes, the patient will respond with a higher level of information retention.

Learner Readiness

Desire to move toward a goal and *readiness to learn* are factors that influence motivation. Desire cannot be imposed on the learner. It can, however, be critically influenced by external forces and be promoted by the nurse. Incentives are specific to the individual learner. An incentive to one individual can be a deterrent to another.

Incentives in the form of reinforcers and rewards can be tangible or intangible, external or internal.

In patient teaching, the nurse offers positive perspectives and encouragement, which shape the desired behavior toward goal attainment. By ensuring that learning is stimulating, making information relevant and accessible, and creating an environment conducive to learning, nurses can facilitate motivation to learn (see Chapter 4 on readiness to learn).

Realistic Goals

Goals that are reasonable and possible to achieve are goals toward which an individual will work. Goals that are beyond one's reach are frustrating and counterproductive. Unrealistic goals that waste valuable time can set the stage for the learner to give up.

Setting realistic goals is a motivating factor. Learning what the learner wants to change is a critical factor in setting realistic goals. Mutual goal setting between the learner and the nurse reduces the negative effects of hidden agendas or the sabotaging of educational plans.

Learner Satisfaction/Success

The learner is motivated by success. Success is self-satisfying and feeds one's self-esteem. When a learner feels good about step-by-step accomplishments, motivation is enhanced. Focusing on successes as a means of positive reinforcement promotes learner satisfaction and instills a sense of accomplishment.

Dialogue about Uncertainty

Uncertainty, as well as certainty, can be a motivating factor in the learning situation. Mishel (1990) views uncertainty as a necessary and natural rhythm of life rather than an adverse experience. Uncertainty influences choices. It can capitalize on readiness for change and influence health behaviors of the learner.

Assessment of Motivation

How does the nurse know when the learner is motivated? Redman (2001) views motivational assessment as a part of general health assessment. Leddy and Pepper (1998) view assessment of motivation in relation to capacity for change. In collecting assessment data the nurse can ask several questions of the learner, such as those focusing on previous attempts, curiosity, goal setting, self-care ability, stress factors, survival issues, and life situations.

TABLE 6-1   Comprehensive Parameters for Motivational Assessment of the Learner

COGNITIVE VARIABLES
- Capacity to learn
- Readiness to learn
  - Expressed self-determination
  - Constructive attitude
  - Expressed desire and curiosity
  - Willingness to contract for behavioral outcomes
- Facilitating beliefs

AFFECTIVE VARIABLES
- Expressions of constructive emotional state
- Moderate level of anxiety

PHYSIOLOGICAL VARIABLES
- Capacity to perform required behavior

EXPERIENTIAL VARIABLES
- Previous successful experiences

ENVIRONMENTAL VARIABLES
- Appropriateness of physical environment
- Social support systems
  - Family
  - Group
  - Work
  - Community resources

TEACHER–LEARNER RELATIONSHIP SYSTEM
- Prediction of positive relationship

Motivational assessment of the learner needs to be comprehensive, systematic, and based on concepts. Cognitive, affective, physiological, experiential, environmental, and learning relationship variables need to be considered. Table 6-1 shows parameters for a comprehensive motivational assessment of the learner.

To assess motivation, several perspectives need to be considered. Bandura's (1986) construction of incentive motivators; Ajzen and Fishbein's (1980) intent and attitude; Becker's (1974) notion of likelihood of engaging in action; Pender's (1996) commitment to a plan of action; and Barofsky's (1978) focus on alliance in the learning situation. These theories guide assessment of learner motivation. If the learner's responses to the parameters in Table 6-1 are positive, then the learner is likely to be motivated.

Assessment of learner motivation involves the nurse's judgment, because teaching-learning is a two-way process. In particular, motivation can be assessed through both subjective and objective means. A subjective means of assessing level of motivation is through dialogue. By using communication skills, the nurse can obtain verbal information from the client such as "I really want to maintain my weight" or "I want to have a healthy baby." Both of these statements indicate a desire toward an expected health outcome. Nonverbal cues can also indicate motivation, such as browsing through lay literature about healthy pregnancy.

Measurement of motivation is another aspect to be considered. Subjective self-reports indicate the level of motivation from the learner's perspective. Behaviors that can be observed as the learner moves toward preset realistic health or practice goals can serve as objective measurements of motivation.

Motivational Strategies

As noted earlier, incentives to motivation can be either intrinsically or extrinsically generated. Incentives and motivation are both stimuli to act. Bandura (1986) associates motivation with incentives. Rarely does motivation occur without extrinsic influence. Green and Kreuter (1999) note that "strictly speaking we can appeal to people's motives, but we cannot motivate them" (p. 30). Motivational strategies for patient learning are extrinsically generated through the use of specific incentives. The critical question for the nurse to ask is, "What specific behavior, under what circumstances, in what time frame, is desired by this learner?"

Strategizing begins with a systematic assessment of learner motivation (see Table 6-1). When applicable incentives are absent or reduced, then the individual is likely to move away from the desired outcome. When considering strategies to improve learner motivation, Maslow's (1943) hierarchy of needs should also be taken into consideration. An appeal can be made to the innate need for the learner to succeed, known as achievement motivation (Atkinson, 1964).

When teaching others, clearly communicating directions and expectations is critical. Organizing material in a way that makes information meaningful to the learner, giving positive verbal feedback, and providing opportunities for success are some examples of motivational strategies (Haggard, 1989). Reducing or eliminating barriers to achieve goals is also an important way to enhance motivation.

One particular model developed by Keller (1987), the Attention, Relevance, Confidence, and Satisfaction (ARCS) Model, focuses on creating and maintaining motivational strategies used for teaching. This model emphasizes strategies that the teacher can use to effect changes in the learner by creating a motivating learning environment.

- **A**ttention introduces opposing positions, uses case studies, and varies the way materials are presented.
- **R**elevance refers to focusing on the learner's experiences, usefulness, needs, and personal choices.
- **C**onfidence of the learner is influenced by learning requirements, level of difficulty, expectations, learner attributes, and sense of accomplishment.
- **S**atisfaction pertains to the ability to use a new skill, the use of rewards, praise, and the extent to which self-evaluation is positive.

COMPLIANCE

Compliance is a term used to describe submission or yielding to predetermined goals. It has a manipulative or authoritative undertone in which the healthcare provider is viewed as the traditional authority, and the consumer or learner is viewed as submissive. This term has not been well received in nursing, perhaps due to the philosophical perspective that clients have the right to make their own healthcare decisions and to not necessarily follow established courses of action as set by healthcare professionals. Ward-Collins (1998) notes that a diagnosis of noncompliance can be highly subjective.

Healthcare literature suggests that compliance is the equivalent of achieving a goal based on a preset regimen. Compliance, as an end unto itself, is different from motivational factors, which are viewed as means to an end. Compliance to a health regimen is an observable behavior and as such can be directly measured. Motivation, by comparison, is a precursor to action that can be indirectly measured through behavioral consequences or results.

Commitment or attachment to a regimen is known as *adherence*, which may be long-lasting. Both compliance and adherence refer to the ability to maintain health-promoting regimens, which are determined largely by a healthcare provider. A subtle difference separates compliance and adherence. It is possible for an individual to comply with a regimen and not necessarily be committed to it. For example, a patient who is experiencing sleep disturbances may comply with medication as directed for a period of one week. The same patient may not continue to adhere to the regimen for an extended period of time, however, even though the sleep disturbances continue. In this situation, there is no commitment to follow through. Both compliance and adherence are terms used in the measurement of health outcomes; for the purpose of this chapter, they are used interchangeably.

COMPLIANCE AND CONTROL

One way to view the issue of control in the learning situation is through the concept of *locus of control* (Rotter, 1954) and health locus of control (Wallston, Wallston, & DeVellis, 1978). Through objective measurement, individuals can be categorized as "internals," whose health behavior is self-directed, or "externals," whereby others are viewed as more powerful in influencing health outcomes. Externals believe that fate is a powerful external force that determines life's course, whereas internals believe that they control their own destiny. For instance, an external might say, "Osteoporosis runs in my family, and it will catch up with me." An internal might say, "Although there is a history of osteoporosis in my family, I will have necessary screenings, eat an appropriate diet, and do weight-bearing exercise to prevent or control this problem."

Hussey and Guilliland (1989) note that both locus of control and functional literacy level influence compliance. Functional literacy level in relation to compliance also needs to be assessed by the nurse (see Chapter 7 on literacy).

Noncompliance describes resistance of the individual to follow a predetermined regimen. Literature indicates high levels of patient noncompliance, with estimates of noncompliance ranging from 30% to 50% (Becker & Green, 1975; Sackett & Haynes, 1976). The question of why clients are noncompliant remains largely unanswered.

The expectation of total compliance at all times is unrealistic. At times, noncompliant behavior may be desirable and could be viewed as a necessary defense to stressful situations. The learner may use "time-outs" as the intensity of the learning situation is maintained or escalates. This mechanism of temporary withdrawal from the learning situation may actually prove beneficial. Following withdrawal, the learner could reengage, feeling renewed and ready to continue with an educational program or regimen. Viewed in this way, noncompliance is not an obstacle to learning and does not carry a negative connotation.

HEALTH BEHAVIORS OF THE LEARNER

Motivation and compliance are concepts relevant to health behaviors of the learner. The nurse focuses on health education as well as the expected health behaviors. Health behavior frameworks are blueprints that can be used to maintain desired patient behaviors or promote changes. As a consequence, a familiarity with models and theories that describe, explain, or predict health behaviors will increase the range of health-promoting strategies for patient education. The principles inherent in each can be used either to facilitate motivation or to promote compliance to a health regimen. This chapter presents an overview of several models and theories: Health Belief

Model, Health Promotion Model, Self-Efficacy Theory, Stages of Change Model, and Therapeutic Alliance Model.

Health Belief Model

The original Health Belief Model was developed in the 1950s to examine why people did not participate in health-screening programs (Rosenstock, 1974). This model was modified by Becker (1974) to address compliance to therapeutic regimens. Becker (1990) notes two major premises of the model that need to be present: (1) the client's willingness to participate in disease prevention and curing regimens, and (2) the belief that health is highly valued.

Figure 6-1 shows the direction and flow of three components, each of which is further divided into subcomponents:

1. The individual perceptions component comprises perceived susceptibility or perceived severity of a specific disease.
2. The modifying factors component consists of demographic variables (age, sex, race, ethnicity), socio-psychological variables (personality, locus of control, social class, peer and reference group pressure), and structural variables (knowledge about and prior contact with disease). These variables, in conjunction with cues to action (mass media, advice, reminders, illness, reading material), influence the subcomponent of perceived threat of the specific disease.
3. The likelihood of action component consists of the subcomponents of perceived benefits of preventive action minus perceived barriers to preventive action.

All of the components are directed toward the likelihood of taking recommended preventive health action as the final phase of the model. In sum, individual perceptions and modifying factors interact. An individual appraisal of the preventive action occurs, which is followed by a prediction of the likelihood of action.

The Health Belief Model has been the predominant explanatory model since the 1970s for uncovering differences in preventive health behaviors as well as differences in preventive use of health services (Langlie, 1977). The model has also been widely used to study patient behaviors in relation to preventive behaviors and acute and chronic illnesses.

Janz and Becker (1984) reviewed the Health Belief Model literature over a 10-year period and found that the model was robust in predicting health behaviors, with perceived barriers being the most influential factor. Therefore, the nurse needs to take into consideration the availability of barrier-free educational resources, such as using printed materials for teaching that the patient can understand.

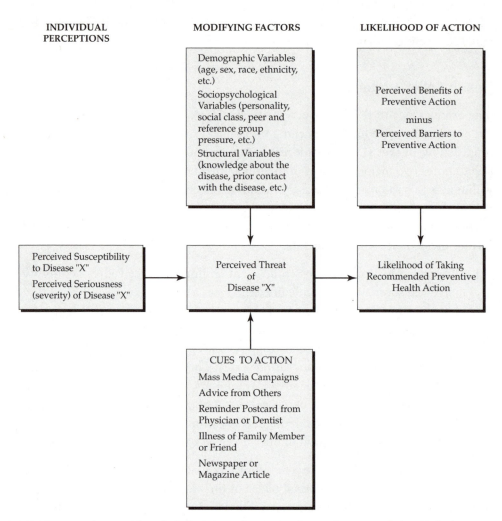

FIGURE 6-1   The Health Belief Model used as a predictor of preventive health behavior
Source: From M. Becker, R. Drachman, and J. Kirscht, A new approach to explaining sick-role behavior in low-income populations. (1974). *American Journal of Public Health, 64*(3), 206. Copyright by American Public Health Association. Reprinted with permission.

Health Promotion Model (Revised)

The Health Promotion Model, developed in 1987 and revised by Pender (1996), has been primarily used in the discipline of nursing (Figure 6-2). The emphasis on actualizing health potential and increasing the level of well-being using approach behaviors

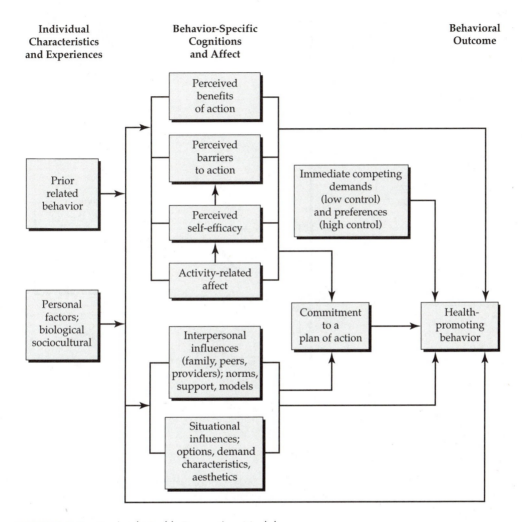

FIGURE 6-2   Revised Health Promotion Model
Source: From N. Pender, *Health Promotion in Nursing Practice*, 3rd ed., p. 67, 1996. Reprinted by permission of Pearson Education, Inc., Upper Saddle River, NJ.

rather than avoidance of disease behaviors distinguishes this model as a health promotion rather than a disease prevention model.

The three major components are as follows:

1. Individual characteristics and experiences, which consist of two variables—prior related behavior and personal factors

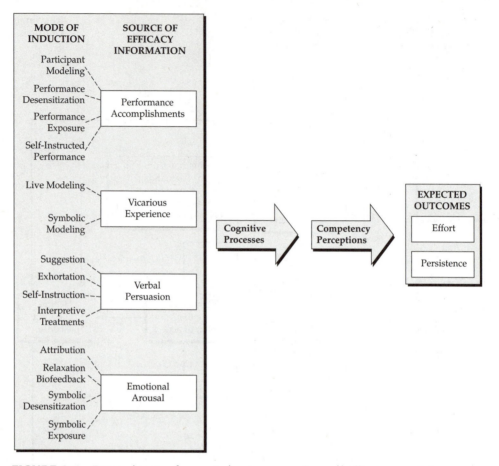

FIGURE 6-3   Determinants of expected outcomes using self-efficacy perceptions
Source: From A. Bandura, *Social Learning Theory*, © 1977, p. 80. Reprinted by permission of Prentice Hall, Upper Saddle River, NJ.

2. Behavior-specific cognitions and affect, which consist of perceived benefits of action, perceived barriers to action, perceived self-efficacy, activity-related affect, interpersonal influences, and situational influences
3. Behavioral outcome, which consists of health-promoting behavior

The Health Belief Model and the Health Promotion Model share several similarities, seen in a comparison of Figures 6-1 and 6-2. Both models describe the use of factors or components that impact on perceptions, but the Health Belief Model targets the likelihood of engaging in preventive health behaviors, whereas the revised Health Promotion Model targets positive health outcomes.

Self-Efficacy Theory

Self-Efficacy Theory is based on a person's expectations relative to a specific course of action (Bandura, 1977a, 1977b, 1986). It is a predictive theory in the sense that it deals with the belief that one is competent and capable of accomplishing a specific behavior. Figure 6-3 shows an adaptation of Bandura's efficacy expectations model extended to include expected outcomes. In this adapted model, self-efficacy is used as an outcome determinant. According to Bandura (1986), self-efficacy is cognitively appraised and processed through four principal sources of information:

1. Performance accomplishment evidenced in self-mastery of similarly expected behaviors
2. Vicarious experiences such as observing successful expected behavior through the modeling of others
3. Verbal persuasion by others who present realistic beliefs that the individual is capable of the expected behavior
4. Emotional arousal through self-judgment of physiological states of distress

Bandura (1986) notes that the most influential source of efficacy information is that of previous performance accomplishment. Self-efficacy has proved useful in predicting the course of health behavior. Indeed, nursing literature has addressed linkages between self-efficacy and self-care.

The use of the Self-Efficacy Theory is particularly relevant in developing educational programs. The behavior-specific predictions of the theory can be used for understanding the likelihood of individuals to participate in existing or projected educational programs. Educational strategies such as modeling, demonstration, and verbal reinforcement parallel modes of self-efficacy induction.

Stages of Change Model

Another model that informs the phenomenon of health behaviors of the learner is the Stages of Change Model (Prochaska & Di Clemente, 1982). This model (see Table 6-2) was developed around addictive and problem behaviors. Prochaska (1996) notes six distinct stages of change: precontemplation, contemplation, preparation, action, maintenance, and termination.

Motivation and readiness to change are seen as important constructs. It is useful in nursing to stage the client's intentions and behaviors for change, as well as strategies that will enable completion of each stage (Saarman, Daugherty, & Riegel, 2000).

TABLE 6-2   **Six Stages of Change**
Precontemplation The individual makes no plans to change. Teaching strategy—discussion.
Contemplation The individual identifies the problem and contemplates change. Teaching strategy—clarify issue and need to change.
Preparation The individual plans to make a change soon. Teaching strategy—develop plan of action.
Action The individual actively changes behavior. Teaching strategy—create environment conducive to change.
Maintenance The individual maintains new behavior over time. Teaching strategy—maintain environment conducive to change.
Termination No further risk of relapse to old behavior.

Therapeutic Alliance Model

Barofsky's (1978) Therapeutic Alliance Model addresses a shift in power from the provider to a learning partnership in which collaboration and negotiation with the patient are key. A therapeutic alliance is formed between the caregiver and receiver in which both participants are viewed as having equal power. The patient is viewed as active and responsible, with an outcome expectation of self-care. Self-determination and control over one's own life is fundamental to this model (Figure 6-4).

The Therapeutic Alliance Model uses the components of compliance, adherence, and alliance. According to Barofsky (1978), change is needed in the way nurses and patients interact. The nurse–patient relationship must change from coercion in compliance and from conforming in adherence to collaboration in alliance. The power in the relationship between the participants is equalized by alliance. In alliance, the role of the patient is neither passive nor rebellious, but rather active and responsible. The expected outcomes are not compliant dependence or counterdependence, but responsible self-care.

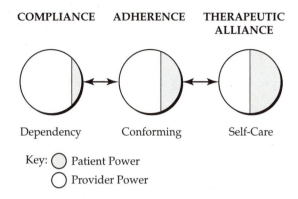

COMPLIANCE ADHERENCE THERAPEUTIC
ALLIANCE

Dependency   Conforming   Self-Care

Key: Patient Power
Provider Power

Figure 6-4 Continuum of the Therapeutic Alliance Model

This interpersonal partnership model is appropriate in the educational process when shifting the focus from the patient as a passive-dependent learner to one of an active learner. The nurse as teacher and the patient as learner form a collaborative alliance with the goal of self-care. Luker and Caress (1989) support the notion of therapeutic alliance in patient education, arguing that "nurses have resisted equalizing their role with patients" (p. 715). They encourage the transfer of responsibility for learning from nurse to patient.

SUMMARY

Components of this chapter have included a discussion of concepts of motivation and compliance, assessment of the level of learner motivation, identification of incentives and obstacles that affect motivation and compliance, and discussion of axioms of motivation relevant to learning. Strategies that facilitate motivation and compliance have been outlined and theories have been presented that influence motivation and/or compliance.

When information is imparted, accepted, and applied, the foundation is set for change in health behaviors. When people are motivated and know that they can make a difference in their own lives, then a barrier to health has been lifted.

REVIEW QUESTIONS

1. How are the terms *motivation*, *compliance*, and *adherence* defined?
2. How do the terms defined in Question 1 relate to one another?

3. What are the three major motivational factors?

4. Which axioms (premises) are involved in promoting motivation of the learner?

5. What are the six parameters for a comprehensive motivational assessment of the learner?

6. What are the basic concepts particular to each model or theory?

REFERENCES

Ajzen, I. & Fishbein, M. (1980). Understanding attitudes and predicting social behavior. Englewood Cliffs, NJ: Prentice-Hall.

Atkinson, J. W. (1964). An introduction to motivation. Princeton, NJ: Van Nostrand.

Bandura, A. (1977a). Self-efficacy: Toward a unifying theory of behavioral change. *Psychological Review, 84*(2), 191–215.

Bandura, A. (1977b). Social learning theory. Upper Saddle River, NJ: Prentice Hall.

Bandura, A. (1986). Social foundations of thought and action: A social cognitive theory. Upper Saddle River, NJ: Prentice Hall.

Barofsky, I. (1978). Compliance, adherence and the therapeutic alliance: Steps in the development of self-care. *Social Science and Medicine, 12,* 369–376.

Becker, M. (ed.). (1974). The health belief model and personal health behavior. Thorofare, NJ: Slack.

Becker, M. (1990). Theoretical models of adherence and strategies for improving adherence. In S. A. Shumaker, E. B. Schron, & J. K. Ockene (eds.), *The handbook of human health behavior* (pp. 5–43). New York: Springer.

Becker, M. W., Drachman, R. H., & Kirscht, J. P. (1974). A new approach to explaining sick-role behavior in low-income populations. *American Journal of Public Health, 64*(3), 205–216.

Becker, M. H. & Green, L. W. (1975). A family approach to compliance with medical treatment: A selective review of the literature. *International Journal of Health Education, 18,* 173–182.

deTornay, R. & Thompson, M. A. (1987). *Strategies for teaching nursing* (3rd ed.). New York: Wiley.

Eraker, S. A., Kirscht, J. P., & Becker, M. H. (1984). Understanding and improving patient compliance. *Annals of Internal Medicine, 100,* 258–268.

Green, L. W. & Kreuter, M. W. (1999). *Health promotion planning: An educational and ecological approach* (3rd ed.). Mountain View, CA: Mayfield.

Haggard, A. (1989). *Handbook of patient education.* Rockville, MD: Aspen.

Hussey, L. C. & Guilliland, K. (1989). Compliance, low literacy, and locus of control. *Nursing Clinics of North America, 24*(3), 605–610.

Janz, N. K. & Becker, M. H. (1984). The health belief model: A decade later. *Health Education Quarterly, 11*(1), 1–47.

Keller, J. M. (1987). Development and use of the ARCS model of instructional design. *Journal of Instructional Development, 10*(3), 2–10.

Kort, M. (1987). Motivation: The challenge for today's health promoter. *Canadian Nurse, 83*(9), 16–18.

Langlie, J. K. (1977). Social networks, health beliefs, and preventive health behavior. *Journal of Health and Social Behavior, 18*, 244–260.

Leddy, S. K. & Pepper, J. M. (1998). *Conceptual bases of professional nursing*. Philadelphia: Lippincott.

Luker, K. & Caress, A. L. (1989). Rethinking patient education. *Journal of Advanced Nursing, 14*, 711–718.

Lusk, S. L., Kerr, M. J., & Ronis, D. L. (1995). Health promoting lifestyles of blue-collar, skilled trade, and white-collar workers. *Nursing Research, 44*(1), 20–24.

Maslow, A. H. (1943). A theory of human motivation. *Psychological Review, 50*(4), 371–396.

Miller, J. (1999). Stages of change theory and the nicotine-dependent client: Direction for decision making in nursing practice. *Clinical Nurse Specialist, 13*(1), 18–22.

Mishel, M. H. (1990). Reconceptualization of the uncertainty in illness theory. *Image: Journal of Nursing Scholarship, 22*(4), 256–262.

Moore, E. J. (1990). Using self-efficacy in teaching self-care to the elderly. *Holistic Nursing Practice, 4*(2), 22–29.

Pender, N. (1987). *Health promotion in nursing practice* (2nd ed.). Norwalk, CT: Appleton-Lange.

Pender, N. (1996). *Health Promotion in Nursing Practice* (3rd ed.). Upper Saddle River, NJ: Pearson Education.

Peplau, H. E. (1979). *The psychotherapy of Hildegard E. Peplau*. Texas: Atwood.

Prochaska, J. O. (September 1996). Just do it isn't enough: Change comes in stages. *Tufts University Special Report Diet and Nutrition Letter*.

Prochaska, J. O. & Di Clemente, C. C. (1982). Transtheoretical therapy: Towards a more integrative model of change. *Psychotherapy, Theory, and Practice, 19*(3), 276–288.

Redman, B. K. (2001). *The practice of patient education* (9th ed.). St. Louis: Mosby.

Rosenstock, I. M. (1974). Historical origins of the health belief model. In M. H. Becker (ed.), *The health belief model and personal health behavior*. Thorofare, NJ: Slack.

Ross, M. W. & Rosser, B. R. (1989). Education and AIDS risks: A review. *Health Education Research, 4*(3), 273–284.

Rotter, J. B. (1954). *Social learning theory and clinical psychology*. Upper Saddle River, NJ: Prentice Hall.

Saarman, L., Daugherty, J., & Riegel, B. (2000). Patient teaching to promote behavior change. *Nursing Outlook, 48*(6), 281–287.

Sackett, D. L. & Haynes, R. B. (1976). *Compliance with therapeutic regimens*. Baltimore: Johns Hopkins University Press.

Sands, D. S. & Holman, E. H. (1985). Does knowledge enhance patient compliance? *Journal of Gerontological Nursing, 11*(4), 23–29.

Shillinger, F. (1983). Locus of control: Implications for nursing practice. *Image: Journal of Nursing Scholarship, 15*(2), 58–63.

Wallston, K. A., Wallston, B. S., & DeVellis, R. (Spring 1978). Development of the multidimensional health locus of control (MHLC) scales. *Health Education Monographs*, 160–170.

Ward-Collins, D. (1998). Noncompliant: Isn't there a better way to say it? *American Journal of Nursing, 98*(5), 17–31.

CHAPTER 7

Literacy in the Adult Patient Population

Susan B. Bastable

CHAPTER HIGHLIGHTS

KEY TERMS

comprehension
functional illiteracy
health literacy
illiteracy
literacy

low literacy
numeracy
readability
reading

After completing this chapter, the reader will be able to

1. Define the terms *literacy, illiteracy, health literacy, low literacy, functional illiteracy, readability, reading, comprehension*, and *numeracy*.
2. Explain the magnitude of the literacy problem in the United States.
3. Identify the population groups at risk for illiteracy and low literacy.
4. Discuss common myths and assumptions about people who are illiterate.
5. Identify clues that indicate reading and writing deficiencies.
6. Recognize the impact of illiteracy and low literacy on patient motivation and compliance with healthcare regimens.
7. Recognize the ethical and legal responsibility of the nurse in providing education materials that patients can read and understand.
8. Use specific formulas and tests to analyze readability of printed materials and to test comprehension and reading skills of patients.
9. Describe specific guidelines for writing effective education materials.
10. Outline various teaching strategies useful in educating clients with marginal literacy skills.

The rate of illiteracy and low literacy is a major problem in this country despite public and private efforts at all levels to address the issue. Today, the fact remains that many adults do not have the basic literacy abilities to function effectively in our technologically complex society. Many individuals have difficulty reading and comprehending information well enough to be able to perform such common tasks as filling out job and insurance applications, interpreting bus schedules and road signs, completing tax forms, or registering to vote.

In 1992, the U.S. Department of Education conducted the National Adult Literacy Survey (NALS). The NALS findings revealed a shockingly high rate of illiteracy and low literacy in this country (Kirsch, Jungeblat, Jenkins, & Kolstad, 1993). In 2002, a more extensive follow-up survey, known as the NAALS (National Assessment of Adult Literacy Survey), was carried out. Although the final results have not yet been released, early findings indicate that the literacy problem in the United States has worsened over the past decade.

The levels of illiteracy and low literacy, once thought to be mainly a problem in developing countries, has taken on new meaning for the welfare of our nation (Lasater & Mehler, 1998). Recently, nursing and medical literature has begun to focus significant attention on the effects of patient illiteracy on health outcomes. Today, the emphasis is on health literacy—that is, the extent to which Americans can read and comprehend well enough to follow prescribed regimens of care. If patients with low literacy abilities cannot fully benefit from the type and amount of information they are typically given, then they cannot be expected to maintain health and manage independently. The result is a significant negative impact on the cost of health care and the quality of life (Brez & Taylor, 1997; Brownson, 1998; Fisher, 1999). People with poor reading and comprehension skills have higher medical costs and more physical and psychosocial problems than do literate persons (Jenks, 1992). A great deal more needs to be understood about the causes and effects associated with poor health literacy as well as the methods available to screen and teach patients (Ad Hoc Committee, 1999; Fetter, 1999).

Traditionally, health providers have relied heavily on printed education materials as a cost-effective and time-efficient means to communicate health messages. For years, nurses and physicians have assumed that the written materials commonly distributed to patients were sufficient to ensure informed consent for tests and procedures, to promote compliance with treatment regimens, and to guarantee adherence to discharge instructions. Only recently have they begun to recognize that the medical terminology used in printed information is hardly understood by the majority of patients. Unless education materials are written at an appropriate level, patients cannot be expected to be able or willing to accept responsibility for self-care. Even though illiteracy and low literacy are quite prevalent in the U.S. population, problems with literacy frequently continue to go undiagnosed (Doak, Doak, & Root, 1996).

This chapter examines the magnitude of the illiteracy problem, the factors that influence readability and comprehension of written health educational materials, the important role nurses play in assessing patients' literacy skills, and the effects of illiteracy on the health and well-being of the public. In addition, the formulas and tests used to evaluate readability and the comprehension and reading skills of patients are reviewed, specific guidelines are put forth for writing effective health education materials, and teaching strategies are recommended as a means for breaking down the barriers of illiteracy and low literacy.

DEFINITION OF TERMS

The word *literate* is defined in Webster's Collegiate Dictionary (1999) as "an educated person," one who is "able to read and write" (p. 680). More specifically, to be literate is to understand information commonly encountered in daily living. In 1993, the U.S. Department of Education defined literacy as "the ability to use print and written information to function in society, to achieve one's goals, and to develop one's knowledge and potential" (p. 6). Others have defined literacy based on the number of grade levels of school completed. However, the reported number of years of schooling attended has been found to be an inadequate predictor of a person's reading and writing skills (Adams-Price, 1993; Davis et al., 1990; Doak et al., 1996; French & Larrabee, 1999; Jackson et al., 1991; Kelly, 1999; and Winslow, 2001).

The commonly accepted definition of *literacy* is the ability to read, understand, and interpret information written at the eighth grade level or above. On the other end of the spectrum, *illiteracy* is the inability to read or write, which until now has been relatively rare in our society (Doak et al., 1996).

Literacy can be categorized into three general kinds of tasks (Adams-Price, 1993; Fisher, 1999):

- Prose tasks, which measure reading comprehension and the ability to find themes in newspapers, magazines, poems, and books
- Document tasks, which assess the ability to interpret documents such as insurance reports, consent forms, and transportation schedules
- Quantitative tasks, which assess the ability to calculate or interpret numbers on such things as restaurant bills, income tax forms, paycheck stubs, or a nutrition checklist of calories.

Health literacy refers to how well an individual can read, interpret, and comprehend health information to maintain an optimal level of wellness. The Ad Hoc Committee on Health Literacy for the Council on Scientific Affairs of the American Medical Association (1999) defined health literacy as "a constellation of skills, including the ability to perform basic reading and numerical tasks required to function in the health care environment" (p. 553). This committee identified the scope and consequences of poor health literacy in the United States. It concluded that an individual's health literacy is likely to be significantly worse than his or her general literacy skills. One reason is because of the complex medical and technical terms used in patient education materials.

As managed care requires individuals to take more responsibility for self-care and symptom management, health literacy is becoming an important determinant of health status. Poor health literacy may lead to serious negative consequences, such as increased morbidity and mortality, when a person is unable to read and comprehend instructions for medications, follow-up appointments, diet, procedures, and other regimens. Patients cannot be expected to be independent in self-care if they do not have the ability to follow the instructions they are given (Fetter, 1999). Health knowledge, health status, and the use of health services are all related to literacy levels.

Low literacy, also referred to as marginally literate or marginally illiterate, is the ability of adults to read, write, and comprehend information between the fifth- and eighth-grade levels of difficulty. Low-literate persons have trouble reading and writing common information to meet their everyday needs such as understanding a TV schedule, taking a telephone message, or filling out a relatively simple application form (Doak et al., 1996).

Functional illiteracy means that adults have reading, writing, and comprehension skills below the fifth-grade level. That is, they lack the basic education skills needed to manage effectively in today's society. Functionally illiterate persons have very limited ability to communicate via the written and sometimes even the spoken word. They do not understand basic printed instructions or audiovisual aids, and may even have difficulty with tape recordings. Such individuals are unable to read well enough to understand and interpret what they have read or use the information as it was intended (Doak et al., 1996). For example, functionally illiterate persons may be able to read the words on a label of a can of soup that directs "Pour soup into pan. Add one can water. Heat until hot." However, they cannot comprehend the meaning and sequence of the words to carry through with these directions.

Although an individual may have poor reading skills, this does not necessarily imply a lack of intelligence. Low literacy or illiteracy does not equal low IQ (Hussey & Guilliland, 1989). A person can be illiterate or low literate, yet intellectually be within at least normal IQ range (Doak et al., 1996).

Reading, readability, and comprehension are also terms frequently used when determining levels of literacy. Fisher (1999) defines *reading*, or word recognition, as "the process of transforming letters into words and being able to pronounce them correctly" (p. 57). *Readability* is defined as how well printed or written materials can be read based on a measure of a number of different variables within a given text of information.

Comprehension, on the other hand, is the degree to which individuals understand what they have read (Fisher, 1999; Hirsch, 2001). It is the ability to grasp the meaning of a message—to get the gist of it. Nurses can determine comprehension by noting whether patients are able to correctly demonstrate or recall in their own words the messages contained in printed health instruction materials. Comprehension is affected by the amount, clarity, and complexity of the information presented. The ability to read does not alone guarantee comprehension. For example, illness or other disruptive life situations have been found to significantly interfere with understanding and remembering information that has been read.

Another term used when discussing literacy is *numeracy*, which is the ability to read and interpret numbers. Most often, those with limited literacy also have limited skills in numeracy (Doak et al., 1996; Fisher, 1999; Morgan, 1993; Williams et al., 1995).

Literacy Relative to Computer Instruction

Recently, computer literacy has become an increasingly popular topic and a new dimension of the issue of literacy. There is a bright future for the use of computers as educational tools, but this potential is only beginning to be fully realized or appreciated.

As healthcare organizations and agencies invest more resources in computer technology and software programs, computer literacy in the patient population will become an issue of increasing concern. More and more, computers are being used as an instructional tool as well as a way to access additional sources of information for patient education (see Chapter 13 on technology in education). The opportunity to expand patients' knowledge base by using technology will require nurses in their role as teachers to pay attention to computer literacy levels much in the same way they have begun to recognize the limited value in using print materials with patients who are illiterate or low literate (Doak et al., 1996).

SCOPE AND INCIDENCE OF THE PROBLEM

Based on available statistics, it is evident that the United States has a significant literacy problem. The 1992 National Adult Literacy Survey (NALS) is considered to be the most accurate, detailed, and recent profile on literacy in the United States. NALS took a representative sample of 26,000 individuals, aged 16 years and older, to assess their skills in three areas: prose, document, and quantitative literacy. Scores ranged from Level 1, being the lowest level, to Level 5, being the highest level. The results were that 21–23%, or approximately 40 to 44 million of the 191 million adults in the country, scored in the lowest levels of the three skill areas. Those that fell into Level 1 are considered to be functionally illiterate. Another 25% to 28%, or approximately 50 million adults, scored in the Level 2 category. That is, they are considered to have low literacy skills.

Thus, the total number of illiterate and low-literate adults in the United States conservatively is estimated to be approximately 90 million. This figure means that about one-half of the adult population in this country has deficiencies in reading, writing, and math skills (Fisher, 1999; Williams, Counselman, & Caggiano, 1996). NALS did not specifically test health literacy levels (Ad Hoc Committee, 1999), but the survey did find that those individuals with poor literacy skills are more often from minority populations, from lower socioeconomic groups, and with poorer health status (Fisher, 1999; TenHave et al., 1997).

Thus, at least one out of every four to five Americans lacks the literacy skills and knowledge to cope with the requirements of day-to-day living. For example, one needs to be able to read at the sixth-grade level to understand a driver's license manual, at the eighth-grade level to follow directions on a frozen dinner package, and at the tenth-grade level to read instructions on a bottle of aspirin (Doak, Doak, & Root, 1985).

Because few people with limited reading skills admit to having such difficulty, the scope of the literacy problem may be much greater than reported (Brownson, 1998; Jolly, Scott, Feied, & Sandford, 1993). Many people read two to four grade levels below the number of years of school attended. This is because schools have a tendency to promote students for social and age-related reasons rather than for academic achievement alone. Also, patients may report inaccurate histories of years of school attended, and reading skills may be lost over time through lack of practice (Davidhizar & Brownson, 1999; Jackson et al., 1991; Miller & Bodie, 1994; Stephens, 1992; Yasenchak & Bridle, 1993). The average literacy level is at the eighth grade of reading ability. Medicaid enrollees, on average, read at the fifth-grade level (Winslow, 2001).

The trend is toward an increased proportion of Americans with literacy levels that are inadequate for active participation in our advanced technological society. A greater number of people are beginning to fall behind, unable to keep up with our increasingly sophisticated world. The literacy problem most likely is due to factors such as the following (Baydar, Brooks-Gunn, & Furstenberg, 1993; Hayes, 2000; Hirsch, 2001; Weiss, Reed, & Kligman, 1995):

- A rise in the number of immigrants
- The aging of the population
- The increasing complexity of information
- More people living in poverty
- Changes in policies and funding for public education
- A disparity in the literacy achievements of minority versus nonminority populations

Levels of literacy are often seen as indicators of the well-being of individuals. The literacy problem also has greater implications for the social and economic status of the country as a whole. Low levels of literacy have been associated with marginal productivity, high unemployment, minimum earnings, high costs of health care, and high rates of welfare dependency (Baydar et al., 1993; Kelly, 1999; Winslow, 2001; Ziegler, 1998). Illiteracy is considered to be an element contributing to many of the grave social issues confronting the United States today, such as homelessness, teen pregnancy, unemployment, delinquency, crime, and drug abuse (Fleener & Scholl, 1992). Deficiencies in basic literacy skills compound to create a social burden that is extremely costly for the American people. Reports indicate that poor basic literacy skills are evident in 69% of all those arrested, 85% of unwed mothers, 79% of welfare recipients, 85% of dropouts, and 72% of unemployed people (Johnson & Layng, 1992).

THOSE AT RISK

Illiteracy has been portrayed "as an invisible handicap that affects all classes, ethnic groups, and ages" (Fleener & Scholl, 1992, p. 740). It has been termed the "silent epidemic," the "silent barrier," and the "silent disability" (Doak & Doak, 1987; Kefalides, 1999). Illiteracy knows no boundaries and exists among persons of every race and ethnic background, socioeconomic class, and age category (Duffy & Snyder, 1999; Weiss et al., 1995). It is true, however, that illiteracy is rare in the higher socioeconomic classes, for example, and that certain segments of the U.S. population are more likely to be affected than others by lack of literacy skills. Populations that have been identified as having poorer reading and comprehension skills than the average American include the following (Cole, 2000; Hayes, 2000; Jackson et al., 1991; Lasater & Mehler, 1998; Winslow, 2001):

- The economically disadvantaged
- Older adults
- Immigrants (particularly illegal ones)
- Racial minorities
- High school dropouts
- The unemployed
- Prisoners
- Inner-city and rural residents
- Southerners (Louisiana, Texas, and Mississippi report the highest rates of illiteracy in the nation)
- Those with poor health status due to chronic mental and physical problems

Statistics indicate that 38 million Americans are presently living in poverty and that nearly half of all adults with low literacy live in poverty (Kelly, 1999). Although the disadvantaged represent many diverse cultural and ethnic groups, including millions of poor white people, one-third of the disadvantaged in this country are minorities (see Chapter 8 on cultural attributes). In the twenty-first century, the major growth in the population will come from the ranks of minority groups. By 2010, one out of every three people in the United States is projected to belong to a racial or ethnic minority (Robinson, 2000). In 1996, the U.S. Census Bureau reported that 1 in every 10 people living in this country was born in another country. Since 1980, the number of people speaking a language at home other than English has risen by 43% to 28.3 million people (Denboba, Bragdon, Epstein, Garthright, & Goldman, 1998).

Many minority and economically disadvantaged people, as well as the prison population—which has the highest concentration of adult illiteracy (Duffy & Snyder, 1999)—do not benefit from the typical health education activities, which often fail to reach them. Many lack reading skills good enough to make use of written health material used for patient education (Denboba et al., 1998; Morra, 1991). Areas with the highest percentage of minorities and high rates of poverty and immigration also have the highest percentage of functionally illiterate people. When these people need medical care, they tend to require more resources, have longer hospital stays, and have a greater number of readmissions (Davis et al., 1990; TenHave et al., 1997).

Also, of those Americans older than 65 years of age, two out of five adults (approximately 40%) are considered functionally illiterate (Brooks, 1998; Davidhizar & Brownson, 1999). Individuals older than 85 years of age make up the fastest growing age group in the country (Gollop, 1997). Today, the illiteracy problem in the older adult population is due to the fact that not only did these individuals have less education in the past, but also their reading skills have declined over time because of disuse. If a person does not use a skill, he or she loses the skill (Brownson, 1998). In addition, intellectual functioning is affected by aging (Jackson, Davis, Murphy, Bairnsfather, & George, 1994; Pearson & Wessman, 1996; Weinrich & Boyd, 1992; Weiss et al., 1995). The majority of older people have some degree of cognitive changes and vision impairments, and about one-fourth have serious hearing loss. Along with these normal physiological changes, many suffer from chronic diseases, and large numbers are taking prescribed medications. All of these conditions can interfere with the ability to learn, which contributes to the high incidence of illiteracy in this population group.

Cultural diversity, although not considered to be directly related to illiteracy, may also serve as a barrier to effective client education (Wilson, 1995). According to Davidhizar and Brownson (1999), most illiterate adults in this country are white, native-born, English-speaking Americans. However, when examining the proportion of the population that has poor literacy skills, minority ethnic groups are at higher risk. It is estimated that 44% of African Americans and 56% of Hispanic Americans are illiterate or marginally illiterate. According to the NALS report, adults belonging to the four major cultural groups (Black American, Hispanic American, Native

American, and Asian/Pacific Islander) were more likely than Caucasians to perform at the two lowest literacy levels (Kirsch et al., 1993).

In communicating with clients from different cultures, it is important to be aware that even though people may speak the English language, the meanings of words and the understanding of facts may vary significantly based on life experiences, family background, and culture of origin, especially if English is the client's second language (Davidhizar & Brownson, 1999). Nurses must be aware of these potential barriers to communication when interacting with clients from other cultures whose literacy skills may be limited (see Chapter 8 on cultural attributes). Given the increasing diversity of the U.S. population, most currently available written materials are inadequate based on the literacy level of minority groups.

This profile of the various population groups with literacy problems is not intended to stereotype people. Instead, it is offered to give a broad picture of who most likely is lacking in literacy skills. It is essential that nurses and other healthcare providers be aware of those individuals susceptible to having literacy problems when carrying out assessments on their patient populations. Also, the challenge now and in the future will be to find improved ways of communicating with these population groups and to develop innovative teaching strategies in the delivery of medical and nursing care (Denboba et al., 1998; Morra, 1991; Robinson, 2000).

MYTHS, STEREOTYPES, AND ASSUMPTIONS

Rarely do people voluntarily admit that they are illiterate. Illiteracy is a stigma that creates feelings of shame, inadequacy, fear, and low self-esteem (Parikh et al., 1996). Most individuals with poor literacy skills have learned that it is dangerous to reveal their problem because of fear that others, such as family, strangers, friends, or employers, would consider them dumb or incapable of functioning responsibly. In fact, the majority of people with literacy problems have never told their spouse or children of their disability (Kelly, 1999; Murphy & Davis, 1997; Parikh et al., 1996; Quirk, 2000).

People also tend to underreport their limited reading abilities because of embarrassment or lack of insight about the extent of their limitation. The NALS report revealed that the majority of adults performing at the two lowest levels of literacy skill describe themselves as good at being able to read and/or write English (Kirsch et al., 1993). Because self-reporting is so unreliable and because illiteracy and low literacy are so common, many experts suggest that screening of all patients should be done to identify clients who have reading difficulty to determine the extent of their impairment (Lasater & Mehler, 1998; Wilson, 1995).

Most people with limited literacy abilities are masters at concealment. Typically, they are ashamed by their limitation and attempt to hide the problem in clever ways. Many have discovered ways to function quite well in society without being able to read. They memorize signs and instructions, make intelligent guesses, or find employment opportunities that are not heavily dependent on reading and writing skills. As Fain (1994) points out, illiterate patients "become very good actors, practiced in misdirection and evasion" (p. 16B). In fact, people would rather tell you they have a venereal disease than let you know that they can't read (Doak et al., 1996).

An important thing to remember is that there are many myths about illiteracy. It is very easy for health providers to fall into the trap of wrongly labeling someone as illiterate or, for that matter, assuming that they are literate based on stereotypical images. Some of the most common myths include the following (Brooks, 1998; Doak et al., 1996; Lasater & Mehler, 1998; Mayeaux et al., 1996; Walker, 1987; Winslow, 2001):

Myth #1: Illiterate people are stupid and slow learners or incapable of learning at all. (In fact, many have normal or above-normal IQs.)

Myth #2: Illiterate people can be recognized by their appearance. (In fact, appearance alone is not a good basis for judgment because some very articulate, well-dressed people suffer from illiteracy, and some who do not speak well and are poorly dressed are, in fact, literate.)

Myth #3: The number of years of schooling completed is a good indicator of literacy skills. (In fact, grade-level achievement does not correspond well to reading ability. The number of years of schooling attended overestimates reading levels by up to four grade levels.)

Myth #4: All illiterate people are foreigners, poor, of ethnic or racial minority, and/or from the South. (In fact, illiterate people come from very diverse backgrounds.)

Myth #5: Most illiterate people will freely admit that they do not know how to read or do not understand. (In fact, most try to hide their reading deficiencies and will go to great lengths to avoid discovery, even when directly asked about their possible limitations.)

ASSESSMENT OF THE LITERACY PROBLEM

So the question remains: How does one recognize a person who is illiterate or low literate? Identifying a literacy problem is not easy because there is no stereotypical pattern. It is easy to overlook illiteracy or low literacy because the problem has no particular face, age, socioeconomic status, or nationality (Cole, 2000; Hayes, 2000). Nurses, because of their highly developed assessment skills and frequent contact with patients, are in an ideal position to determine the literacy levels of their clients. Due to the prevalence of illiteracy, nurses should never assume that their patients are literate.

Because illiterate or semiliterate patients often have had many years of practice at disguising the problem, they will go to elaborate lengths to hide it. There are so many instances when a patient does not fit the stereotypical image of an illiterate or low-literate person that nurses and physicians have never even considered the possibility. Overlooking the problem has the potential for grave consequences in treatment outcomes, and has resulted in frustration for both the patient and the caregiver (Cole, 2000; Rudolph, 1994). If healthcare providers become aware of a patient's literacy problem, they must convey sensitivity and maintain confidentiality to prevent increased feelings of shame (Parikh et al., 1996; Quirk, 2000).

There are a number of informal clues to watch out for that indicate reading and writing deficiencies. The caveat is not to rely on the obvious, but to look for the unexpected. During assessment, the nurse should take note of the following clues that illiterate patients may demonstrate (Brooks, 1998; Fain, 1994; Lasater & Mehler, 1998; Loughrey, 1983; Meade & Thornhill, 1989):

- Reacting to complex learning situations by withdrawal, complete avoidance, or repeatedly not being compliant
- Using the excuse that they were too busy, too tired, too sick, or too sedated with medication to maintain attention span when given a booklet or instruction sheet to read
- Claiming that they just did not feel like reading, that they gave the information to their spouse to take home, or that they lost, forgot, or broke their glasses
- Surrounding themselves with books, magazines, and newspapers to give the impression they are able to read
- Insisting on taking the information home to read or having a family member or friend with them when written information is presented
- Asking you to read the information for them with the excuse that their eyes are bothersome, they lack interest, or they do not have the energy to learn
- Showing nervousness as a result of feeling stressed by the threat of the possibility of "getting caught" or having to confess to illiteracy
- Acting confused, talking out of context, or holding reading materials upside down

- Showing a great deal of frustration and restlessness when attempting to read, often mouthing words aloud or moving lips silently, substituting words they cannot read with meaningless words, pointing to words or phrases on a page, or showing facial signs of bewilderment or defeat
- Standing in a location clearly designated for "authorized personnel only"
- Listening and watching very attentively to observe and memorize how things work
- Demonstrating difficulty with following instructions about relatively simple activities such as operating the electric bed, call light, and other simple equipment, even when the instructions are clearly printed on them
- Failing to ask any questions about the information they received

These clues from the patient in the form of puzzled looks, inappropriate behaviors, excuses, or irrelevant statements are indications to the nurse that the message being communicated is neither received nor understood. Not only do illiterate patients become confused and frustrated in their attempts to deal with written and verbal information, but they also become stressed in their efforts to cover up their disability.

Nurses, in turn, can feel frustrated when patients with undiagnosed literacy problems seem at face value to be unmotivated and noncompliant in following self-care instructions. Many times nurses wonder why patients make care-giving so difficult for themselves as well as for the provider. It is not unusual for nurses to conclude, "He's too stubborn for his own good," "She's in denial," or "He's just noncompliant—it's a control issue." Nurses must go beyond their own assumptions and look beyond a patient's appearance and behavior. They must seek out the less than obvious by conducting a thorough initial assessment to uncover the possibility that a literacy problem exists (Rudolph, 1994). An awareness of this possibility and good skills at observation are key to diagnosing illiteracy or low literacy in the patient population. Early diagnosis will enable nurses to intervene appropriately to avoid disservice to illiterate patients, who do not need condemnation, but support and encouragement from every nurse.

IMPACT OF ILLITERACY ON MOTIVATION AND COMPLIANCE

In addition to the fact that poor literacy skills affect the ability to read, understand, and interpret the meaning of written and also often verbal instruction, an illiterate or semiliterate person struggles with other significant limitations in communication that negatively influence healthcare teaching (Doak, Doak, Friedell, & Meade, 1998; Murphy & Davis, 1997).

People with poor reading skills have difficulty analyzing instructions, taking in and organizing new information, problem solving, and formulating questions (Brooks, 1998). They may be reluctant to ask questions because they probably do not know what to ask or they are afraid other people will think of them as ignorant or lacking in intelligence. Even when questioned about their understanding of information, people with low literacy skills will most likely claim they understood something even when they did not (Doak et al., 1996).

For example, a young pregnant girl was prescribed antiemetic suppositories to control her nausea. When she had no relief of symptoms, questioning by the nurse revealed that she was swallowing the medication. Obviously, not only did she misunderstand how to take the medicine, but she also probably had never seen a suppository and was not even able to read the word. She did not ask what it was, probably because she did not know what to ask in the first place, and she may have been reluctant to question the treatment out of fear that she would be regarded as stupid (Hussey & Guilliland, 1989).

People with poor literacy skills also tend to think in only concrete, specific, and literal terms. An example of this limitation is the diabetic patient whose glucose levels were out of control even when the patient insisted he was taking his insulin as instructed—injecting the orange and then eating the fruit (Brooks, 1998; Hussey & Guilliland, 1989).

The illiterate or semiliterate person may also experience difficulty handling large amounts of information. For example, patients who need to take several different medications at various times and in different dosages may either become confused with the schedule or ignore the instruction. If asked to change their daily medication routine, a great deal of retraining may be needed to convince them of the benefits of the new regimen.

Another major factor in noncompliance is the lack of simple instructions about prescribed treatments. Unfortunately, poor literacy skills are seldom assessed by nurses when teaching patients. For instance, a patient with a literacy problem has limited ability to understand the complex instructions regarding medication labels, dosage scheduling, adverse reactions, drug interactions, and complications. No wonder those who lack vocabulary, organized thinking, and the ability to formulate questions become confused and easily frustrated to the point of taking medications incorrectly or refusing to take them at all.

Nurses and physicians often overestimate an individual's ability to understand instructions and are quick to label someone as uncooperative. In reality, the underlying problem may be limited ability to comprehend and follow written and oral communication (Lasater & Mehler, 1998). What is often mistaken for noncompliant behavior is, instead, the simple inability to comply. Although approximately 21% to 23% of adult patients are functionally illiterate, this statistic is overlooked by many health professionals. It is, however, a major factor in noncompliance with prescribed regimens, follow-up appointments, and measures to prevent medical complications (Doak et al., 1996). A number of studies have correlated literacy levels with noncompliance (Doak et al., 1998; Hussey, 1994; Hussey & Guilliland, 1989; Jolly et al., 1993). Individuals with poor literacy skills have difficulty following instructions and providing accurate and complete health histories, which are vital to the delivery of good health care. The burden of illiteracy leads patients to behave in ways that seem uncooperative. Often, it is not because they are unwilling to comply, but rather because they are unable to do so (Hayes, 2000; Williams et al., 1996).

ETHICAL AND LEGAL CONCERNS

Printed education materials (PEMs), distributed primarily by nurses and physicians, are the major sources of information for patients participating in health programs in many settings. Materials that are too difficult to read or comprehend serve little purpose. Unless patients are competent in reading and comprehending the literature given to them, these tools are useless for health education. They are neither a cost-effective nor a time-efficient means for teaching and learning. Materials that are widely distributed, but little or not at all understood, pose not only a health hazard for the patient, but also an ethical and legal liability for health providers (Ad Hoc Committee, 1999; French & Larrabee, 1999). Patient education cannot be considered to have taken place if the patient has not gained enough knowledge and skills necessary for self-care (Fisher, 1999; Winslow, 2001).

Initial standards for health education put forth by the Joint Commission for Accreditation of Healthcare Organizations (JCAHO) require that "the patient and/or, when appropriate, his/her significant other(s) are provided with education that can enhance their knowledge, skills, and those behaviors necessary to fully benefit from the health care interventions provided by the organization" (JCAHO, 1993, p. 1030). In 1996, JCAHO identified additional standards specifying that patient education must be provided by an interdisciplinary healthcare team, with special consideration being given to the client's literacy level, educational level, and language. All clients must have an assessment of their readiness to learn and an identification of any obstacles to learning. Furthermore, education must be "understandable" and culturally appropriate to the patient and/or significant others. Therefore, PEMs must be written in ways that assist patients to undertake self-care regimens such as medications, diet, exercise therapies, and use of medical equipment (Bernier, 1993; Davidhizar & Brownson, 1999; Fisher, 1999).

In addition, the federally mandated Patient's Bill of Rights has established the right of patients to receive complete and current information regarding their diagnoses, treatments, and prognoses in terms they can understand (Duffy & Snyder, 1999). Therefore, the reading levels of PEMs must match the patients' reading abilities.

Given the trends in health care today, such as early discharge and increased complexity of treatments, patient education has assumed an even more vital role in assisting patients to independently manage their own healthcare needs. Because there is not always sufficient opportunities for patients in various healthcare settings to receive the necessary education they need for self-management after discharge, nurses are relying to a greater extent than ever before on PEMs to supplement their teaching (Owen, Porter, Frost, O'Hare, & Johnson, 1993; Stephens, 1992; Zimm, 1998). The burden has fallen on nurses to safeguard the lives of their clients by becoming better, more effective communicators of written health information (Osborne, 1999).

Only recently, however, have written health education materials been examined from the perspective of patients' literacy skills. As a result, some basic questions must be asked:

- Do patients read the education literature provided them?
- Are they capable of reading it?
- Can they comprehend what they read?
- Are written materials appropriately used to provide information needed by patients?

The potential for inadequate information or misinterpretation of instructions can adversely affect treatment. Also, serious concerns arise about professional liability when information is written at a level beyond the reading level and comprehension of many patients (French & Larrabee, 1999). Thus, properly informing the consumer is both a legal and an ethical concern in health care today.

READABILITY OF PRINTED EDUCATION MATERIALS

A substantial body of evidence indicates that there is a significant gap between patients' reading and comprehension levels and the level of reading difficulty of PEMs (Winslow, 2001). Nurses are beginning to recognize that the written materials relied on by so many of them to convey health information to consumers are essentially useless to the illiterate patient (Morgan, 1993). For example, look at the lines below:

Laeyo aoiou dxpo quto a uoixyo mnstr. Mnstr laeyo dxpo guto tzny auoibxgo.

Do they make sense, or are you confused? If they appear unreadable, that is exactly what written instructions look like to someone who cannot read (Loughrey, 1983).

A number of researchers have assessed specific population groups in a variety of healthcare settings based on the ability of patients to meet the literacy demands of written materials related to their care. Their findings revealed:

- Emergency department instructional materials (which average tenth-grade readability) are written at a level of difficulty that cannot be understood by most patients (Duffy & Snyder, 1999; Jolly et al., 1993; Lerner, Jehle, Janicke, & Moscati, 2000; Williams et al., 1996).
- Government documents essential to helping people gain access to health-related services offered through local, state, and federal government programs, such as Medicare and Medicaid, are written well beyond the reading ability of the majority of patients (Glanz & Rudd, 1990; Holt, Hollon, Hughes, & Coyle, 1990; Owen, Porter et al., 1993; Swanson et al., 1990; Williams-Deane & Potter, 1992; Winslow, 2001).
- The readability demand of PEMs used in ambulatory care settings do not match the average patient reading comprehension levels (Davis et al., 1990; Lerner et al., 2000).
- Standard institutional consent forms require college-level reading comprehension (Davis et al., 1990; Doak et al., 1998).
- An analysis of more than 2,000 healthcare publications used in hospitals, clinics, and private doctors' offices are written in medical school language, which is at a level that cannot be comprehended by the average reader (Doak et al., 1996; Jenks, 1992).
- More than half of the American Cancer Society PEMs commonly used to deliver messages about cancer detection methods, lifestyle risks, and treatment recommendations are written at the twelfth-grade level or higher (Brownson, 1998; Doak et al., 1998; Meade, Dieckmann, & Thornhill, 1992).

Thus, PEMs are written at grade levels that far exceed the reading ability of the majority of patients. Most patient education literature is written above the eighth-grade level, with the average level falling between the tenth and twelfth grades. Many PEMs exceed this upper range, even though the average reading level of adults is at the eighth-grade level and millions of people in our population read at considerably lower levels (Brownson, 1998; Doak et al., 1998). Furthermore, people typically read at least two to four grade levels below their highest level of schooling and prefer materials that are written below their school level. In fact, contrary to popular belief, good readers also prefer simplified PEMs when ill and even when well due to the demands of their busy schedules (Lasater & Mehler, 1998; Winslow, 2001).

The conclusion to be drawn is that complex and lengthy PEMs serve no useful teaching purpose if patients are unable to understand them or unwilling to read them. If the readability of education materials matches the patients' literacy levels, consumers may be better able to understand and comply with treatment regimens, thereby reducing the number of readmissions and improving quality of life (Ad Hoc Committee, 1999).

The Internet is an excellent resource for nurses to locate easy-to-read PEMs. The Web site http://www.oshu.edu/bicc-Library/patiented/links.shtml is a helpful place to locate low-literacy education materials. The Food and Drug Administration also has a Web site at http://www.fda.gov/opacom/lowlit/7lowlit.html for publications with low reading-grade levels (Duffy & Snyder, 1999).

MEASUREMENT TOOLS TO TEST THE READABILITY OF WRITTEN MATERIALS

Because nurses rely heavily on PEMs to convey necessary information to their clients, the appropriateness of these materials in terms of readability must be determined. Today, more than 40 formulas are available to measure the readability levels of PEMs.

Readability formulas are mathematical equations that measure the correlation between an author's style of writing and a reader's skill at decoding words as printed symbols (Doak et al., 1996). Most of them predict a grade level of reading difficulty of material based on an analysis of sentence structure and the length of words. The following guidelines are important to remember:

- Readability formulas should not be the only tool used for assessing the difficulty level of PEMs.
- Readability formulas should be selected that have been validated on the reader population for whom the PEM is intended. Several formulas are geared to specific types of materials or population groups.

- At least two formulas should be applied to any given piece of written material and the results should be averaged to yield an overall reading grade level score (Ley & Florio, 1996).

Because so many readability formulas are available for assessment of reading levels of PEMs, only those that are relatively simple to work with, are accepted as reliable and valid, and are in widespread use have been chosen for review here.

Flesch Formula

This formula was developed to measure readability of materials between grade five and college level. It has been used for more than 50 years to assess news reports, adult education materials, and government publications. The Flesch formula is based on a count of two basic language elements: average sentence length in words and average word length measured as syllables per word in selected samples. The reading ease (RE) score is calculated by combining these two variables (Flesch, 1948; Spadero, 1983; Spadero, Robinson, & Smith, 1980). See Appendix A for the method of formula analysis.

Fog Index

This formula is appropriate for determining readability of materials from fourth grade to college level. It is calculated based on average sentence length and the percentage of multisyllabic words in a 100-word passage. The Fog index is considered one of the easier methods because it is based on a short sample of words (100), it does not require counting syllables of all words, and the rules are simple (Gunning, 1968; Spadero, 1983; Spadero et al., 1980). See Appendix A for the method of formula analysis.

Fry Readability Graph-Extended

The Fry formula tests materials at the level of grade one through college. A few simple rules can be applied to estimate the readability of a wide range of reading materials, especially books, pamphlets, and brochures. This formula plots two language elements—the number of syllables and the number of sentences in three 100-word selections (Fry, 1968, 1977; Spadero et al., 1980). See Appendix A for directions on how to use the Fry Readability Graph.

SMOG Formula

This formula has been used extensively to judge grade-level readability of patient education materials. It is the most popular measurement tool because of its reputation for reading-level accuracy, its simple directions, and its speed of use (Meade & Smith, 1991). Also, it can measure the reading grade level of materials that contain as few as 10 sentences. The SMOG formula measures readability of PEMs from grade four to college level based on the number of multisyllabic (or polysyllabic) words (three or more syllables) within a set number of sentences to define the grade level of the material (McLaughlin, 1969). The SMOG formula is recommended because it is one of the most valid tests of readability (Doak et al., 1996). Whereas other methods base the calculation of grade level on 50% to 75% comprehension, the SMOG method is based on 100% comprehension of material read. That is, if the SMOG formula tests reading material at grade seven, it means all readers able to read at a seventh-grade level should fully comprehend the material. Thus, when using the SMOG formula to calculate the grade level of material, it is important to remember that the SMOG results are usually about two grades higher than the grade levels calculated by the other methods (Spadero, 1983). See Appendix A for the method of formula analysis and for an example of how to apply the SMOG formula to a short passage.

It is critically important to determine the readability of all written materials at the time they are developed or adopted by using one or more of the many available formulas. Doak et al. (1996) state that "you cannot afford to fly blind" by using health materials that are untested for readability difficulty. Pretesting PEMs before distribution is the way to be sure they fit the literacy level of the audience for which they are intended. The formulas chosen to measure grade-level readability of PEMs must be appropriate for the word length of materials being tested in relation to the grade level of the target reader (see Table 7-1).

Computerized Readability Software Programs

The recent availability of computerized programs has helped tremendously in calculating the grade level of printed material in a matter of seconds. Some software programs are capable of applying a number of formulas to analyze one text selection. In addition, some packages are able to identify difficult words in written passages that may not be understood by patients, but may be only one or two syllables in length. Dozens of user-friendly commercial software packages can automatically calculate reading levels as well as provide advice on how to simplify text (Doak et al., 1996;

TABLE 7-1 Appropriate Readability Formula Choice					
Formula	**Materials with Less Than 100 Words**	**Materials with 100–299 Words**	**Materials with 300 Words or More**	**Entire Piece**	**Grade Level**
Flesch formula	No	No	Yes	Yes	5 to college
Fog formula	No	Yes	Yes	Yes	4 to college
Fry graph	No	No	Yes	Yes	1 to college
SMOG formula	Yes	Yes	Yes	Yes	4 to college

Source: Adapted from Spadero (1980), p. 216.

Mailloux, Johnson, Fisher, & Pettibone, 1995). Computerized assessment of readability is fast and easy, and it provides a high degree of reliability, especially when several formulas are used. Determining readability by computer programs rather than manually is also more accurate in calculating reading levels because it eliminates human error in scoring and because entire articles, pamphlets, or books can be scanned (Duffy & Snyder, 1999). It is advisable to take an average across several pieces of literature, using several different formulas and software programs, when calculating estimates of readability (Mailloux et al., 1995).

MEASUREMENT TOOLS TO TEST COMPREHENSION

In addition to the four readability formulas described in the previous section, a number of standardized tests have proved reliable and valid to measure comprehension skills of patients, a relatively new concept in health education (Doak et al., 1996). The two most popular tools are the Cloze test and the listening test. These tests can be used to assess how much a patient understands from reading or listening to a passage of text.

Cloze Test

The Cloze test (derived from the term closure) has been specifically recommended to assess a patient's understanding of health education literature. Because it takes more time and resources to test comprehension levels than it does to test readability levels of materials, it is recommended that this test be administered to only a representative sample of clients rather than to every patient in a particular setting. However, the Cloze test can be used on individual patients who demonstrate difficulty comprehending health materials used for instruction. The Cloze test should be used only with patients whose reading skills are at sixth grade or higher. Otherwise, it is likely that the test will prove too difficult and frustrating for them to take (Doak et al., 1996).

The reader may or may not be familiar with the material being tested. This procedure is designed so that every fifth word is systematically deleted from a portion of a text. The reader is asked to fill in the blanks with the *exact* word replacements. One point is scored for every missing word guessed correctly. The Cloze score is the total number of blanks filled in correctly by the reader. To be successful, the reader must demonstrate sensitivity to clues related to grammar and vocabulary. How well the reader is able to fill in the blanks with appropriate words indicates how well the material has been comprehended (Dale & Chall, 1978; Doak et al., 1996). The underlying theory is that the more readable a passage is, the better it will be understood even when words are omitted.

A score for the Cloze test is obtained by dividing the number of exact word replacements (the raw score) by the total number of blank spaces in the passage. A score of 60% or better indicates that the passage was sufficiently understood by the patient. A score of 40% to 59% indicates a moderate level of difficulty, where additional teaching is required for the patient to understand the message. A score of less than 40% indicates the material is too difficult to be understood and is not suitable to be used for teaching (Doak et al., 1996).

Instead of using packaged Cloze tests available from commercial sources, it is suggested that educators devise their own tests from material used for patient education so that the scores obtained will indicate a patient's comprehension of these instructions. Then problem words or sentences within these PEMs can be revised accordingly to make them more understandable. See Appendix A for an outline of the steps for constructing a Cloze test, test scoring methodology, and a sample test.

Because the Cloze procedure is a test of patients' ability to understand what they have read, be sure to be honest about the purpose of the test. You might state that it is important for them to know what they are to do when on their own after discharge, so you want to be sure they understand the written instructions they will need to follow. Doak et al. (1996) found that most patients are willing to participate in the testing activity. They suggest that the following guidelines should be given to patients before taking the Cloze test:

1. Encourage them to read through the entire test passage before attempting to fill in the blanks.
2. Inform them that only one word should be written in each blank.
3. Let them know that it is all right to guess, but that they should try to fill in every blank with the word they think belongs there.

4. Reassure them that spelling errors are okay just as long as the word they have put in the blank can be recognized.

5. Let them know that this exercise is not a timed test. (If patients struggle to complete the test, tell them not to worry, that it is not necessary for them to fill in all the blanks, and set the test aside to go on to something else less frustrating or less threatening.)

Listening Test

This test also measures a reader's comprehension skills. Unlike the Cloze test, which may be too difficult for patients who read below the sixth-grade level, the listening test is a good approach to determine what a low-literate or illiterate patient understands and remembers when listening (Doak et al., 1996).

The procedure for administering the listening test is to select a passage from instructional materials that takes about 3 minutes to read aloud and is written at approximately the fifth-grade level. Formulate 8 to 10 questions relevant to the content of the passage by selecting key points of the text. Read the passage to the patient at a normal rate. Ask the listener the questions orally and record the answers. To determine the percentage score, divide the number of questions answered correctly by the total number of questions.

The instructional material will be appropriate for the patient's comprehension level if the score is approximately 75% (some additional assistance when teaching the material may be necessary for full comprehension). A score of 90% or higher indicates that the material is too easy for the patient and can be fully comprehended independently. A score of less than 75% means that the material is too difficult and simpler instructional material will need to be used when teaching the patient. Doak et al. (1996) provide examples of a sample passage and questions for a listening comprehension test.

MEASUREMENT TOOLS TO TEST READING SKILLS _____

The two most popular standardized methods to measure reading skill are the WRAT and the REALM tests. The TOFHLA is a newer test for the same purpose.

WRAT (Wide Range Achievement Test)

The WRAT is a word recognition screening test that takes about 5 minutes to administer. It is used to assess a patient's ability to recognize and pronounce a list of words out of context as a criterion for measuring reading skills. Although it does not test other aspects of reading, such as vocabulary and comprehension of text material, this test is nevertheless useful for determining a patient's level of literacy. As designed, it should be used to test only people whose native language is English.

The WRAT tests on two levels: Level I is designed for children 5 to 12 years of age, and Level II is intended for testing persons older than age 12. The WRAT consists of 100 words, listed from the most simple to the most complex. The individual administering the test listens carefully to the patient's responses. Next to those words that are mispronounced, a checkmark should be placed. When three consecutive words are missed, indicating that the patient has reached his or her limit, the test is stopped. To score the test, the number of words pronounced incorrectly or not tried is subtracted from the list of words on the master score sheet to get a raw score. Then a table of raw scores is used to find the equivalent grade rating (GR). For more information on this test, see Doak et al. (1996) and Quirk (2000).

REALM (Rapid Estimate of Adult Literacy in Medicine)

The REALM test is another reading skills measure that has advantages over the WRAT and other word tests because it measures a patient's ability to read medical and health-related vocabulary, it takes less time to administer, and the scoring is simpler (Duffy & Snyder, 1999; Foltz & Sullivan, 1998). Although it has established validity, this test offers less precision than other word tests (Hayes, 2000). The raw score is converted to a range of grade levels rather than an exact grade level, but this result correlates well with the WRAT reading scores.

Sixty-six medical and health-related words are arranged in three columns, beginning with short, easy words such as *fat*, *flu*, *pill*, and *dose*, and ending with more difficult words such as *anemia*, *obesity*, *osteoporosis*, and *impetigo*. Patients are asked to begin at the top of the first column and read down, pronouncing all the words that they can from the three lists. The total number of words pronounced correctly is their raw score, which is converted to a grade ranging from third grade and below to ninth grade and higher. For the REALM test and scoring guide, see Doak et al. (1996).

TOFHLA (Test of Functional Health Literacy in Adults)

This test is a relatively new instrument for measuring patients' literacy skills using actual hospital materials, such as prescription labels, appointment slips, and informed consent documents. The test consists of two parts: reading comprehension and numeracy. It has demonstrated reliability and validity, requires approximately 20 minutes to administer, and is available in a Spanish version (TOFHLA-S) as well as English (Parker, Baker, Williams, & Nurss, 1995; Quirk, 2000; Williams et al., 1995).

INSTRUMENT FOR SUITABILITY
ASSESSMENT OF MATERIALS (SAM)

In addition to using formulas to determine readability and tests to measure comprehension and reading skills, Doak et al. (1996) have designed the SAM instrument to assess the suitability of instructional materials for a given population of patients. Not only can the SAM be used with print material and illustrations, but also it has been designed to be applied to video- and audiotaped instructions. SAM yields a numerical (percent) score, with materials tested falling into one of three categories: superior, adequate, or not suitable. The SAM can assess specific factors, such as content, literacy demand, graphics, layout, and cultural characteristics to determine the appropriateness of instructional materials being developed or already in use. For directions, a score sheet, and a description of the evaluation criteria, see Doak et al. (1996).

SIMPLIFYING THE READABILITY
OF PRINTED EDUCATION MATERIALS

Even though printed materials are the most commonly used form of media, as currently written, they remain the least effective means for reaching a large proportion of the adult population who have marginal literacy skills. Despite the well-documented potential of written materials to increase knowledge, compliance, and satisfaction with care, printed education materials are often too difficult for even motivated patients to read (Glanz & Rudd, 1990). What the nurse in the role of teacher must strive to achieve when designing or selecting PEMs is a good and proper fit between the material and the reader.

Certainly the best solution for improving the overall comprehension and reading skills of patients would be to strengthen their basic general education, but this process will require decades to accomplish (Jackson et al., 1991). Since most available health education materials are written at high readability levels, often requiring college-level reading skills to fully comprehend, they need to be simplified (Winslow, 2001). What is needed now are ways in which to write or rewrite educational materials that match the current comprehension and reading skills of patients.

Nathaniel Hawthorne was once reported to have said, "Easy reading is damned hard writing" (Pichert & Elam, 1985). He was correct that clear and concise writing is a task that takes effort and practice. It is possible, though, to reduce the literacy demand of written instructional materials to equal the actual reading level of patients. This requires attention to some basic linguistic, motivational, organizational, and content principles. *Linguistics* refers to the type of language and grammatical style used. *Motivation principles* focus on those elements that stimulate the reader, such as appeal of the material. *Organizational factors* deal with layout and clarity. *Content principles* relate to amount and concept density of information (Bernier, 1993). These elements must be examined when designing or revising instructional materials for the marginally literate reader.

Prior to writing or rewriting a text for easier reading, however, some preliminary planning steps need to be taken to ensure that the final written material will be geared to the target audience (Doak et al., 1996):

1. Decide what the patient should do or know. In other words, what is the purpose of the instruction? What outcomes do you hope the patient will achieve?
2. Choose information that is needed by the patient to accomplish the behavioral objectives. Limit or cut out altogether extraneous and "nice to know" information such as the history or detailed physiological processes of a disease. Include only survival skills and essential main ideas of who, what, where, and when that builds on information the reader already knows. **Remember: A person does not have to know how an engine works to drive a car.**
3. Select other media to supplement the written information, such as pictures, models, audiotapes, and videotapes. Even poor readers will benefit from written material if it is combined with other forms of delivering a message. Consider the field of advertising, for example. Advertisers get their message across with words but often in combination with strong, action-packed visuals.
4. Organize topics into chunks that follow a logical sequence. Put the most important information first. If topics are of equal importance, start with the more general as a basis on which to build to the more specific. Begin with a statement of purpose. Place key facts at the beginning and the end, because readers best remember information presented first and last.
5. Determine what the reading grade level of the material should be. If readers have been tested, preferably write two to four grades below their reading grade–level score. If the audience has not been tested, a group of patients is likely to display a wide range of reading skills. When in doubt, write instructional materials at the fifth- or sixth-grade level (Estey, Musseau, & Keehn, 1991), keeping in mind that the average reading level of the population is approximately eighth grade. It is also possible to develop two sets of instruc-

---

TABLE 7-2   Example of Lowered Readability Level

NINTH-GRADE LEVEL

Smoking contributes to heart disease in the following ways:

1. When you smoke, you inhale carbon monoxide and nicotine, which causes your blood vessels to narrow, your heart rate to increase, and your blood pressure to go up. All of these factors increase the workload for your heart.

2. Carbon monoxide stimulates your body to produce more red blood cells. The presence of more red cells means that your blood will clot more readily, leading to increased risk of coronary artery disease and stroke.

3. Carbon monoxide and nicotine may also increase your risk of atherosclerotic buildup by causing damage to your artery walls.

4. Smoking raises blood cholesterol level and has been known to cause irregular heartbeats.

FOURTH-GRADE LEVEL

Smoking hurts your heart in many ways:

1. Smoking makes your heart beat faster, raises your blood pressure, and makes your blood vessels smaller. All these things cause your heart to work harder.

2. Smoking makes your blood clot easier. This increases your chance of having a heart attack or a stroke.

3. Smoking makes your cholesterol level go up. It may also damage your blood vessels.

4. Smoking may make your heartbeat less regular.

Source: From Martha Wong, "Self-Care Instructions: Do Patients Understand Educational Materials?" Reprinted with permission of American Association of Critical-Care Nurses from *Focus on Critical Care, 19*(1), February 1992.

---

tions—one at a higher grade level and one at a lower grade level—to meet the needs of patients with a wide range of reading skills. See Table 7-2 for an example of the same information written at different levels of difficulty.

6. Once the reading grade level of a piece of written material is determined, it should be printed on the back of the document in coded form for easy reference. For example, the reading level (RL) of a PEM at the 7th grade would be RL7 or RL = 7.

A number of recommendations have been put forth for developing written instructions that can be more easily understood by a wide audience (Bernier, 1993; Brooks,

1998; Brownson, 1998; Buxton, 1999; Doak & Doak, 1987; Doak et al., 1996, 1998; Duffy & Snyder, 1999; Wong, 1992). The key to simplifying written health information for patients with low literacy skills is to write in plain, familiar language using an easy visual format. The following general guidelines include the basic linguistic, motivational, organizational, and content principles for writing effective PEMs:

1. Write in a conversational style using the personal pronoun *you* and the possessive pronoun *your*. Write in an active voice, which uses the present tense, rather than a passive voice, which uses the past or future tense. A message delivered in an active voice is more personalized, more direct, and easier to understand; for example, write "Take your medicine . . ." instead of "Medicine should be taken. . . ." This rule is considered to be one of the most important techniques to reduce the level of reading difficulty and to improve comprehension of what is read. Speaking personally to the reader engages their attention to the message being conveyed. For example:

    LESS EFFECTIVE

    People who sunburn easily and have fair skin with red or blond hair are most prone to develop skin cancer. The amount of time spent in the sun affects a person's risk of skin cancer.[1]

    MORE EFFECTIVE

    If you sunburn easily and have fair skin with red or blond hair, you are more likely to get skin cancer. How much time you spend in the sun affects your risk of skin cancer.

2. Use short words with only one or two syllables as much as possible. Rely on common words recognized by almost everyone. The key is to choose words that sound familiar and natural and are easy to read and understand, like *shot* rather than *injection* and *use* instead of *utilize*. Avoid compound words, such as *stomachache*, and words with prefixes or suffixes, such as *reoccur* or *emptying*, that create multisyllable words. Also, try to avoid technical words and medical terms by substituting lay terms such as *stroke* instead of *cerebrovascular accident*. Select substitutions carefully, because they may have a different meaning for some people than for others. For example, if the word *medicine* is replaced with the

---

[1]*Fry Now, Pay Later*. American Cancer Society pamphlet, No. 2611, 1985.

word *drug*, the substitute word may be interpreted as the illegal variety. Using simple, everyday language is not considered "talking down" to patients; it is considered "talking to" them at a more comfortable level.

3. Spell words out rather than using abbreviations or acronyms. *That is* should be used instead of *i.e.* and *for example* instead of *e.g.* Abbreviations for the months of the year (*Sept.* for *September*) or the days of the week (*Wed.* for *Wednesday*) are a real problem for patients with limited vocabulary. Also, avoid acronyms, such as *CVA* or *NPO*, unless these medical terms are clearly defined the first time they are used in the text.

4. Organize information into "chunks," which improves recall. Use numbers only when absolutely necessary. Statistics are usually meaningless and are another source of confusion for the low-literate reader. Limit the number of items in any list to no more than seven. Beyond that number, people have a difficult time remembering them (Baddeley, 1994). Also, a question-and-answer format using the patient's point of view is an effective way to summarize information in single units using a conversational style. The following example is adapted from the American Cancer Society pamphlet entitled *Fry Now, Pay Later* (1985):

Q: Am I likely to get skin cancer?

A: If you have spent a lot of time in the sun, if you sunburn easily, and if you have fair skin with red or blond hair, you have a greater chance of getting skin cancer than people with dark skin or people who have stayed out of the strong sunlight.

Q: How can I tell if I have skin cancer?

A: The only way to know for certain if you have a skin cancer is to see your doctor. Your doctor may want to take a sample of skin to test for cancer if you have a problem such as red, scaly patches, a mole that has changed, or an area of the skin that does not heal.

Q: How can I prevent skin cancer?

A: Stay out of direct sunlight between 11 a.m. and 2 p.m. When in the sun, cover up with clothing, wear a wide-brimmed hat, and use sunscreens that block out the sun's harmful rays.

5. Keep sentences short, limiting them to 20 words or less if possible, because they are easier to read and understand for readers with short-term memories. Avoid using commas, colons, or dashes that make for long, complex sentences, which "turn off" the reader. Titles also should be brief (no more than 10 words) and convey the purpose and meaning of the material that follows.

6. Clearly define any technical or unfamiliar words by using parentheses to explain the meaning—for example, bacteria (germ). A glossary of terms is a helpful tool, but defining the terms and spelling out difficult words phonetically (by how they sound) immediately following the unfamiliar word within the text is most recommended, for example, "Alzheimer's (pronounced Altz-hi-merz)." New vocabulary words should be taught in small amounts and reviewed frequently (Byrne & Edeani, 1984; Spees, 1991). The meaning of some words that the patient will see or hear often, such as *hypertension* or *diabetes*, can be simplified to *high blood pressure* or *high blood sugar*. Or, any technical terms used should be taught to the reader prior to introducing the instructional material to increase comprehension (Standal, 1981).

7. Use words consistently throughout the text. Avoid interchanging of words such as *diet* with *meal plan*, *menu*, *food schedule*, and *dietary prescription*, which merely confuses the reader and can lead to misunderstanding of instruction. Repetition is good and the same words should be used over and over again as necessary. This technique may seem monotonous to you, but repeating the exact same words for poor readers increases their comprehension.

8. Avoid value judgment words such as *excessive* and *regularly*. How much pain or bleeding is excessive? How often is regularly? Use exact terms to describe what you mean by using, for example, a scale of 1–5 or explaining frequency in terms of minutes, hours, or days.

9. Put the most important information first by prioritizing the "need to know." Avoid including "nice to know" information, which just overwhelms the reader.

10. Use advance organizers (topic headings or headers) and subheadings. They clue the reader in to what is going to be presented and help focus the reader's attention on the message.

11. Limit the use of connective words, such as *however*, *consequently*, *even though*, and *in spite of*, that lengthen sentences and make them more complex.

12. Make the first sentence of a paragraph the topic sentence, and, if possible, make the first word the topic of the sentence. For example:

LESS EFFECTIVE

Even though overexposure to the sun is the leading cause, it isn't necessary to give up the outdoors in order to reduce your chances of developing skin cancer.[1]

MORE EFFECTIVE

Enjoying the outdoors is still possible if you take steps to reduce your risk of skin cancer when in the sun.

or

Your chance of skin cancer can be reduced even when enjoying the outdoors.

13. Reduce concept density by limiting each paragraph to a simple message or action and include only one idea per sentence. In the following example, the first paragraph contains at least six concepts. As rewritten, the second paragraph has been reduced to four concepts (and is written using the second person pronoun, which is a much more personalized approach):

> A person who has had a stroke may or may not be able to return to his or her former level of functioning, depending on the extent and location of brain damage. Mental attitude, efforts of the rehabilitation team, and the understanding of family and friends also affect the patient's progress. Recovery must be gradual, but it should begin the moment the patient is hospitalized. After the patient is tested to determine the extent of brain damage, rehabilitation such as physical, speech, and occupational therapy should begin. Family and friends should be told how to handle special problems the stroke victim may have, such as irrational behavior or difficulty communicating.[2]

> Returning to your normal life after a stroke is an important part of your recovery. Each stroke patient is different and your progress depends on where and how much the brain is damaged. Your rehabilitation must be gradual and therapy will begin to meet your needs while you are in the hospital. Your mental attitude, the treatment you are given, and the caring of your family and friends will help you handle special problems.

14. Keep density of words low by not exceeding 30–40 characters (letters) per line.
15. Allow for plenty of white (blank) space in margins, and use generous spacing between paragraphs and double spacing between sentences to reduce density of words. Less crowded pages are not as overwhelming to the reader with low literacy skills.
16. Keep right margins unjustified (jagged) to help distinguish one line from another. In this way, the eye does not have to adjust to different spacing between letters and words as it does when justified margins are used.

---

[2] Adapted from American Heart Association. (1983). *An Older Person's Guide to Cardiovascular Health*, National Center, 7320 Greenville Avenue, Dallas, TX 75321. The information from this booklet is not current and is used for illustrative purposes only.

17. Design layouts that encourage eye movement from left to right, as in normal reading. In simple drawings and diagrams, using arrows, numbers, or circles help give direction to the reader.

18. Select a simple type style (serif) and a large font (12 as minimum and 14–16 print size is preferable) in the body of the text for ease of reading and to increase motivation to read. A sans serif font (without little hooks at the top and bottom of letters) should be used only for titles to give style to the handout. Avoid *italics*, *fancy lettering*, or all CAPITAL letters. Low-literate readers are not fluent with the alphabet and need to look at each letter to recognize a word. To help poor readers decode words in titles, headings, and subheadings, use upper- and lowercase letters, which provide reading cues given by tall and short letters on the type line. Avoid using a large stylized letter, as shown below, to begin a new paragraph.

> T his looks attractive, but it is confusing to a poor reader who cannot decode the meaning of the word minus the first letter.

19. Highlight important ideas or terms with bold type or underlining.

20. If using color, apply it consistently throughout the text to emphasize key points or to organize topics. Color, if used appropriately, attracts the reader. Bright, bold colors are more eye-catching and easier to read than light, pastel colors.

21. Create a simple cover page with a title that clearly and briefly states the topic to be addressed.

22. Limit the entire length of a document—the shorter, the better. It should be long enough just to cover the essential information. Too many pages will "turn off" even the most eager and capable reader.

23. Select paper that is attractive and on which the typeface is easy to read. Black print on white paper is most easily read and most economical. Dull finishes reduce the glare of light, while high-gloss paper reflects light into the eyes of the reader. Appearance must match the informal tone of your message.

24. Use bold line drawings and simple, realistic diagrams. Basic visuals aid the reader to better understand the text information. Cartoon characters can be used, but be careful that they don't make the message appear childlike. Graphic designs that are for decoration purposes only should never be used because they are distracting and confusing. Also, never overlay words on a background design because it makes reading the letters of the words very difficult. Only illustrations that help to increase understanding of the text and that relate specifically to the message should be used.

Be careful to use pictures that convey positive rather than negative messages. For example, avoid using a picture of a pregnant woman smoking or drinking alcohol because this negative message is dependent on careful reading of the text to understand the meaning. The visuals should clearly show only those actions that you want the reader to do and remember.

Use simple subtitles and captions for each picture. Be careful that visuals do not communicate cultural bias. Also, be sure drawings can be easily recognized by the reader. For instance, if you draw a picture of the lungs, be certain they are within the outline of the person's body to accurately depict the location of the organ. The low-literate person may not know what they are looking at if the lungs are not put in context with the body's torso.

25. Include a summary paragraph to review in a different form what has already been presented. Ask for feedback after patients have read your instructions. Either have patients explain the information in their own words or have them demonstrate the desired behavior. If patients can do so correctly, it is a good indication that the information is understood. Do not ask questions such as "Do you understand?" because you are likely to get only a "yes" or "no" answer, not a more complete response.

26. Put the reading level (RL) on the back of a written or revised PEM for future reference—for example, "Skin Cancer" (RL = 6).

27. Determine readability by applying at least two formulas. Also, comprehension and reading skills can be measured by the standardized tests. These formulas and tests have been described previously in the Measurement Tools sections and in Appendix A.

It does not take a great deal of effort to improve the readability and comprehension level of instructional materials, just know-how and common sense (see Table 7-3 for a summary of guidelines). The benefits are significant in terms of compliance and quality of care when marginally literate patients are given PEMs that effectively communicate messages they can read and understand.

Always remember to pilot-test any new materials before printing and distributing them. Not only will this effort save the cost of printing handouts that might not be useful, but also patients will have the opportunity to participate in the evaluation process (Brownson, 1998). As Doak and Doak (1987) so aptly summarize, "With so much to be gained, the investments of a little time and thoughtful attention to the materials provided to patients can pay back dividends too important to ignore" (p. 8).

TABLE 7-3   Summary of Guidelines for Designing Effective Low-Literacy Printed Materials

CONTENT

Clearly define the purpose of the material.

Decide when and how the information will be used.

Use behavioral objectives that cover the main points.

Check the accuracy of content with experts.

Give "how to" information for the learner to achieve objectives.

Present only the most essential information (three to four main ideas: who, what, where, and when).

Relate new information to what the audience already knows.

Present content relevant to the audience and avoid cultural bias in writing and in graphics.

ORGANIZATION

Keep titles short, yet use words that clearly convey the meaning of the content.

Provide a table of contents for lengthy material and a summary to review content presented.

Present the most important information first.

Use topic headings (advance organizers).

Make the first sentence of each paragraph the topic sentence.

Include only a few concepts per paragraph.

Use short, simple sentences that convey only one idea at a time; limit the length of the entire text.

Limit lists to no more than seven items.

Present each idea in logical sequence.

LAYOUT/GRAPHICS

Select large, easily read print (minimum 12-point type) and use nonglossy paper.

Write headings and subheadings in both lower- and uppercase letters; avoid fancy lettering.

Use bold type or underlining to emphasize important information.

Use lots of white space between segments of information.

Use generous margins and keep right-hand margins unjustified.

Provide a question-and-answer format for patient–nurse interaction.

Select double spacing (between lines of type), simple type style (serif), and large font (print size)
   for ease of reading.

Design a colorful, eye-catching cover that suggests the message contained in the text.

LINGUISTICS

Keep sentences short (20 words or less).

Write in the active voice, using the present tense and the pronouns *you* and *your* to engage
   the reader.

Use one- to two-syllable words as much as possible; avoid multi-syllabic (polysyllabic) words.

Use words familiar and understandable to the target audience.

Avoid complex grammatical structures (i.e., use few commas, colons, and semicolons).

Limit the number of concepts.

Focus content on what the audience should do as well as know.

TABLE 7-3	Summary of Guidelines for Designing Effective Low-Literacy Printed Materials (*continued*)

LINGUISTICS

Use positive statements; avoid negative messages.

Use questions throughout the text to encourage active learning.

Provide examples the audience can use to relate to personal experiences/circumstances.

Avoid using double negatives and value judgment words.

Clearly define terms likely to be unclear to audience.

VISUALS

Include simple, culturally sensitive illustrations and pictures.

Use simple drawings, but only if they improve the understanding of essential information.

Choose illustrations and photographs free of clutter and distractions.

Convey a single message or point of information in each visual.

Use visuals that are relevant to the text and meaningful to the audience.

Use drawings recognizable to the audience that reflect familiar images.

Use adult rather than childlike images (use cartoons sparingly).

Use captions to describe illustrations.

Use cues such as arrows, underlines, circles, and color to give direction to ideas and to highlight the most important information.

Use appealing and appropriate colors for the audience (for older adults, use black and white, and avoid pastel shades, especially blue, green, and violet hues).

READABILITY AND COMPREHENSION

Perform analysis with formulas and tests to determine the level of readability and comprehension of the material.

Write materials two to four grade levels below the estimated literacy level of the audience.

Pilot-test the material to determine readability, comprehension, and appeal before its widespread use.

Source: Adapted from Bernier (1993), p. 42, and from papers from the 16th Annual Conference on Patient Education, Nov. 17–20, 1994, Orlando, FL—sponsored by American Academy of Family Physicians and Society of Teachers of Family Medicine.

TEACHING STRATEGIES FOR LOW-LITERATE PATIENTS

Working with marginally literate patients requires more than designing simple-to-read instructional materials. It also calls for using alternative and innovative teaching strategies to break down the barriers of illiteracy (Mayeaux et al., 1996). Teaching clients with poor reading skills does not have to be viewed as a problem, but rather can be seen as a challenge (Dunn, Buckwalter, Weinstein, & Palti, 1985). By the way, highly literate patients also can benefit from some of these same teaching strategies. Many authors (Austin et al., 1995; Brez & Taylor, 1997; Byrne & Edeani, 1984; Doak et al., 1998; Dunn et al., 1985; Fain, 1994; Hussey, 1991; Lerner et al., 2000; Mayeaux et al., 1996; Meade & Thornhill, 1989; Murphy & Davis, 1997; Spees, 1991; Walker, 1987; Wallerstein, 1992; Winslow, 2001) suggest the following tips as useful strategies to meet the logic, language, and experience of the patient who has difficulty with reading and comprehension:

1. **Establish a trusting relationship before beginning the teaching-learning process.** Start by getting to know the patients and helping to reduce their anxiety. Because many poor readers have a history of being defensive, the nurse educator must attempt to overcome their defense mechanisms. Cast aside myths and stereotypes about illiteracy. Focus on the patients' strengths, be open and honest about what specifically needs to be learned, and build up their confidence in their ability to perform self-care activities. Show patience and provide guidance and support to encourage learning.

2. **Use the smallest amount of information possible to accomplish the behavioral objectives.** Stick to the essentials by focusing on the "need to know" rather than the "nice to know" information. Prioritize information by selecting only one or two concepts to discuss in any one session. Explain what you are going to teach before giving any new information. Because patients with poor reading and comprehension skills are easily overwhelmed, keep teaching sessions short, limiting them to no more than 20 to 30 minutes.

3. **Make points of information as vivid and explicit as possible.** Explain information in simple terms, using everyday language and personal examples relevant to the patient's background. For example, a sign reading "NOTHING BY MOUTH" or, worse yet, "NPO" should be changed to "Do Not Eat or Drink Anything" (remember to avoid using all-capital letters and abbreviations). Visual aids, such as signs and pictures, should be large with readable print. Each visual should contain only one message. Underlining, highlighting, color coding, and arrows help give direction to the reader and draw attention to important information.

4. **Teach one step at a time.** Teaching information in small amounts and organizing information into chunks help to reduce anxiety, frustration, and confusion. Pace instruction to allow enough time for patients to understand each item and to ask questions before moving on to the next unit of information. Reward them with words of encouragement and praise, and reinforce information every step of the way.

5. **Use multiple teaching methods and tools requiring few literacy skills.** Oral instruction, which contains cues such as tone, gestures, and expressions, should be used first. Next, follow up by using visual resources such as simple lists, pictures, audiotapes, and videotapes to improve comprehension and reduce learning time. These media forms can also be sent home to reinforce health messages.

6. **Allow patients the chance to restate information in their own words and to demonstrate any procedures being taught.** Encouraging patients to explain something in their own words can reveal gaps in knowledge or misconceptions of information. Return demonstration and question and answer sessions provide you with feedback as to the patient's level of functioning. Remember, do not ask questions that will elicit only a "yes" or "no" response, because patients will likely respond that they understand, even when they have no clue as to what you are talking about. Patients are unlikely to ask questions of you for fear they will appear ignorant. Asking open-ended questions, such as "Tell me what you understand about . . . ," provides feedback from patients to verify their comprehension. Encouraging patients to repeat instructions in their own words or physically demonstrate an activity is an effective approach to determine what the patient really understands.

7. **Keep motivation high.** Illiterate and low-literate persons may feel like failures when they cannot work through a problem. Reassure patients that it is normal to have trouble with new information, that they are doing well, and encourage them to keep trying. Recognize any progress made, even if it is small, to maintain a patient's interest and willingness to learn. Rewards—not punishments—are excellent motivators.

8. **Coordinate procedures to fit into everyday routines.** A way to facilitate learning is to simplify information by using the principles of tailoring and cuing. *Tailoring* refers to coordinating patients' regimens into their daily schedules rather than forcing them to adjust their lifestyles to regimens imposed on them. Tailoring allows new tasks to be associated with old behaviors. It personalizes the message so that instruction is individualized to meet the patient's learning needs. For example, setting up a medication schedule to coincide with patients' meal times does not drastically alter everyday lifestyles and tends to increase motivation and compliance. *Cuing* focuses on using prompts and reminders to get a person to perform a routine task. For example, placing medications where they best can be seen on a frequent basis or keeping a simple chart to check off each time a pill is taken serves as a reminder to comply with treatments as prescribed.

9. **Use repetition to reinforce information.** Repetition, at appropriate intervals, is a key strategy to use with low-literate clients. Review information often, and set aside time to remind learners of what has already been learned and to prepare them for what is to follow. Repetition, in the form of saying the same thing in different ways, is one of the most powerful tools to increase understanding.

All of these teaching strategies are especially well suited to the individual needs of patients with low literacy skills. Creating an open, trusting, and accepting environment that makes it acceptable for the client to say "I don't understand" is the cornerstone of effective communication (Cole, 2000). It is always a challenge to teach patients who, because of illness or a threat to their well-being, may be anxious, frightened, depressed, in denial, or in pain. Patient teaching is even more of a special challenge when illiteracy or low literacy interferes with the ability of a significant portion of the adult population to understand information vital to their health and welfare.

SUMMARY

The prevalence of functional illiteracy and low literacy is a major problem in the adult population of this country. Nurses, in the role of teachers and interpreters of health information, must always be alert to the potentially limited capacity of patients to grasp the meaning of written and oral instruction. Nurses need to know how to identify patients with literacy problems, assess their needs, and choose appropriate teaching strategies that help patients with poor reading and comprehension skills to better and more safely care for themselves. An awareness of the effects that literacy levels have on motivation and compliance is key to understanding the barriers to communication between nurses and patients.

The first half of this chapter focused on the definition of literacy terms, the scope and incidence of the literacy problem, the populations at risk, the myths and stereotypes associated with poor literacy skills, and the assessment of literacy levels. In addition, the impact of illiteracy on motivation and compliance and ethical and legal concerns were discussed. The remainder of the chapter examined the readability of patient education materials, the measurement tools available to test the readability of PEMs as well as the comprehension and reading skills of patients, guidelines for writing effective education materials, and specific teaching strategies to be used to match the logic, language, and experience of the low-literate patient.

Written materials are an important source of health information to reinforce and complement other methods and tools of instruction. PEMs have the potential to be cost-effective and time-efficient means to communicate health messages. However, a large discrepancy has been found between the average reading skills of patients and the readability level required with written instructional aids. Unless this gap is narrowed, printed sources of information will serve no useful purpose for functionally illiterate and low-literate adult clients.

Nurses are in an ideal position to select and design PEMs and choose teaching strategies appropriate for patients with marginal literacy skills. It is the mandated responsibility of nurses to convey information in understandable terms so that patients can fully benefit from our healthcare interventions.

REVIEW QUESTIONS

1. What are the definitions of the terms *literacy, illiteracy, health literacy, low literacy,* and *functional illiteracy?*
2. Approximately how many million Americans are considered to be illiterate or functionally illiterate? This represents what percentage of the U.S. population?
3. Why are the rates of low literacy and illiteracy on the rise in the United States?
4. Why is the number of years of schooling a poor indicator of someone's literacy level?
5. What population groups in the United States are more likely to be at risk for having poor reading and comprehension skills?
6. Why is the literacy problem greater in older adults than in younger age groups?
7. What are three common myths about persons who are illiterate?
8. What are seven clues that an individual is illiterate?
9. What impact does illiteracy or low literacy have on a person's level of motivation and compliance?
10. How does reliance on printed education materials pose an ethical or legal liability for nurses?
11. Which measurement tools are used specifically to test readability, comprehension, and reading skills?
12. What are 10 general guidelines to simplify written teaching materials?
13. What five teaching strategies can be used by nurses to make health information more understandable for clients with poor reading and comprehension skills?

REFERENCES

Adams-Price, C. E. (1993). Age, education, and literacy skills of adult Mississippians. *Gerontologist,* *33*(6), 741–746.

Ad Hoc Committee on Health Literacy for the Council on Scientific Affairs, American Medical Association. (1999). Health literacy: Report of the Council on Scientific Affairs. *Journal of the American Medical Association, 281*(6), 552–557.

American Cancer Society. (1985). *Fry now, pay later.* No. 2611, Author.

Austin, P. E., Matlock, R., Dunn, K. A., Kesler, C., & Brown, C. K. (1995). Discharge instructions: Do illustrations help our patients understand them? *Annals of Emergency Medicine, 25*(3), 317–320.

Baddeley, A. (1994). The magical number seven: Still magic after all these years? *Psychological Review, 101*(2), 353–356.

Baydar, N., Brooks-Gunn, J., & Furstenberg, F. F. (1993). Early warning signs of functional illiteracy: Predictors in childhood and adolescence. *Child Development, 64*(3), 815–829.

Bernier, M. J. (1993). Developing and evaluating printed education materials: A prescriptive model for quality. *Orthopedic Nursing, 12*(6), 39–46.

Brez, S. M. & Taylor, M. (1997). Assessing literacy for patient teaching: Perspectives of adults with low literacy skills. *Journal of Advanced Nursing, 25,* 1040–1047.

Brooks, D. A. (1998). Nurse educator: Techniques for teaching ED patients with low literacy skills. *Journal of Emergency Nursing, 24*(6), 601–603.

Brownson, K. (1998). Education handouts: Are we wasting our time? *Journal for Nurses in Staff Development, 14*(4), 176–182.

Buxton, T. (1999). Effective ways to improve health education materials. *Journal of Health Education, 30*(1), 47–50, 61.

Byrne, T. & Edeani, D. (1984). Knowledge of medical terminology among hospital patients. *Nursing Research, 33*(3), 178–181.

Cole, M. R. (2000). The high risk of low literacy. *Nursing Spectrum, 13*(10), 16–17.

Dale, E. & Chall, J. S. (1978). The Cloze procedure: Measuring the readability of selected patient education materials. *Health Education, 9,* 8–10.

Davidhizar, R. E. & Brownson, K. (1999). Literacy, cultural diversity, and client education. *Health Care Manager, 18*(1), 39–47.

Davis, T. C., Crouch, M. A., Wills, G., Miller, S., & Abdehou, D. M. (1990). The gap between patient reading comprehension and the readability of patient education materials. *Journal of Family Practice, 31*(5), 533–538.

Denboba, D. L., Bragdon, J. L., Epstein, L. G., Garthright, K., & Goldman, T. M. (1998). Reducing health disparities through cultural competence. *Journal of Health Education, 29*(5), 47–51.

Doak, C. C., Doak, L. G., Friedell, G. H., & Meade, C. D. (1998). Improving comprehension for cancer patients with low literacy skills: Strategies for clinicians. *CA-A Cancer Journal for Clinicians, 48*(3), 151–162.

Doak, C. C., Doak, L. G., & Root, J. H. (1985). *Teaching patients with low literacy skills* (1st ed.). Philadelphia: Lippincott.

Doak, C. C., Doak, L. G., & Root, J. H. (1996). *Teaching patients with low literacy skills* (2nd ed.). Philadelphia: Lippincott.

Doak, L. G. & Doak, C. C. (1987). Lowering the silent barriers to compliance for patients with low literacy skills. *Promoting Health,* July/August, 6–8.

Duffy, M. M. & Snyder, K. (1999). Can ED patients read your patient education materials? *Journal of Emergency Nursing, 25*(4), 294–297.

Dunn, M. M., Buckwalter, K. C., Weinstein, L. B., & Palti, H. (1985). Teaching the illiterate client does not have to be a problem. *Family & Community Health, 8*(3), 76–80.

Estey, A., Musseau, A., & Keehn, L. (1991). Comprehension levels of patients reading health information. *Patient Education and Counseling, 18*, 165–169.

Fain, J. A. (1994). When your patient can't read. *American Journal of Nursing, 94*(5), 16B, 16D.

Fetter, M. S. (1999). Recognizing and improving health literacy. *MEDSURG Nursing, 8*(4), 226.

Fisher, E. (1999). Low literacy levels in adults: Implications for patient education. *Journal of Continuing Education in Nursing, 30*(2), 56–61.

Fleener, F. T. & Scholl, J. F. (1992). Academic characteristics of self-identified illiterates. *Perceptual and Motor Skills, 74*(3), 739–744.

Flesch, R. (1948). A new readability yardstick. *Journal of Applied Psychology, 32*(3), 221–233.

Foltz, A. & Sullivan, J. (1998). Get real: Clinical testing of patients' reading abilities. *Cancer Nursing, 21*(3), 162–166.

French, K. S. & Larrabee, J. H. (1999). Relationships among educational material readability, client literacy, perceived beneficence, and perceived quality. *Journal of Nursing Care Quality, 13*(6), 68–82.

Fry, E. (1968). A readability formula that saves time. *Journal of Reading, 11*, 513–516, 575–579.

Fry, E. (1977). Fry's Readability Graph: Clarifications, validity, and extension to level 17. *Journal of Reading, 21*, 242–252.

Glanz, K. & Rudd, J. (1990). Readability and content analysis of print cholesterol education materials. *Patient Education and Counseling, 16*,109–118.

Gollop, C. J. (1997). Health information-seeking behavior and old African American women. *Bulletin of the Medical Library Association, 85*(2), 141–146.

Gunning, R. (1968). The Fog Index after 20 years. *Journal of Business Communications, 6*, 3–13.

Hayes, K. S. (2000). Literacy for health information of adult patients and caregivers in a rural emergency department. *Clinical Excellence for Nurse Practitioners, 4*(1), 35–40.

Hirsch, E. D. (2001). Overcoming the language gap. *American Educator, 4*, 6–7.

Holt, G. A., Hollon, J. D., Hughes, S. E., & Coyle, R. (1990). OTC labels: Can consumers read and understand them? *American Pharmacy, NS30*(11), 51–54.

Hussey, L. C. (1991). Overcoming the clinical barriers of low literacy and medication noncompliance among the elderly. *Journal of Gerontological Nursing, 17*(3), 27–29.

Hussey, L. C. (1994). Minimizing effects of low literacy on medication knowledge and compliance among the elderly. *Clinical Nursing Research, 3*(2), 132–145.

Hussey, L. C. & Guilliland, K. (1989). Compliance, low literacy, and locus of control. *Nursing Clinics of North America, 24*(3), 605–611.

Jackson, R. H., Davis, T. C., Bairnsfather, L. E., George, R. B., Crouch, M. A., & Gault, H. (1991). Patient reading ability: An overlooked problem in health care. *Southern Medical Journal, 84*(10), 1172–1175.

Jackson, R. H., Davis, T. C., Murphy, P., Bairnsfather, L. E., & George, R. B. (1994). Reading deficiencies in older patients. *American Journal of the Medical Sciences, 308*(2), 79–82.

Jenks, S. (1992). Researchers link low literacy to high health care costs. *Journal of the National Cancer Institute, 84*(14), 1068–1069.

Johnson, K. R. & Layng, T. V. J. (1992). Breaking the structuralist barrier: Literacy and numeracy with fluency. *American Psychologist, 47*(11), 1475–1490.

Joint Commission on Accreditation of Healthcare Organizations. (1993). *Accreditation manuals for hospitals—1993.* Chicago: Author.

Jolly, T., Scott, J. L., Feied, C. F., & Sandford, S. M. (1993). Functional illiteracy among emergency department patients: A preliminary study. *Annals of Emergency Medicine, 22*(3), 573–578.

Kefalides, P. T. (1999). Illiteracy: The silent barrier to health care. *Annals of Internal Medicine, 130*(4), 333–336.

Kelly, C. K. (1999). Helping low-literacy patients: What they don't know can hurt them. *Professional Medical Assistant,* Jan.–Feb., 8–13.

Kirsch, I. S., Jungeblat, A., Jenkins, L., & Kolstad, A. (1993). *Adult literacy in America: A first look at results of the National Adult Literacy Survey.* Washington, DC: National Center for Education Statistics, U.S. Department of Education.

Lasater, L. & Mehler, P. S. (1998). The illiterate patient: Screening and management. *Hospital Practice, 33*(4), 163–165, 169–170.

Lerner, E. B., Jehle, D. V. K., Janicke, D. M., & Moscati, R. M. (2000). Medical communication: Do our patients understand? *American Journal of Emergency Medicine, 18*(7), 764–766.

Ley, P. & Florio, T. (1996). The use of readability formulas in health care. *Psychology, Health & Medicine, 1*(1), 7–28.

Loughrey, L. (1983). Dealing with the illiterate patient . . . You can't read him like a book. *Nursing, 13*(1), 65–67.

Mailloux, S. L., Johnson, M. E., Fisher, D. G., & Pettibone, T. J. (1995). How reliable is computerized assessment of readability? *Computers in Nursing, 13*(5), 221–225.

Mayeaux, E. J., Murphy, P. W., Arnold, C., Davis, T. C., Jackson, R. H., & Sentell, T. (1996). Improving patient education for patients with low literacy skills. *American Family Physician, 53*(1), 205–211.

McLaughlin, G. H. (1969). SMOG-grading: A new readability formula. *Journal of Reading, 12,* 639–646.

Meade, C. D., Diekmann J., & Thornhill, D. G. (1992). Readability of American Cancer Society patient education literature. *Oncology Nursing Forum, 19*(1), 51–55.

Meade, C. D. & Smith, C. F. (1991). Readability formulas: Cautions and criteria. *Patient Education and Counseling, 17,* 153–158.

Meade, C. D. & Thornhill, D. G. (1989). Illiteracy in healthcare. *Nursing Management, 20*(10), 14–15.

Miller, B. & Bodie, M. (1994). Determination of reading comprehension level for effective patient health-education materials. *Nursing Research, 43*(2), 118–119.

Morgan, P. P. (1993). Illiteracy can have major impact on patients' understanding of health care information. *Canadian Medical Association Journal, 148*(7), 1196–1197.

Morra, M. E. (1991). Future trends in patient education. *Seminars in Oncology Nursing, 7*(2), 143–145.

Murphy, P. & Davis, T. C. (1997). When low literacy blocks compliance. *RN, 60*(10), 58, 60–63.

Osborne, H. (1999). In other words . . . Getting through . . . Lives can depend on simplifying the written word. *On-Call, 2*(9), 42–43.

Owen, P. M., Johnson, E. M., Frost, C. D., Porter, K. A., & O'Hare, E. (1993). Reading, readability, and patient education materials. *Cardiovascular Nursing, 29*(2), 9–13.

Owen, P. M., Porter, K. A., Frost, C. D., O'Hare, E., & Johnson, E. (1993). Determination of the readability of educational materials for patients with cardiac disease. *Journal of Cardiopulmonary Rehabilitation, 13*(1), 20–24.

Parikh, N. S., Parker, R. M., Nurss, J. M., Baker, D. W., & Williams, M. V. (1996). Shame and health literacy: The unspoken connection. *Patient Education and Counseling, 27*, 33–39.

Parker, R., Baker, D., Williams, M., & Nurss, J. (1995). The test of functional health literacy in adults (TOFHLA): A new instrument for measuring patients' literacy skills. *Journal of General Internal Medicine, 10*, 537–545.

Pearson, M. & Wessman, J. (1996). Gerogogy. *Home Healthcare Nurse, 14*(8), 631–636.

Pichert, J. W. & Elam, P. (1985). Readability formulas may mislead you. *Patient Education and Counseling, 7*, 181–191.

Quirk, P. A. (2000). Screening for literacy and readability: Implications for the advanced practice nurse. *Clinical Nurse Specialist, 14*(1), 26–32.

Robinson, J. H. (2000). Increasing students' cultural sensitivity: A step towards greater diversity in nursing. *Nurse Educator, 25*(3), 131–135, 144.

Rudolph, R. S. (1994). What Mr. Connor couldn't say. *Nursing, 24*(6), 47–48.

Spadero, D. C. (1983). Assessing readability of patient information materials. *Pediatric Nursing, 4*, 274–278.

Spadero, D. C., Robinson, L. A., & Smith, L. T. (1980). Assessing readability of patient information materials. *American Journal of Hospital Pharmacy, 37*, 215–221.

Spees, C. M. (1991). Knowledge of medical terminology among clients and families. *Image: Journal of Nursing Scholarship, 23*(4), 225–229.

Standal, T. C. (1981). How to use readability formulas more effectively. *Social Education, 45*, 183–186.

Stephens, S. T. (1992). Patient education materials: Are they readable? *Oncology Nursing Forum, 19*(1), 83–85.

Swanson, J. M., Forrest, K., Ledbetter, C., Hall, S., Holstine, E. J., & Shafer, M. R. (1990). Readability of commercial and generic contraceptive instructions. *Image: Journal of Nursing Scholarship, 22*(2), 96–100.

TenHave, T. R., VanHorn, B., Kumanyika, S., Askov, U., Matthews, Y., & Adams-Campbell, L. L. (1997). Literacy assessment in a cardiovascular nutrition education setting. *Patient Education and Counseling, 31*, 139–150.

United States Department of Education. (1993). *Adult literacy in America: National Adult Literacy Survey*. Washington, DC: Author.

Walker, A. (1987). Teaching the illiterate patient. *Journal of Enterostomal Therapy, 14*(2), 83–86.

Wallerstein, N. (1992). Health and safety education for workers with low-literacy or limited-English skills. *American Journal of Industrial Medicine, 22*(5), 751–765.

Webster's Collegiate Dictionary, 10th ed. (1999). Springfield, MA: Merriam Webster.

Weinrich, S. P. & Boyd, M. (1992). Education in the elderly. *Journal of Gerontological Nursing, 18*(1), 15–20.

Weiss, B. D., Reed, R. L., & Kligman, E. W. (1995). Literacy skills and communication methods of low-income older persons. *Patient Education and Counseling, 25,* 109–119.

Williams, D. M., Counselman, F. L., & Caggiano, C. D. (1996). Emergency department discharge instructions and patient literacy: A problem of disparity. *American Journal of Emergency Medicine, 14*(1), 19–22.

Williams, M. V., Parker, R. M., Baker, D. W., Parikh, W. S., Pitkin, K., Coates, W. C., & Nurss, J. R. (1995). Inadequate functional health literacy among patients at two public hospitals. *Journal of the American Medical Association, 274*(21), 1677–1682.

Williams-Deane, M. & Potter, L. S. (1992). Current oral contraceptive use instructions: An analysis of patient package inserts. *Family Planning Perspectives, 24*(3), 111–115.

Wilson, F. L. (1995). Measuring patients' ability to read and comprehend: A first step in patient education. *Nursing Connections, 8*(4), 17–25.

Winslow, E. H. (2001). Patient education materials: Can patients read them, or are they ending up in the trash? *American Journal of Nursing, 101*(10), 33–38.

Wong, M. (1992). Self-care instructions: Do patients understand educational materials? *Focus on Critical Care, 19*(1), 47–49.

Yasenchak, P. A. & Bridle, M. J. (1993). A low-literacy skin care manual for spinal cord injury patients. *Patient Education and Counseling, 22*(1), 1–5.

Ziegler, J. (1998). How literacy drives up healthcare costs. *Business & Health, 16*(4), 53–54.

Zimm, A. (1998). The need to understand: Addressing issues of low literacy and health. *On-Call, 1*(4), 20–23.

CHAPTER 8

Gender, Socioeconomic, and Cultural Attributes of the Learner

Susan B. Bastable

CHAPTER HIGHLIGHTS

Gender Characteristics
    Teaching Strategies
Socioeconomic Characteristics
    Teaching Strategies
Cultural Characteristics
    Definition of Terms
    Approaches to Delivering Culturally
        Sensitive Care
    Cultural Assessment
    General Assessment and Teaching
        Interventions

    Use of Translators
    The Four Major Culture Groups
        Hispanic American Culture
        Black American Culture
        Asian/Pacific Islander Culture
        Native American Culture
Preparing Nurses for Diversity Care
Stereotyping: Identifying the Meaning, the
    Risks, and the Solutions

KEY TERMS

acculturation
assimilation
cultural assessment
cultural competence
culture
ethnocentrism

gender-related cognitive abilities
poverty circle (cycle of poverty)
socioeconomic status (SES)
stereotyping
transcultural nursing

OBJECTIVES

After completing this chapter, the reader will be able to

1. Identify gender-related characteristics in the learner based on social and hereditary influences on brain functioning, cognitive abilities, and personality attributes.
2. Recognize the influence of socioeconomics in determining health status and health behaviors.
3. Define the various terms associated with diversity.
4. Examine cultural assessment from the perspective of different models of care.

5. Distinguish between the beliefs and customs of the four major cultural groups in the United States.
6. Suggest teaching strategies specific to the needs of learners belonging to each of the four cultural groups.
7. Examine ways in which transcultural nursing can serve as a framework for meeting the learning needs of various cultural populations.
8. Identify the meaning of stereotyping, the risks involved, and ways to avoid stereotypical behavior.

Gender, socioeconomic level, and cultural background have a significant influence on a learner's willingness and ability to respond to and make use of the teaching-learning situation. In recent years, these factors have been the focus of increased attention with respect to their effects on learning. Understanding those characteristics among learners related to gender, socioeconomics, and cultural diversity are of major importance when designing and implementing education programs to meet the needs of an increasingly unique population of learners.

First, this chapter explores how individuals respond differently to healthcare interventions due to gender-related variations resulting from heredity or social conditioning that affect how the brain functions for learning. Second, the influence of the environment on the learner from a socioeconomic viewpoint is examined. Third, consideration is given to the significant effects cultural norms have on the behaviors of learners from the perspective of the four major culture groups in the United States. In addition, models for cultural assessment and the planning of care are highlighted. This chapter also includes ways to prepare nurses for diversity care and to deal with the issue of stereotyping.

GENDER CHARACTERISTICS

Most of the information on gender variations with respect to learning can be found in the educational psychology literature. Nursing literature contains very little information about this subject from a teaching-learning perspective. There are, however, characteristics of male and female orientations that affect learning and need to be addressed more closely. One well-established fact exists: Studies that compare the sexes seldom are able to separate genetic differences from environmental influences on behavior (Gage & Berliner, 1998; Ormrod, 1995; Woolfolk, 1998).

There remains a gap in knowledge of how males and females might think and behave if they were not influenced by their environment right from birth. For example, our U.S. culture exposes girls and boys, respectively, to pink and blue blankets in the nursery, dolls and trucks in preschool, ballet and basketball in the elementary grades, and cheerleading and football in high school. These social influences continue to affect the sexes throughout the life span (Gorman, 1992).

Of course, men and women are different. But the question is: Are they different or the same when it comes to learning and to what can the similarities and differences be attributed? The fact remains that there are sex characteristics as to how males and females act, react, and perform in situations affecting every aspect of life. For example, when it comes to human relationships, intuitively women tend to pick up subtle tones of voice and facial expressions, whereas men tend to be less sensitive to these communication cues. In navigation, women tend to have difficulty finding their way, while men seem to have a better sense of direction. Scientists are beginning to believe that gender differences have as much to do with the biology of the brain as with the way people are raised (Gorman, 1992; Baron-Cohen, 2005).

Some would argue that these examples are representative of stereotyping. But as generalizations these statements seem to hold enough truth that neuroscientists have begun to detect structural as well as functional differences in the brains of males and females. These early findings have led to an upsurge in research into the mental lives of men and women.

Exploring how the human brain works is just beginning to yield some understanding of the types of sensory input that wire the brain and how they affect it. Circuits in different regions of the brain are thought to mature at different stages of development. These circuits are critical "windows of opportunity" at different ages for the learning of math, music, language, and emotion. Brain development is much more sensitive to life experiences than once believed (Begley, 1996; Hancock, 1996). A baby's brain is like "a work in progress, trillions of neurons waiting to be wired . . . to be woven into the intricate tapestry of the mind" (Begley, 1996, pp. 55–56). Some of the neurons of the brain have been hard-wired by genes, but others are waiting to be connected by the influence of environment. The first three years of life, it is being discovered, are crucial in the development of the mind. The wiring of the brain, a process of both nature and nurture, forms the connections that determine what and how people learn (Nash, 1997).

Thanks to modern technology, functional magnetic resonance imaging (FMRI) is being used to observe human brains in the very act of thinking, feeling, or remembering (Kawamura, Midorikawa, & Kezuka, 2000; Monastersky, 2001; Speck et al., 2000; Yee et al., 2000). Amazing discoveries through brain scanning have been made, such as where the emotion of love resides in the brain. Although machines can measure blood flow in the brain that supports nerve activity, no machines have been developed to date that can "read" or "interpret" a person's thoughts. The field of brain scanning still has far to go, but experts consider its potential to be incredible.

The trend in current studies is to focus on how separate parts of the brain *interact* while performing different tasks rather than focusing on only isolated regions of the brain associated with certain tasks (Monastersky, 2001). Researchers have already reported that men and women use different clusters of neurons when they read than when their brains are "idling." For example, in a study by Speck et al. (2000) of verbal working memory, the amount of brain activity increased with task difficulty. Interestingly, male subjects demonstrated right-sided hemispheric dominance whereas females showed more left-sided hemispheric dominance, with higher accuracy and slightly slower reaction times than males. The results revealed significant gender differences in the functional brain organization for working memory.

In general, the brains of men and women seem to operate differently. New studies are revealing that women engage more of their brains than men when thinking sad thoughts. When men and women subjects were asked to recall sad memories, the front of the limbic system in the brain of women glowed with activity eight times more than in men. Although men and women were able to perform equally well in math problems, tests indicated that they seemed to use the temporal lobes of the brain differently to figure out problems. Also, it has been found that men and women use different parts of their brains to figure out rhymes. These results are just a few examples of some of the tentative, yet fascinating, findings from research. Along with genetics, life experiences and the choices men and women make in the course of a lifetime help to mold personal characteristics and determine the very way the sexes think, sense, and respond (Begley, Murr, & Rogers, 1995).

In comparing how men and women feel, act, process information, and perform on cognitive tests, scientists have been able to identify only a few gender differences in the actual brain structure of humans (Table 8-1). Most differences that have been uncovered are quite small and are not as significant as, for example, the disparity found between male and female height. There seems to be, in fact, a great deal of overlap. Otherwise, "women could never read maps and men would always be lefthanded. That flexibility within the sexes reveals just how complex a puzzle gender actually is, requiring pieces from biology, sociology, and culture" (Gorman, 1992, p. 44).

With respect to brain functioning, there is likely a mix between the factors of heredity and environment that accounts for gender characteristics. The following is a comparison of cognitive abilities between the genders (Gage & Berliner, 1998; Ormrod, 1995; Woolfolk, 1998):

TABLE 8-1 Gender Differences in Brain Structure		
	Men	**Women**
TEMPORAL LOBE Region of the cerebral cortex that helps to control hearing, memory, and a person's sense of self and time.	In cognitively normal men, a small region of the temporal lob has about 10% fewer neurons than it does in women.	More neurons are located in the temporal region where language, melodies, and speech tones are understood.
CORPUS CALLOSUM The main bridge between the left and right brain contains a bundle of neurons that carry messages between the two brain hemispheres.	This part of the brain in men takes up less volume than in women, which suggests less communication between the two brain hemispheres.	The back portion of the callosum in women is bigger than in men, which may explain why women use both sides of their brains for language.
ANTERIOR COMMISSURE This collection of nerve cells, smaller than the corpus callosum, also connects the brain's two hemispheres.	The commissure in men is smaller than in women, even though men's brains are, on average, larger in size than women's brains.	The commissure in women is larger than in men, which may be a reason why their cerebral hemispheres seem to work together on tasks from language to emotional responses.
BRAIN HEMISPHERES The left side of the brain controls language, and the right side of the brain is the seat of emotion.	The right hemisphere of men's brains tends to be dominant.	Women tend to use their brains more holistically, calling on both hemispheres simultaneously.
BRAIN SIZE Total brain size is approximately 3 pounds.	Men's brains, on average, are larger than women's.	Women have smaller brains, on average, than men because the anatomical structure of their entire bodies is smaller. However, they have more neurons than men (an overall 11%) crammed into the cerebral cortex.

Source: Adapted from Begley, Murr, & Rogers (March 27, 1995). Gray Matters. *Newsweek* p. 51.

General intelligence: Various studies have not yielded consistent findings on whether males and females differ in general intelligence. On IQ tests, during preschool years, girls score higher; in high school, boys score higher on these tests. Differences may be due to greater dropout rates in high school for low-ability boys. Thus, overall the sexes have been found on average to be equal on measures of general intelligence.

Verbal ability: Girls learn to talk, use sentences, and use a greater variety of words earlier than boys. In addition, girls speak more clearly, read earlier, and do consistently better on tests of spelling and grammar. However, recent research has found that this early superiority of females in the verbal domain does not always persist. When boys and girls are tested in later years on verbal reasoning, verbal comprehension, and vocabulary, the findings are not consistent about gender differences.

Mathematical ability: During the preschool years, there appears to be no gender-related differences in ability to do mathematics. By the end of elementary school, however, boys show signs of excelling in mathematical reasoning, and the differences in math abilities of boys over girls become even greater in high school. Recent studies reveal that any male superiority likely is related to the way math is traditionally taught—as a competitive individual activity rather than as a cooperative group learning endeavor. When the approach to teaching math is taken into consideration, only about a 1% variation in quantitative skills is seen in the general population. In our culture, math achievement differences may result from different role expectations. The findings on math ability and achievement can also be extended to science achievement, as these two subjects are related.

Spatial ability: The ability to recognize a figure when it is rotated, to detect a shape embedded in another figure, or to accurately replicate a three-dimensional object is consistently better for males than for females. Of all possible gender-related differences in intellectual activity, the spatial ability of males is consistently higher than that of females, and probably has a genetic origin. Interestingly, women surpass men in the ability to discern and later recall the location of objects in a complex, random pattern. Scientists have reasoned that historically men may have developed strong spatial skills so as to be successful hunters, while women may have needed other types of visual skills so as to excel as gatherers and foragers of food (Gorman, 1992).

Problem solving: The complex concepts of problem solving, creativity, analytical skill, and cognitive styles, when examined, have led to mixed findings regarding gender differences. Men tend to try new approaches in problem solving and are less likely to be influenced by irrelevant cues and more focused on common features in certain learning tasks. Males also show more curiosity and significantly less conservatism than women in risk-taking situations. In the area of human relations, however, women perform better at problem solving than do men.

School achievement: Without exception, girls get better grades on average than boys, particularly at the elementary school level. Scholastic performance of girls is more stable and less fluctuating than that of boys.

Although no compelling evidence proves significant gender-linked differences in the areas of cognitive functioning mentioned above, some findings do reveal sex differences when it comes to personality characteristics (Gage & Berliner, 1998; Ormrod, 1995; Woolfolk, 1998). Most of the observed differences between the sexes in personality behaviors are thought to be largely determined by culture but are, to some extent, a result of mutual interaction between environment and heredity:

Aggression: Males of all ages and in most cultures are generally more aggressive than females. The role of the gender-specific hormone testosterone is being investigated as a possible cause of the more aggressive behavior demonstrated by males. However, scientists continue to disagree about whether aggression is biologically based or environmentally influenced. Regardless, male and female roles differ widely in most cultures, with males usually being more dominant, assertive, energetic, active, hostile, and destructive.

Conformity and dependence: Females have been found generally to be more conforming and more influenced by suggestion. The gender biases of some studies have made these findings open to suspicion, however.

Emotional adjustment: The emotional stability of the sexes is approximately the same in childhood. But differences do arise in how emotional problems are manifested. Some evidence indicates that adolescent girls and adult females have more neurotic symptoms than males. However, this tendency may reflect how society defines mental health in ways that coincide with male roles or the fact that tests to measure mental health usually have been designed by men and, therefore, may be biased.

Values and life goals: In the past, men have tended to show greater interest in scientific, mathematical, mechanical, and physically active occupations. Women have tended to choose literary, social service, and clerical occupations and to express stronger aesthetics, social sense, and religious values. These differences have become smaller over time as women have begun to think differently about themselves, have more freely pursued career and interest pathways, and society has begun to take a more "equal opportunity" viewpoint for both sexes.

Achievement orientation: Females are more likely to express achievement motivation in social skills and social relations, whereas men are more likely to try to succeed in intellectual or competitive activities. This difference is thought to be due to sex-role expectations that are strongly communicated at very early ages.

How do these observations on gender characteristics in intellectual functioning and personality relate to the process of teaching clients? It is very difficult to differentiate between biological and environmental influences simply because these two factors are intertwined and influence each other.

The behavioral differences that are well documented include the fact that females have an accelerated biological timetable and, in general, are more prone to have verbal ability. Conversely, males lag behind females in biological development and attention span but tend to excel in visual-spatial ability and mathematical pursuits. With respect to gender differences in aging, men are biologically weaker, as suggested by lifespan mortality rates. White females have a life expectancy of approximately 80 years compared to approximately 73 years for white males (U.S. Census Bureau, 2000). However, less is known about women's health because women's health issues have been underrepresented in research efforts, although this trend is changing.

Overall, women are likely to seek health care more often than men do. It is suspected that one of the reasons women have more contact with the healthcare system is that they traditionally have tended to be the primary caretakers of their children, who need pediatric services. In addition, during childbearing years, women seek health services for care surrounding pregnancy and childbirth. Perhaps the reason that men tend not to rely as much as women on care from health providers is because of the sex-role expectation by our society that men should be stronger. They also have a tendency to be risk takers and to think of themselves as more independent. It is known that men are less likely to pursue routine health care for purposes of health and safety promotion and disease and accident prevention. Yet, they typically face a greater number of health hazards, such as a higher incidence of automobile accidents, use of drugs and alcohol, suicide, heart disease, and engaging in dangerous occupations.

Teaching Strategies

As health educators, nurses must become aware of the extent to which social and heredity-related differences between the genders affect health-seeking behaviors and influence individual health needs. As stated previously, in some areas males and females display different orientations and learning styles. The differences seem to depend on their interests and past experiences in the biological and social roles of men and women in our society.

Women and men are part of different social cultures, too. They use different symbols, belief systems, and ways to express themselves, much in the same manner that different ethnic groups have distinct cultures (Tear, 1995). In the future, these gender characteristics may become less pronounced as the sex roles become more blended. Nurses are encouraged to use versatile teaching style strategies so as not to perpetuate stereotypical approaches to teaching and learning with the two genders.

SOCIOECONOMIC CHARACTERISTICS

Socioeconomic status (SES), in addition to gender characteristics, influences the teaching-learning process. SES is considered to be the single most important determinant of health in our society (Crimmins & Saito, 2001; Pappas, Queen, Hadden, & Fisher, 1993). Socioeconomic class is an aspect of diversity that must be addressed in the process of teaching and learning. Class is the "unmentionable five-letter word" (Rhem, 1998, p. 1). Many people are hesitant to categorize themselves according to class. They also are reluctant to discuss the issue of class differences because of the widespread idea that the United States should be a classless society (Rhem, 1998). It is a myth, though, that America is a country without classes (McGoldrick, 1995). The question remains as to whether class depends on income level or educational level, on having a rural or an urban background, on the kind of work your parents do, or on the inner sense of one's status. Class, as universal as race or gender, "hides in the shadows." Those who are privileged feel embarrassed about their advantages just as much as those who are poor feel embarrassed about their disadvantages (Rhem, 1998).

Social and economic levels of individuals have been found to be significant variables affecting health status and in determining health behaviors (Crimmins & Saito, 2001; Pappas et al., 1993). Millions of Americans are living in poverty, including more than one in four American children under the age of 18 years. By 2020, the total number of children living in poverty is expected to reach 20 million (Woolfolk, 1998). Disadvantaged people—those with low incomes, low educational levels, and/or social deprivation—come from many different ethnic groups, including millions of poor White people (Morra, 1991; Woolfolk, 1998). The variables of family income, educational level, and family structure (Gage & Berliner, 1998; Woolfolk, 1998) seem to affect health beliefs, health practices, and readiness to learn.

Patients belonging to lower social classes have higher rates of illness, more severe illnesses, and reduced rates of life expectancy. People with low SES, as measured by indicators such as income, education, and occupation, have increased rates of mortality compared to those with higher SES. An inverse relationship exists between SES and morbidity and mortality; that is, individuals who have higher incomes and are better educated live longer and healthier lives than those who are of low income and poorly educated (Crimmins & Saito, 2001; Pappas et al., 1993). Thus, the level of socioeconomic well-being is a strong indicator of health outcomes. This raises serious questions about health differences among our nation's people as a result of unequal access to health care due to SES.

Social class is measured by one or more of the following: occupation of parents, income of family, location of residence, and educational level of parents (Gage & Berliner, 1998). Woolfolk (1998) explains that many factors, including poor health care for mothers and children, limited resources, family stress, discrimination, and low-paying jobs, maintain the cycle by which generation after generation are born into poverty. Whatever the factors that keep particular groups from achieving at higher levels, these groups are likely to remain on the lower end of the occupational structure. This cycle has been coined the *poverty circle* (Gage & Berliner, 1998; Nagoshi, Johnson, & Honbo, 1993) or the *cycle of poverty* (Woolfolk, 1998). The poverty circle is described as follows:

> Parents low in scholastic ability and consequently in educational level create an envi-
> ronment in their homes and neighborhoods that produces children who are also low
> in scholastic ability and academic attainment. These children grow up and become
> parents, repeating the cycle. Like them, their children are fit only for occupations at
> lower levels of pay, prestige, and intellectual demand. (Gage & Berliner, 1992, p. 61)

In addition, Baydar, Brooks-Gunn, & Furstenberg (1993) point out that illiteracy and marginal literacy have been linked to low productivity, high unemployment, low earnings, high rates of welfare dependency, and teenage parenting. All of these factors are common measures of a society's economic well-being.

The alarming verbal and reading gap between rich and poor students "represents the single greatest failure in American public schooling" (Hirsch, 2001, p. 5). Many low-income children entering kindergarten have heard only half the words and understand only half the meanings of language that the high-income child has heard and understands. This gap continues to widen as students progress in each succeeding grade in school. Standards need to be developed for every grade to make sure each child meets these expectations before being allowed to progress in school.

The lower socioeconomic classes have been studied more than others. This is probably because the health views of this group differ the most from those viewpoints of health professionals who care for this group of individuals. People of lower social status have been characterized as being indifferent to the symptoms of illness until poor health interferes with their lifestyle and independence. Their view of life is one of a sense of powerlessness, meaninglessness, and isolation from middle-class knowledge of health and the need for preventive measures, such as vaccination for their children (Lipman, Offord, & Boyle, 1994; Winkleby, Jatulis, Frank, & Fortmann, 1992).

The high cost of health care may well be a major factor affecting health practices of people in the lower socioeconomic classes. Individuals with inadequate financial and emotional resources are unable to purchase services. Also, they usually do not have support systems to sustain them during chronic illness or during recovery from acute illness. Individuals deprived of monetary and psychosocial resources are at a much greater risk for failing to reach an optimal level of health and well-being.

Just as SES can have a negative effect on illness, so too can illness have a devastating effect on a person's socioeconomic well-being. A catastrophic or chronic illness can lead to unemployment, loss of health insurance coverage or ineligibility for health insurance benefits, enforced social isolation, and a strain on social support systems. Without the socioeconomic means to counteract these threats to their well-being, individuals of low SES may be powerless to improve their situation. These multiple losses tax the individual, their families, and the healthcare system.

Teaching Strategies

The nurse plays a key role in educating the consumer about avoiding health risks, reducing illness episodes, establishing healthful environmental conditions, and accessing healthcare services. Patient education by nurses for those who are socially and economically deprived have the potential for yielding short-term benefits in meeting these individuals' immediate healthcare needs. However, more research must be done to determine whether teaching can ensure the long-term benefits of helping deprived people develop the skills needed to reach and sustain independence in self-care management.

Nurses must be aware of the likely effects of low SES on an individual's ability to learn as a result of poor intellectual functioning, poor academic achievement, low literacy, high susceptibility to illness, and breakdown of social support systems. Low-income people are at greater risk for these factors that can interfere with learning. However, it cannot be assumed that everyone at the poverty or near-poverty level is equally influenced by these threats to their well-being. To avoid stereotyping, it is essential that each individual or family be assessed to determine their particular strengths and weaknesses for learning. In this way, teaching strategies unique to each person's circumstances can be designed to assist socioeconomically deprived individuals in meeting their needs for health care.

Nevertheless, it is well documented that individuals with low SES are likely to have poor self-esteem, feelings of helplessness and hopelessness, and low expectations. They also tend to think in concrete terms, are more focused on satisfying immediate needs, have a more external locus of control, and have decreased attention spans. They have difficulty in problem solving and in analyzing and synthesizing large amounts of information (Gage & Berliner, 1998; Woolfolk, 1998). With these individuals, the nurse will most likely have to rely on specific teaching methods and tools similar to those identified as appropriate for intervening with clients who have low literacy abilities (see Chapter 7 on literacy).

CULTURAL CHARACTERISTICS

At the beginning of the 21st Century, the composition of the U.S. population was 71.3% Whites, 12.2% Blacks, 11.2% Hispanics, 3.8% Asian/Pacific Islanders, 0.7% American Indians, and 0.8% others. Thus, more than one-quarter (28.7%) of the U.S. population consists of people from culturally diverse groups (U.S. Census Bureau, 2000). By 2010, one out of every three people in the United States is projected to belong to a racial or ethnic minority (Robinson, 2000) and these minority groups will become the majority in 53 of the 100 largest cities (Morra, 1991). By 2080, it is predicted that people of diversity will account for more than half (51%) of the U.S. total population, which will be the first time in U.S. history that minority subgroups will become the majority of the total population. If the present demographic trends continue, by 2080 the racial and ethnic composition of this country will be 23.4% Hispanics, 14.7% Blacks, and 12% Asian and others (Morra, 1991).

To keep pace with a society that is increasingly more culturally diverse, nurses will need to have sound knowledge of the cultural values and beliefs of specific ethnic groups (Price & Cordell, 1994; Price & Cortis, 2000; Rooda & Gay, 1993; Spicer et al., 1994). In the past, health providers have experienced difficulties in caring for clients whose cultural beliefs differ from their own, because beliefs about health and illness vary considerably among cultural groups. Lack of cultural sensitivity by health professionals has resulted in millions of dollars wasted annually through misuse of healthcare services, the alienation of large numbers of people, and the misdiagnosis of health problems with often tragic and dangerous consequences.

In addition, certain underrepresented groups are beginning to demand health care that respects their cultural rights and includes their specific beliefs and practices in the delivery of care. This expectation is in direct conflict with the unicultural, Western, biomedical paradigm taught in many nursing and other healthcare provider programs across the country. A serious problem exists within the nursing profession because nurses are presumed to understand and be able to meet the healthcare needs of a culturally diverse population, but many of them do not have the formal educational preparation to do so (Andrews, 1992).

Definition of Terms

Before examining the four major cultural groups within the United States, it is important to define the following terms commonly used in dealing with the subject of culture:

Acculturation: A willingness to modify one's own culture as a result of contact with another culture (Purnell & Paulanka, 1998).

Assimilation: The willingness of a person settling in a new country to adopt characteristics of that new culture (Purnell & Paulanka, 1998).

Cultural assessment: A systematic appraisal of beliefs, values, and practices to determine client needs so that nursing interventions can be tailored to meet those specific needs (Tripp-Reimer & Afifi, 1989).

Cultural competence: Recognizing, accepting, and respecting cultural beliefs and practices about wellness and illness in the delivery of care by adapting interventions to be in harmony with the client's culture (Denboba et al., 1998; Purnell & Paulanka, 1998).

Culture: Includes knowledge, beliefs, values, morals, customs, traditions, and habits characteristic of a population of people that guide their thinking and decision making (Purnell & Paulanka, 1998).

Ethnocentrism: A concept describing "the universal tendency of human beings to think that their ways of thinking, acting, and believing are the only right, proper, and natural ways. . . . Ethnocentrism perpetuates an attitude that beliefs that differ greatly from one's own are strange, bizarre, or unenlightened, and therefore wrong" (Purnell & Paulanka, 1998, p. 3).

Transcultural nursing: An analysis of different cultures with respect to health and illness beliefs, values, and practices with the goal of using this knowledge as a framework to provide culture-specific care to people to meet the health needs of diverse groups and individuals (Leininger, 1978).

Approaches to Delivering Culturally Sensitive Care

Given increases in immigration and birth rates in the United States, our system of health care must respond by shifting from a dominant monocultural, ethnocentric focus to a more multicultural, transcultural focus. The major question is: "How can nurses competently respond to and effectively care for people from diverse cultures who act, speak, and behave in ways different than their own?" (Leininger, 1994). Health professionals are often unaware of the complex factors influencing clients' responses to health care. In conducting a nursing assessment, six cultural phenomena need to be taken into consideration: communication, personal space, social organization, time, environmental control, and biological variations (Figure 8-1).

According to Anderson (1990), the cultural meanings that shape clients' experiences are not being taken into account when care is planned by practitioners. Strategies must be implemented to enhance the profession's ability to deliver care to

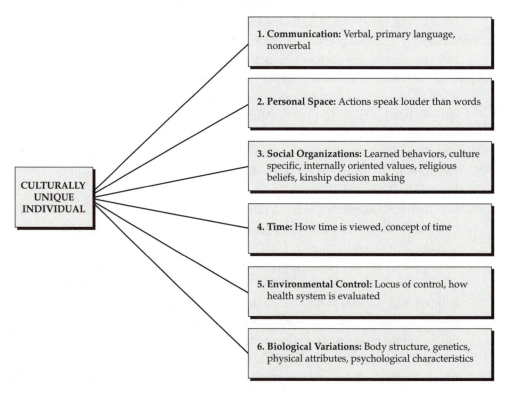

Figure 8-1 Six Cultural Phenomena
Source: Adapted from Giger, J. N. & Davidhizar, R. E. (1995). *Transcultural Nursing: Assessment and Intervention* (2nd ed.), p. 9. St. Louis: Mosby-Year Book.

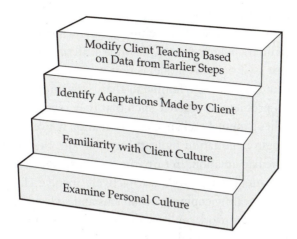

Figure 8-2 Four-Step Approach to Providing Culturally Sensitive Care
Source: Reprinted with permission from Price, J. L. & Cordell, B. (1994). Cultural diversity and patient teaching. *Journal of Continuing Education in Nursing, 25*(4), 164.

culturally diverse populations in the United States as well as abroad (Hahn, 1995). Price and Cordell (1994) outlined a four-step approach to help nurses provide culturally sensitive patient teaching (Figure 8-2).

Cultural Assessment

The *Nurse-Client Negotiations Model* has been developed for the purpose of cultural assessment and planning for care of culturally diverse people. This model recognizes differences that exist between notions of the nurse compared with those of the client about health, illness, and treatments. It attempts to bridge the gap between the scientific perspectives of the nurse and the popular perspectives of the client.

The Nurse-Client Negotiations Model serves as a framework to attend to the "culture of the nurse" as well as the "culture of the client." In addition to the professional culture, each nurse has his or her own personal beliefs and values, which may operate without the nurse being fully aware of them. These beliefs and values may influence nurses' interactions with patients and families. Explanations of the same phenomena may yield different interpretations based on the cultural perspective of the layperson or the professional. For example, putting lightweight covers on a patient may be interpreted by family members as placing their loved one at risk for "getting a chill," whereas the nurse will use this technique to prevent or reduce a fever. As another example, a Jehovah's Witness family considers a blood transfusion for their child as contamination of the child's body, whereas the nurse and other healthcare team members believe a transfusion is a lifesaving treatment (Anderson, 1987). The important aspect of this model is that it can open lines of communication between the nurse and the patient/family so that each understands how the other interprets or values a problem or practice such that they respect one another's goals.

Negotiation implies a mutual exchange of information between the nurse and client. The nurse should begin negotiation by learning from the clients about their understanding of their particular situation. In turn, the nurse explains to the clients about the professional scientific model. The goal is to actively involve clients in the learning process so as to acquire healthy coping mechanisms and styles of living. Together, the nurse and client then need to work out how the popular and scientific perspectives can be meshed to achieve goals related to the individual client's interests (Anderson, 1990).

General areas to assess when first meeting the client include the following:

1. The client's perceptions of health and illness
2. His or her use of traditional remedies and folk practitioners
3. The client's perceptions of nurses, hospitals, and the care delivery system
4. His or her beliefs about the role of family and family member relationships
5. His or her perceptions of and need for emotional support (Anderson, 1987; Jezewski, 1993).

According to Anderson (1990), the following are some questions that can be used as a means for understanding the client's perspectives or viewpoints and can serve as the basis for negotiation:

*   What do you think caused your problem?
*   Why do you think the problem started when it did?
*   What major problems does your illness cause you?
*   How has being sick affected you?
*   How severe is your illness? Will it have a short- or long-term course?
*   What kinds of treatments do you think you should receive?
*   What are the most important results you hope to obtain from your treatments?
*   What do you fear most about your illness?

The *Culturally Competent Model of Care* proposed by Campinha-Bacote (1995) is another model for conducting a thorough and sensitive cultural assessment. Cultural competence is defined as a set of behaviors, attitudes, and policies that enable a professional to work effectively in a cross-cultural situation. Through this model, cultural competence is seen as a continuous process involving four components: cultural awareness, cultural knowledge, cultural skill, and cultural encounter.

Cultural awareness is the process of becoming sensitive to interactions with other cultural groups. It requires nurses to examine their biases and prejudices toward others of another culture or ethnic background. *Cultural knowledge* is the process in which nurses become educated about various cultural world views. *Cultural skill* involves the process of learning how to conduct an accurate cultural assessment. *Cultural encounter* encourages nurses to expose themselves in practice to cross-cultural interactions with clients of diverse cultural backgrounds. All four components are essential if one is to deliver culturally competent nursing care (Figure 8-3).

Nurses who are competent in cultural assessment and negotiation will be able to assist their colleagues in working with clients who may be considered "uncooperative," "noncompliant," or "difficult." Also, they can help identify potential areas of cultural conflict and select teaching interventions that minimize conflict. Nurses must understand how the reactions of practitioners influence labeling of clients' behaviors and, therefore, eventually influence nurse–client interactions (Anderson, 1987, 1990). There is one very important caveat to remember:

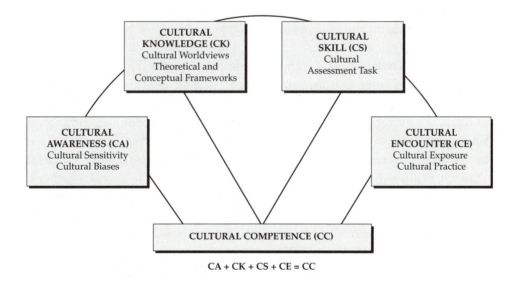

Figure 8-3 Culturally Competent Model of Care
Source: Reprinted with permission from Campinha-Bacote, J. (1995). The quest for cultural competence in nursing care. *Nursing Forum, 30*(4), 20.

Nurses must be especially careful not to over-generalize or stereotype clients on the basis of their cultural heritage. Just because someone belongs to a particular ethnic group does not necessarily mean they adhere to all the beliefs, values, customs, and practices of that ethnic group.

Cultural stereotyping can occur when nurses use "a recipe-like approach to clients from specific cultural groups. . . . There is a tendency by the nurse to view all members of a group homogenously and to expect certain beliefs or practices . . . that may or may not apply to the client" (Andrews & Boyle, 1995, p. 50). Knowledge of cultural variations should serve only as a cue for obtaining additional information about an individual through assessment.

General Assessment and Teaching Interventions

As the first step in the teaching process, assessment should attempt to determine health beliefs, values, and practices. Nurses need to be aware of the established customs that influence the behavior one is attempting to change (Tripp-Reimer & Afifi, 1989). The nurse should, however, keep in mind that belonging to an ethnic group does not always mean a person follows or "buys into" all of the traditions or customs of the group to which they belong. Given that culture affects the way someone perceives a health problem and understands its course and possible treatment options, it is essential to carry out a thorough assessment prior to establishing a plan of action for long-term behavioral change. The nurse in the role of teacher must implement successful teaching interventions using the universal skills of establishing rapport, assessing readiness to learn, and using active listening to understand problems.

Different cultural backgrounds not only create different attitudes and reactions to illness, but also can influence how people express themselves, both verbally and nonverbally, which may prove difficult to interpret. For example, asking a patient to explain what they believe is the cause of a problem will help to reveal whether the patient thinks it is due to a spiritual intervention, a hex, an imbalance in nature, or other culturally based beliefs. The nurse should accept the client's explanation (most likely reflecting the beliefs of the support system as well) in a nonjudgmental manner.

Culture also guides the way an ill person is defined and treated. For example, some cultures believe that once the symptoms disappear, illness is no longer present. This belief can be harmful for individuals suffering from an acute illness such as a streptococcal infection, when a one- or two-day course of antibiotic therapy relieves the soreness in the throat. This belief also can be a problem for the individual afflicted with a chronic disease that is manifested by periods of remission or exacerbation.

In addition, readiness to learn must be assessed from the standpoint of a person's culture. Patients and their families, for instance, may follow a recommended medical regimen while in the hospital setting but fail to follow through with the guidelines once they return to their homes. In addition, the nurse and other health providers must be careful not to assume that the values adhered to by professionals are equally important to the patient and significant others. Consideration also must be given to barriers that might exist, such as time, financial, and environmental variables, which may interfere with readiness to learn (see Chapter 4 on readiness to learn). Finally, the client needs to believe that new behaviors are not only possible, but also beneficial if behavioral change is to be maintained over the long term.

The following specific guidelines for assessment should be used regardless of the particular cultural orientation of the client (Anderson, 1987):

1. **Observe the interactions between patient and family members and among family members.** Determine who makes the decisions, how decisions are made, who is the primary caregiver, what type of care is given, and what foods and other objects are important to the patient and family.
2. **Listen to the patient.** Find out what the patient wants, how the patient's wants differ from what the family wants, and how these wants differ from what you think is appropriate.
3. **Consider communication abilities and patterns.** Be aware of the patient's primary language (which may be different from your own), manners of speaking (rate of speech), and nonverbal behaviors (expressions used) that can enhance or hinder understanding.
4. **Explore customs or taboos.** Observe behaviors and ask to clarify beliefs and practices that may interfere with care or treatment.
5. **Determine the notion of time.** Become oriented to the patient's and family's sense of time and importance of time frames.
6. **Be aware of cues for interaction.** Determine the symbolic objects or the traditions that provide comfort and security to patients and family members.

These guidelines will assist in the exchange of information between the nurse and patient/family. The patient–nurse relationship is one in which the nurse is both learner and teacher and the client is also both learner and teacher. The goal of negotiation is to arrive at a way of working together to solve a problem or to determine a course of action (Anderson, 1987).

Use of Translators

If the client speaks a foreign language, whenever possible the client's primary language should be used. When the nurse does not fluently speak the same language, it is necessary to secure the assistance of a translator. Translators may be family members, neighbors and friends, other healthcare staff, or professional interpreters.

For many reasons, the use of family or friends for translation of messages is not as desirable as using professionally trained interpreters. First, family members and friends may not be sufficiently fluent to assume the role. Second, they may choose to omit portions of the content they believe to be unnecessary or unacceptable. Third, their presence may violate the patient's right to privacy and confidentiality (Baker et al., 1996; Poss & Rangel, 1995). Thus, it is best if professionally trained interpreters can be used. They can translate instructional messages accurately, and they work under an established code of ethics and confidentiality. If there is no bilingual person available to facilitate communication, the AT&T Language Line provides 24-hour access to translators who are fluent in 144 languages (Duffy & Snyder, 1999).

When no translator is used, the following strategies are recommended (Poss & Rangel, 1995; Tripp-Reimer & Afifi, 1989) to help the nurse teach clients who are only partially fluent in English:

- Speak slowly and clearly, allowing for twice as much time as a typical teaching session would take.
- Use simple sentences, relying on an active rather than a passive voice.
- Avoid technical terms (e.g., use *heart* rather than *cardiac*, or *stomach* rather than *gastric*), medical jargon (e.g., use *blood pressure* rather than *BP*), and American idioms (e.g., *red tape* or *I heard it straight from the horse's mouth*).
- Organize instructional material in the sequence in which the plan of action should be carried out.
- Make no assumptions that the information given has been understood. Ask for clients to explain in their own words what they heard, and, if appropriate, request a return demonstration of a skill that has been taught.

THE FOUR MAJOR CULTURE GROUPS

Given the fact that there are hundreds of ethnic minority subgroups in the United States, and many more worldwide, it is impossible to address the cultural characteristics of each one of them. The following is a review of the beliefs and health practices of the four major cultural groups in this country identified by the U.S. Census

Bureau—Hispanics, Blacks, Asian/Pacific Islanders, and American Indians—who account for more than one quarter (28.7%) of the U.S. population.

It must be remembered that one of the most important roles of the nurse as teacher is to serve as an advocate for clients. If nurses are to assume this role, then their efforts should be directed at making the healthcare setting as similar to the client's natural environment as possible. To do so, they must be aware of clients' customs, beliefs, and lifestyles.

The following references have been used for information on the four cultures to be discussed and are recommended as sources of additional information on particular tribes or subgroups not identified: Cantore (2001), Caudle (1993), Chachkes and Christ (1996), Chideya (1999), Cohen (1991), Galanti (1991), Gollop (1997), Horton and Freire (1990), Jackson (1993), Kelley and Fitzsimmons (2000), Kniep-Hardy and Burkhardt (1977), Lowe and Struthers (2001), Parker and Kiatoukaysy (1999), Perry (1982), Purnell and Paulanka (1998), Shomaker (1981), Smolan, Moffitt, and Naythons (1990), Spector (1991), and Westberg (1989).

Hispanic American Culture

According to the U.S. Census Bureau (2000), Hispanics are the fastest-growing minority group in the United States. They now represent 11.2% of the total population of the United States. It is projected that in another 100 years Hispanics will make up approximately 25% of the population. There has been a tremendous increase in the number of Hispanics since 1970 as a result of a significant increase in immigration and a higher birthrate in this group than the rest of the population.

Although sometimes referred to as *Latinos*, the term *Hispanic* is used by the U.S. Census Bureau to label this group of Americans with varied backgrounds in culture and heritage who are of Latin American or Spanish decent or who use the Spanish language in their homes (Caudle, 1993). Although Hispanic Americans have many common characteristics, each subgroup has unique characteristics.

The largest group comprises Mexicans (60% of the population), followed by Puerto Ricans, Central and South Americans, and Cubans. Hispanics are more likely to live in metropolitan areas than are non-Hispanics. They are found in every state but are concentrated in just 10 states. California and Texas together have one-half of the Hispanic population, but other large concentrations are found in New York, New Jersey, Massachusetts, Florida, Illinois, Arizona, New Mexico, and Colorado. Nurses who practice in the Southwestern states are most likely to encounter Mexicans, those practicing in the Northeastern states will most likely be caregivers for Puerto Ricans, and nurses in Florida will be delivering care to a large number of Cubans (Caudle, 1993; Purnell & Paulanka, 1998; Spector, 1991; Torres, 1994).

Access to health care by Hispanics is limited both by choice and by unavailability of health services. Approximately 23% of Hispanic families live below the poverty line. Only one-fifth of Puerto Ricans, one-fourth of Cubans, and one-third of Mexicans see a physician during the course of a year. Even when Hispanics have access to the healthcare system, they may not receive the care they need. Difficulty in obtaining services due to language barriers, dissatisfaction with the care provided, and inability to afford the rising costs of medical care are major factors that discourage them from using the healthcare system. In addition, levels of education correlate highly with access to health care; that is, the less education the head of the household has, the poorer the family's health status and access to health care (Purnell & Paulanka, 1998; Spector, 1991; Westberg, 1989). Hispanics are more likely than the general U.S. population to have reading skills in English below the fourth-grade level and to have lower educational attainment than non-Hispanic whites (Massett, 1996).

The health beliefs of Hispanics also affect their decisions to seek traditional care. For example, illnesses of Mexican Americans can be organized into the following categories (Caudle, 1993; Markides & Coreil, 1986; Spector, 1991):

1. **Diseases of "hot" and "cold":** Believed to be due to an imbalanced intake of foods or ingestion of foods at extreme opposites in temperature. In addition, cold air is thought to lead to joint pain, and a "cold womb" results in women not being able to bear children. Heating or chilling is seen as the cure for parts of the body afflicted by disease.
2. **Diseases of dislocation of internal organs:** Believed to be cured by massage or physical manipulation of body parts.
3. **Diseases of magical origin:** Caused by *mal Ojo* or "evil eye," a disorder of infants and children as a result of a woman admiring someone else's child without touching the child, resulting in crying, fitful sleep, diarrhea, vomiting, and fever.
4. **Diseases of emotional origin:** Attributed to sudden or prolonged terror; called *Susto*.

Possible explanations for the relative advantages and disadvantages in the health status of Hispanics involve such factors as cultural practices favoring reproductive success, early and high fertility contributing to low breast cancer but increased rates of cervical cancer, dietary habits linked to low cancer rates but high prevalence of obesity and diabetes, genetic heritage, extended family support reducing the need for psychiatric services, and low socioeconomic status that contributes to increased infectious and parasitic diseases. Alcoholism also represents a crucial health problem for many Hispanic Americans. As the Hispanic population becomes more acculturated, certain risk factors for cardiovascular disease and certain cancers are expected to play larger roles in this group (Markides & Coreil, 1986; Purnell & Paulanka, 1998).

Today, there is little information in the literature about the extent and frequency to which Hispanics use home remedies and folk practices. In the Southwestern United States, 21% of the Hispanic population has been found to use herbs and other home remedies to treat illness episodes—twice the proportion reported in the total U.S. population. The use of folk practitioners has declined and practically disappeared in some Hispanic subgroups. Some Hispanics, though, still place a high degree of reliance on health healers, known as *curenderos* or *esperitistas*, for health advice and treatment. Knowing where people get their health information can provide clues to nurses as to how to reach particular population groups.

Because the family is central in the lives of Hispanic people, the extended family serves as the single most important source of social support to its members. Mexican Americans, in particular, have been found to have low rates of psychiatric problems, probably explained by strong family ties that protect them against stress. Hispanic culture also is characterized by a pattern of respect and obedience to elders as well as a pattern of male dominance. The nurse's focus, therefore, needs to be on the family rather than on the individual. It is likely, for example, that a woman would be reluctant to make a decision about her or her child's health care without consulting her husband first. Changes are occurring, however, as Hispanic women are taking jobs outside the home. Also, children are picking up the English language more quickly than their parents and are ending up in the powerful position of acting as interpreters for their parents. The heavy reliance on family has been linked to low utilization of healthcare services by Hispanics.

Teaching Strategies

Only about 40% of Hispanics have completed 4 years or more of high school, and only 10% have completed college (Purnell & Paulanka, 1998). Both the educational level and the primary language of Hispanic clients need to be taken into consideration when selecting instructional materials for those who have minimal levels of education (Massett, 1996).

The age of the population can also affect health education efforts. Because the Hispanic population is young as a total group (30% are younger than 20 years of age), the school system is an important setting for educating members of the Hispanic community (Massett, 1996). Education programs for Hispanic students in the school system regarding alcohol and drug abuse and cardiovascular disease risk reduction have proved successful if

- cultural beliefs were observed.
- the nurse was first introduced by an individual accepted and respected by the learners.
- family members were included.
- the Hispanic community was encouraged to take responsibility for solving their own health problems.

Morbidity, mortality, and risk factor data also provide clues to the areas in which patient education efforts should be directed. Hispanics have higher rates of diabetes, AIDS, obesity, alcohol-related illnesses, and mortality from homicide than the general population. All of these topics should be targeted for educational efforts at disease prevention and health promotion (Caudle, 1993).

The following general suggestions are useful when designing and implementing patient education for Hispanic Americans (Caudle, 1993; Massett, 1996; Purnell & Paulanka, 1998; Spector, 1991; Westberg, 1989):

1. Identify the Hispanic American subgroups (e.g., Mexicans, Cubans, and Puerto Ricans) in the community whose needs differ in terms of health beliefs, language, and general health status so that teaching can be targeted to meet their distinct ethnic needs.
2. Take into account the special health needs of Hispanic Americans with respect to incidences of diseases and risk factors to which they are vulnerable—diabetes, AIDS, obesity, alcohol-related illnesses, homicide, and accidental injuries.
3. Be aware of the importance of the family so that patient education efforts include all interested family members. Remember that Hispanic families are usually willing to provide support to each other, and decision making usually rests with the male and older adult authority figures in the family.
4. Provide adequate space for teaching to accommodate family members who typically accompany patients seeking health care.
5. Be aware of the importance of the Roman Catholic religion in the lives of Hispanics when dealing with such issues as contraception, abortion, and family planning.
6. Demonstrate cultural sensitivity to health beliefs by respecting ethnic values and taking time to learn about Hispanic beliefs.

7. Consider other sources of care that Hispanics might be using, such as home remedies, before they enter or while they are within the healthcare system.

8. Be aware of the modesty felt by some Hispanics, especially women and girls, who may be particularly uncomfortable talking about sexual issues in mixed company.

9. Display warmth, friendliness, and tactfulness when developing a relationship with Hispanics because they expect health providers to be informal and interested in their lives.

10. Determine whether Spanish is the language by which the client best communicates. Many Hispanics prefer to speak Spanish, but they are not always literate in reading their own language.

11. Speak slowly and distinctly, avoiding the use of technical words and slang if the client has limited ability to understand the English language.

12. Do not assume that a nod of the head or a smile indicates understanding of what has been said. Many Hispanics are not familiar with English, but because they respect authority, it is not uncommon for them to give nonverbal cues that may be misleading or misinterpreted by the nurse. Ask clients to repeat in their own words what they have been told to determine their level of understanding.

13. If interpreters are used, be sure they speak the dialect used by the learner. Be certain that the interpreter "interprets" rather than just "translates" so that the real meaning of instructions gets across. Also, be sure to talk directly to the client rather than to the interpreter.

14. Provide written and audiovisual materials in Spanish that reflect cultural appropriateness. An increasing number of patient education materials are available in Spanish or have been prepared for a bilingual audience.

15. Locate the hotline telephone number in the community that provides a direct link to Spanish-speaking interpreters who can assist health providers in communicating with non-English-speaking patients.

Much more must be learned about the Hispanic American population with respect to their cultural beliefs and their health and education needs. It is evident that many members of this cultural group are not receiving the kind and amount of health services they desire and deserve. Nurses need to extend themselves to Hispanics in a culturally sensitive manner to effectively and efficiently provide patient education to meet the needs of this rapidly growing segment of the U.S. population.

Black American Culture

At the present time, members of the Black American culture make up the largest minority group in the United States, but this situation is expected to change in the near future due to the rapid growth of the Hispanic population. Currently, Black Americans make up 12.2% of the U.S. population (U.S. Census Bureau, 2000).

The cultural origins of Black Americans are quite diverse. Their roots are mainly from Africa and the Caribbean Islands. They speak a variety of languages, including French, Spanish, and African dialects. The one distinguishing factor of this group is the length of time many of these people have had to acculturate to the American "way of life." Many have adapted to a number of the beliefs and practices of Western medicine. Quite a few Black families have ancestors who settled in America many generations ago, when Blacks were held as slaves. Their cultural heritage has been blended into the social fabric of America over time as Blacks were exposed to Whites with whom they lived and served (Purnell & Paulanka, 1998; Spector, 1991).

Unfortunately, a large proportion of people from the Black American culture are disadvantaged. Poverty and low educational attainment have had major consequences for the Black American community in terms of social and medical issues. These factors are strongly correlated with higher incidences of disease, poor nutrition, lower survival rates, and a decreased quality of life in general. In addition, the majority of Blacks reside in inner-city areas where exposure to violence, crowded and noisy living conditions, and pollution puts them at greater risk for disease, disability, and death (Luster & McAdoo, 1994).

The average life span of Black Americans is 6.5 years shorter than that of White Americans due to high death rates from cancer, cardiovascular disease, cirrhosis, diabetes, accidents, homicides, and infant mortality. Also, Blacks are at higher risk for drug addiction, teen pregnancy, and sexually transmitted diseases. Thirty percent of reported cases of AIDS are found in the Black population, even though Black Americans represent less than 13% of the U.S. population (Guralnik et al., 1993).

Increased exposure to hazardous working conditions has also resulted in a greater incidence of occupation-related diseases and illnesses among this population. Black American males, for example, are at increased risk for developing cancer and stress-related diseases such as hypertension and other cardiovascular illnesses associated with low-paying, insecure, dead-end jobs.

Obesity is another major problem among Black Americans. Food to them is a symbol of health and wealth, and a higher than ideal body weight is viewed as positive by this ethnic group.

Purnell & Paulanka (1998) reported findings that the Black American belief system emphasizes three major themes:

1. The world is a hostile and dangerous place to live.
2. The individual is vulnerable to attack from outside forces.
3. The individual is considered helpless with few internal resources to combat the risk factors associated with poor environmental conditions.

Furthermore, many Black Americans tend to be suspicious of health professionals. Often they hold folk practitioners in high esteem and seek the assistance of physicians and nurses only when absolutely necessary.

Common to the Black culture is the concept of extended family, consisting of several households, with the older adults often taking the leadership role within the family. Respect for elders and ancestors is valued, because living a long life indicates that the individual had more opportunities to acquire much experience and knowledge. Decision making regarding health issues is, therefore, often left to the older adults. Family ties are especially strong between grandchildren and grandparents. It is not unusual for grandmothers to want to stay at the hospital bedside when their grandchildren are ill. This extended family network provides emotional, physical, and financial support to members during times of illness and other crises (Purnell & Paulanka, 1998; Spector, 1991).

Black people often have strong religious values, and these religious beliefs may extend to their feelings about illness and health. A majority of Black Americans find inner strength from their trust in God. Some believe that whatever happens is God's will. This belief has led to the perception that Black Americans have a fatalistic view of life (Purnell & Paulanka, 1998) and are governed by a relatively strong external locus of control.

Some Black Americans believe in a folk practice known as voodoo, which consists of beliefs about spirits inhabiting the world. Living and nonliving objects have good or evil spirits. A religious priest, witch doctor, or medicine man has the power to release hostile spirits. Illness, or disharmony, is thought to be caused by evil spirits because a person failed to follow religious rules or the advice of elders. Curing an illness involves finding the cause—a hex or a spell placed on a person by another or the breaking of a taboo—and then finding someone with magical healing powers or witchcraft to get rid of the evil spirit(s). Some Black American families also continue to practice home remedies, such as the use of mustard plasters, taking of herbal medicines and teas, and wearing of amulets to cure or ward off a variety of illnesses and afflictions (Purnell & Paulanka, 1998; Spector, 1991).

Teaching Strategies

In teaching Black Americans disease preventive and health promotion measures, as well as caring for them during acute and chronic illnesses, the nurse must explore the client's value systems. Generally, any folk practices or traditional beliefs should be respected and allowed (if not harmful) and included in the recommended treatment used by Western medicine. The following discussion offers more specific recommendations for providing culturally appropriate care for Black Americans.

Black Americans tend to be very verbal and express feelings openly to family and friends. However, they are much more private about family matters when in the company of strangers. The volume of their voices tends to be louder than in other cultures and they express their thoughts in a more dynamic manner. However, these types of behaviors should not be perceived as necessarily reflecting anger or frustration. Black Americans feel comfortable with less personal space than do some other ethnic groups. Nevertheless, direct eye contact by others outside of their culture can be misinterpreted by Blacks as aggressive behavior. They are also more oriented to the present than to the past or future. Thus, they tend to be more relaxed about specific time frames. Health providers must be careful not to misinterpret nonverbal and verbal behaviors when delivering care. Also, they must be flexible in the timing of appointments, because Blacks will usually keep their appointments but may not always be on schedule.

Even though Black Americans are very informal when they interact among themselves, they prefer to be greeted in a more formal manner. Addressing them by their last name demonstrates the respect and pride they have in their family heritage. Traditionally, the family structure has been matriarchal. This pattern persists to the present day due to a high percentage of households run by a female single parent. It is important that health providers acknowledge the dominant role that Black women play in decision making and the need to share health information directly with them. Grandmothers continue to play a central role in the Black American family and are often involved in providing economic support and child care for their grandchildren.

With respect to types of diseases and health issues specific to this population group, hypertension continues to be the most serious health problem. Approximately 25% of Black Americans are hypertensive. As a whole, Blacks suffer higher morbidity and mortality rates from this disease than do other Americans. Also, Blacks are greater than three times more likely to develop kidney failure associated with hypertension. In addition, they are at higher risk for being victims of violence, accidents, disabilities, obesity, and cancer.

Strong family ties encourage individuals to be treated by the family before seeking care from health professionals. This cultural practice may be a factor contributing to the delay or failure of Blacks to seek treatment of diseases at the early stages of illness. An effective approach to providing care can be to offer health screening programs in conjunction with community and church activities where the entire family is present.

To improve the overall health status of Black Americans, health education must be culturally appropriate. Nurses must concentrate on disease prevention measures, such as early screening for high blood pressure as well as screening for signs and symptoms of other diseases and problems common in this population.

Due to economic factors, Black Americans are likely to have less access to health care services. Lack of culturally sensitive care, perceptions of racial discrimination, and a general distrust of both health professionals and the healthcare system are identified as barriers to Black Americans getting the health care they need. Establishing a trusting relationship, therefore, is an essential first step if Blacks are to receive and accept the health services they require and deserve. Recognizing their unique responses to health and illness based on their spiritual and religious foundations, their strong family ties, and other traditional beliefs is essential if therapeutic interventions by the healthcare team are to be successful.

Asian/Pacific Islander Culture

People of this cultural group come from Asian countries and the Pacific Islands. Mainly as a result of World War II, the Korean War in the 1950s, the fall of the South Vietnam government in 1975, and the social and political upheavals in China and the Philippines, there has been a large influx of Asian/Pacific Islander refugees. Almost three-quarters of a million people of Southeast Asian origin (Vietnam, Cambodia, and Laos) settled, in particular, in the West Coast region of the United States during the decades of the 1970s and 1980s (Kubota & Matsuda, 1982; Schultz, 1982). The states of New York, New Jersey, and Texas have also experienced a large immigrant population of Chinese, Filipino, and Japanese. Presently, more than 10 million Asian/Pacific Islanders (3.8% of the total U.S. population) live in our country (U.S. Census Bureau, 2000).

Although Asian/Pacific Islander people have been classified as a single ethnic group by census takers, the culture of all these people is not the same. In fact, a wide variety of cultural, religious, and language backgrounds are represented. Some similarities exist among members of the Asian/Pacific Islander group, but there are also many differences (Purnell & Paulanka, 1998). By understanding the basic beliefs of their Asian/Pacific Islander clients, nurses and other health practitioners can be better prepared to understand and accept their cultural differences and varied behavior patterns (Kubota & Matsuda, 1982).

The medical system of the Asian/Pacific Islander countries and the culture and religion of these peoples need to be understood to successfully deal with their health issues. The language barrier has proved to be the biggest problem in providing healthcare services to these populations. Many misconceptions can occur because, in particular, the Southeast Asian languages are not as technical as English.

The major orientation of the Southeast Asian people is a blend of four philosophies—Buddhism, Confucianism, Taoism, and Phi. Four common values are strongly reflected in these philosophies (Kubota & Matsuda, 1982):

1. Male authority and dominance
2. "Saving face" (behavior as a result of a sense of pride)
3. Strong family ties
4. Respect for parents, elders, teachers, and other authority figures

The Asian/Pacific Islander culture values harmony in life and a balance of nature. Shame is something to be avoided, families are the center of life, older adults are respected, and ancestors are worshiped and remembered. Children are highly valued because they carry on the family name and are expected to care for aging parents. The woman's role is one of subservience throughout her entire life—follow her parents' advice while unmarried, her husband's advice while married, and her children's advice when widowed. This dependent role is in direct conflict with U.S. social and family values, which expect women to be more independent, assertive, and self-determined.

For people of the Asian/Pacific Islander ethnic group, marked cultural differences confront them when they live in the United States with respect to ways of life, ways of thinking, values orientation, social structure, and family interactions (Chao, 1994). Children may adapt quickly to acculturation, but the older generations tend to have difficulty. Their medical practices, like their other unique cultural practices, differ significantly from Western ways. The health-seeking behaviors of immigrants are crisis oriented, following the pattern in their homelands where medical care was not readily available. They tend to seek health care only when seriously ill. Reinforcement is needed to encourage them to come for follow-up visits after an initial encounter with the healthcare system. Sometimes they are viewed by practitioners as noncompliant when they do not do exactly what is expected of them, when they withdraw from follow-up treatments, or when they do not keep pre-arranged appointments.

Asians make great use of herbal remedies to treat fevers, diarrhea, and coughs. Dermabrasion, often misunderstood by U.S. practitioners, is a home remedy to treat a wide variety of problems such as headaches, cold symptoms, and fever and chills. In their traditional healthcare system, Asian individuals rely on folk medicines from healers, sorcerers, and monks. Western medicine is thought to be "shots that cure," and Asian patients expect to get medicine (injections or pills) whenever they seek medical help in the United States. If no medication is prescribed, the person, if not given an explanation, may feel that care is inadequate and fail to return for future care.

Common to many Southeast Asians is the idea that illnesses, just like foods, are classified as hot and cold, which coincide with the *yin* and *yang* philosophy of the principles of balance. If a disease is considered hot in origin, then giving cold foods is thought of as the proper treatment.

Conflict and fear are the most likely responses to laboratory tests and having blood drawn because of the belief that removing blood makes the body weak and that blood is not replenished. Fear of surgery may result from the belief that souls inhabit the body and may be released. Loss of privacy leading to extreme embarrassment and humiliation is another major fear.

Teaching Strategies

Respect is automatically given to most healthcare providers and teachers because they are seen as knowledgeable. Asians are sensitive and formal people, so making a friendly and nonthreatening approach to them is necessary before giving care. They must be given permission to ask a question but are not offended by questions from others.

Language barriers are usually the first and biggest obstacle to overcome in dealing with people of Asian/Pacific Islander descent. Translators can be used to facilitate interactions. The learning style of Asians is essentially passive—no personal opinions, no confrontations, no challenges, and no outward disagreements. It must be remembered that decision making is a family affair. Consequently, family members need to be included, especially the male authority figure, in the process of deciding the best solution for a situation.

Nurses and other healthcare practitioners should be aware that Asians wish to "save face" for themselves and others. They avoid being disruptive and will agree to what is said so as not to be offensive. They are easily shamed, so patients must be reassured and told what is considered acceptable behavior by Western moral and legal standards. Nods of the head do not necessarily mean agreement or understanding. Questions directed to them need to be asked in several ways to confirm that they understand any instructional messages given.

Native American Culture

The U.S. Census Bureau (2000) has identified more than 2 million people (0.7% of the U.S. population) who are of Native American (American Indian or Native Alaskan) descent living in the United States. Today, the Indian Health Service (IHS) of the U.S. Public Health Service maintains responsibility for providing health care to more than 500 distinct tribes of American Indians and Native Alaskans, including Eskimo and Aleut tribes (Lowe & Struthers, 2001; Mail et al., 1989). The largest of the Native American tribes is the Navajo. Other tribes of significant size are the Cherokee, Sioux, Chippewa, and Pueblo. These tribes reside primarily in the northwestern, central, and southwestern regions of the United States.

Native American culture has the following major characteristics (Cantore, 2001; Lowe & Struthers, 2001; Primeaux, 1977; Purnell & Paulanka, 1998; Spector, 1991):

1. A spiritual attachment to the land and harmony with nature
2. An intimacy of religion and medicine
3. Emphasis on strong ties to an extended family network, including immediate family, other relatives, and the entire tribe
4. The view that children are an asset, not a liability
5. A belief that supernatural powers exist in living as well as nonliving objects
6. A desire to remain Native American and avoid acculturation, thereby retaining one's own culture and language
7. A lack of materialism and time consciousness, and a desire to share with others

Native Americans see a close connection between religion and health. When a family member becomes ill, witchcraft is still perceived by some tribes as the real cause of illness. It also explains personal insecurities, intragroup tensions, fears, and anxieties. Some Native American tribes still practice witchcraft but tend to deny it as a reality because of the negative stereotype and stigma attached to it by outsiders. Other Native American tribal beliefs include the medicine man (shaman) in the system of care given to patients. Native American medicine embraces the notion of a supernatural power. This intimacy between religion and medicine is exhibited in the form of "sing" prayers and ceremonial cure practices. However, few nurses would think of providing space and privacy for several relatives to be able to conduct a ceremony for a hospitalized family member.

To be considered really poor in the Native American world is to have no relatives. The family and tribe are of utmost importance—a belief that children learn from infancy. It is not unusual for many family members, sometimes including groups as large as 10 to 15 people, to arrive at the hospital and camp out on the hospital grounds to be with their sick relative. Talking is unnecessary, but simply being there is highly important for everyone concerned. Hospital personnel often see this behavior as useless and disruptive and frequently label the patient and family as uncooperative.

Children are doted on by family members, and, in turn, they have high regard for their elders. In fact, the older adults in Native American communities are highly respected and looked to for advice and counsel. Grandmothers, in particular, have great importance to a sick child, and they frequently must give permission for a child to be hospitalized and treated. The Native American kinship system, in fact, allows for a child to have several sets of grandparents, aunts, uncles, cousins, brothers, and sisters. Sometimes a number of women substitute as a mother figure for a child, which may cause role confusion for the non-Native American healthcare provider.

Another characteristic of Native Americans is that they generally are not very future oriented. They take one day at a time and do not feel they have control over their own destiny. Time is seen as being on a continuum with no beginning and no end. Native Americans do not tend to live by clocks and schedules. In fact, many of their homes do not have clocks, and family members eat meals and do other activities when they please. They are more casual in their approach to life than many non-Native American people. This lack of time consciousness and pressure is a crucial factor to be remembered by healthcare providers when a prescribed regimen calls for the patient to follow a medication, exercise, or dietary schedule. Inattention to time also can interfere with their keeping scheduled appointments.

Another aspect of time is reflected in their belief that death is just a part of the life cycle. Funerals are accompanied by large feasts and the sharing of gifts with relatives of the deceased. There is no belief in a life hereafter as a reward for a lifetime of good deeds while on earth. Life after death is, instead, viewed as an opportunity to join the world of long-ago ancestors. Their view of death is closely related to their opinion about the appropriate disposal of amputated limbs. Because diabetes is so prevalent in the Native American population, it is important to know that they usually want to reclaim an amputated body part for proper burial.

Sharing is another core value of Native Americans. The concept of "being" is fundamental, and there is little stress on achievement or material wealth. Individuals are valued much more highly than material goods. Overall, Native Americans are a proud, sensitive, cooperative, passive people, devoted to tribe and family, and willing to share possessions and self with others. They are very vulnerable when it comes to their pride and dignity. They can be easily offended by health providers who are insensitive to their cultural beliefs and practices.

In terms of human relationships, it is important to note that Native Americans believe that to look someone in the eye is considered disrespectful. Some tribes feel that looking into the eyes of another person reveals and may even steal someone's soul. As a friendly handshake and eye contact are acceptable and even expected in many cultures, it must be acknowledged that these gestures do not have the same meaning for the Native American. In fact, lack of eye contact should never be misinterpreted to mean that someone is not paying attention, is disinterested, or does not understand instruction being given (Primeaux, 1977).

The health problems faced by Native Americans are undergoing significant change. In the first half of the twentieth century, acute and infectious diseases were prevalent and were the principal cause of death. Today, as a result of increased life expectancy, Native Americans are succumbing to many lifestyle diseases and chronic conditions. Chief among the causes of morbidity and mortality are heart disease, cancer, diabetes, and drug and alcohol abuse—all of which to some extent are amenable to educational intervention.

Teaching Strategies

Patient education by nurses needs to focus on giving information about these diseases and risk factors, emphasizing the teaching of skills related to changes in diet and exercise, and helping clients to build positive coping mechanisms to deal with emotional problems (Hosey & Stracqualursi, 1990). For the most part, acute and infectious diseases, with the exception of a recurrence in tuberculosis, are no longer a major cause of illness and death among Native Americans, thanks to drug therapy, early case findings, and improved sanitary conditions. Another positive influence on Native American health has been the greater availability of community health representatives (CHRs). CHRs are Native American outreach workers who live and work in the community. They play a significant role in case finding, early diagnosis, and reinforcement of patient and other health education recommendations. As Mail et al. (1989) stated: "Involving the CHR in patient education is an important cross-cultural consideration, because this is the individual who will reinforce behavior changes with the community and home" (p. 97).

Although all Native Americans share some of the core beliefs and practices of their culture, each tribe is unique in its customs and language. Finding the ways and means to integrate Western medicine with the traditional Native American folk medicine presents a challenge to the nurses caring for the varied needs of this population group.

PREPARING NURSES FOR DIVERSITY CARE _____

America is no longer the homogeneous society it once was. Today, the United States is made up of many cultures. Also, there is an increasing trend toward global migration of people and globalization of nursing practice. Nurses must be prepared to care for consumers from a variety of cultural backgrounds. The delivery of appropriate health care now and in the future will depend on use of a culturally informed approach that goes beyond simple language translation and an understanding of the characteristics of different cultures. Diversity has the potential to positively affect our profession. As caregivers, we must learn how to relate to people from a variety of cultural backgrounds and appreciate the cultural meaning of various health events (Dreher, 1996; Marquand, 2001; Thomas & Ely, 1996).

As a result of former President Clinton's national leadership to eliminate cultural disparities in health by the year 2010, the U.S. Department of Health and Human Services (DHHS) established the Initiative to Eliminate Racial and Ethnic Disparities in Health. This "2010 Initiative" calls for the nursing profession to eliminate differences in health outcomes among minority populations. The profession needs to do so in both the academic and the practice settings and through clinical research (Carol, 2001).

One important step to assure culturally competent nursing care in this new century is to increase minority representation in nursing. We need to recruit and retain more minority students and faculty to expand diversity within our ranks. Unfortunately, the nursing workforce comprises less than 10% of people from minority groups, whereas more than 28% of the total U.S. population belongs to a variety of cultural subgroups (Robinson, 2000).

Another initiative to break down cultural barriers to health care is to strengthen multicultural perspectives in the curriculum of nursing education programs (Kelley & Fitzsimmons, 2000). This means that nursing education must recognize diverse lifestyles and acknowledge multicultural and multiracial perspectives (Sims & Baldwin, 1995). As Dreher (1996) points out, nurses must not only better understand the cultural characteristics and traits of patients and families from different ethnic backgrounds, but also improve the relationship between nurses and clients from different cultural backgrounds. Nurses must be able to create an environment in which people are encouraged to express themselves and freely describe their needs. As Dreher so aptly states, "Transcending cultural differences is more than an appreciation of cultural diversity. It is transcending one's own investment in the social and economic system as one knows it and lives it" (p. 4). Nurses must concentrate on the cultural strategies that are needed to help individuals and groups negotiate the health-care system.

STEREOTYPING: IDENTIFYING THE MEANING, THE RISKS, AND THE SOLUTIONS

In addressing the diversity issues of gender, socioeconomics, and culture, one must acknowledge the risks of stereotyping when discussing these three attributes of the learner. Throughout this chapter, it has been recognized that differences exist in learning based on gender, socioeconomics, and culture, and these often require alternative approaches to teaching. It is important to realize that differences should not lead to judgments as to what is good or bad, right or wrong. Rather, these differences should be addressed in a sensitive, open, and fair manner. Nurses must relate to each person as an individual. Although each person belongs to a certain group or subgroup, the individual has his or her own abilities, experiences, preferences, and practices that influence lifestyle behaviors.

Nevertheless, given that we all have been socialized in subtle and not so subtle ways, it is important to acknowledge the prejudices, biases, and stereotypical tendencies that can come into play when dealing with others like or unlike ourselves. We must consciously attempt to recognize these possible attitudes and the effect they may have on others in our care.

Stereotyping is defined by Purnell and Paulanka (1998) as "an oversimplified conception, opinion, or belief about some aspect of an individual or group" (p. 490). Stereotyping is a generalization made about the behaviors of any person or people and is used to label someone (Woolfolk, 1998). For example, we, as Americans, think of ourselves as the freedom fighters and liberty lovers of the world. In the same breath, we may describe members of other groups or nationalities as violators of human rights or terrorists. Simple appearance, such as a beard, type of dress, or form of speech, can be the basis of broad and deep prejudices. We particularly tend to use an excuse to classify individuals when we do not like or respect people whose backgrounds, attitudes, abilities, values, or beliefs are different from or opposed to our own or are misunderstood or misinterpreted. Stereotyping, whether we are aware of our biases or not, results in intolerance toward others. It promotes the belief that our way is the only or the right way. In nursing practice, stereotyping by nurses tends to marginalize patients (Corley & Goren, 1998).

Attitudes toward sex-role competencies are considered a type of stereotyping. Gender bias has produced inequality in education, employment, and other social spheres. For example, research in the past 20 years has documented that teachers in school classrooms interact more actively with boys than with girls by asking boys more questions, giving them more feedback (praise and positive encouragement), and providing them with more specific and valuable comments and guidance. In these subtle ways, stereotypical expectations are reinforced (Gage & Berliner, 1998; Woolfolk, 1998). As another example, women have been labelled as attentive listeners and men as poor listeners when, in fact, listening behavior is not a measure of attentiveness but a matter of behavioral style. Men, when listening, move around and make sporadic eye contact, whereas women are likely to remain still and maintain steady eye contact with occasional nodding or smiling. As a result, the listening style of men is often misinterpreted as inattentive or rude, and the style of females is often mistaken for encouraging or agreeing with what is being said. Even though in the twentieth century women made great strides toward equal opportunity, both socially and economically, stereotypical attitudes persist. Much more attention is being paid to this issue, but we have a long way to go to rid our society of gender bias.

Nurses must concentrate on treating the sexes equally when providing access to health education, delivering health and illness care, and designing health education materials that contain bias-free language. For example, choose gender-specific terms that minimize ambiguity in gender identity, unless critical to the content. If at all possible, avoid using the pronoun *he* or *she* and instead use the plural pronoun *they*. Guidelines for nonsexist language can be found in *McGraw-Hill Guidelines for Bias-Free Publishing* or *The Bias-Free Word Finder.*

With respect to age, socioeconomics, culture, or disability, stereotyping most definitely exists. Throughout this chapter, there are many cautions against stereotyping of individuals and groups. For example, just because someone belongs to a specific cultural group does not necessarily mean that the individual adheres to all of the beliefs and practices of that particular culture. A thorough and accurate assessment of the learner is the key to determining the particular abilities, preferences, and needs of each individual. Refer to someone's ethnicity, race, religion, age, and socioeconomic status only when it is essential to the content being addressed. Just as with issues of gender, you should choose words that are accurate, clear, and free from bias whenever speaking or writing about various individuals or groups. For instance, it is more politically and socially correct to use the term *older adult* or *older people* than to refer to them as *the elderly*. Do not label a member of a special population as a *disabled person* but rather as a *person with a disability*. It is more appropriate and more acceptable to refer to a *person with diabetes* rather than a *diabetic* or to a *person with AIDS* rather than an *AIDS victim*.

To avoid stereotyping, nurses should ask themselves the following questions:

- Do I use neutral language when teaching clients and families?
- Do I confront bias when evidenced by other healthcare professionals?
- Do I request information equally from clients regardless of gender, socioeconomic status, age, or culture?
- Are my instructional materials free of stereotypical terminology and expressions?
- Am I an effective role model of equality for my colleagues?
- Do I treat all clients with fairness, respect, and dignity?
- Does someone's appearance influence (raise or lower) my expectations of that person's abilities or affect the quality of care I deliver?
- Do I routinely assess the educational and experiential backgrounds, personal attributes, and economic resources of clients to ensure appropriate health teaching?
- Am I knowledgeable enough of the cultural traditions of various groups to provide sensitive care in our multicultural society?

It is easy to stereotype someone, not purposefully, but out of ignorance. Nurses have a responsibility to keep informed of the most current information about various gender attributes, socioeconomic influences, and cultural traditions that affect teaching and learning. Every day, research in nursing, social science, psychology, and medicine is yielding information that will assist in planning and revising appropriate nursing interventions to meet the needs of our diverse client populations.

SUMMARY

This chapter explored the influence of gender, socioeconomic status, and cultural beliefs on both the ability and willingness of clients to learn healthcare measures. The most important message to remember from this chapter is the care one must take not to stereotype or generalize common characteristics of a group to all members associated with that particular group. If the nurse does not know much about a particular culture, that lack of knowledge is acceptable. The more important point is to ask clients about their beliefs, rather than just assuming they practice those beliefs associated with a certain cultural group. In that way, nurses can avoid offending the learner.

In their role as teachers, nurses must be cautious to treat each learner as an individual. They must determine the extent to which patients and family members ascribe to, exhibit beliefs in, or adhere to ways of doing things that might affect learning.

Both men and women live in a double environment—an outer layer of social and cultural experiences and an inner layer of innate strengths and weaknesses—that affects how they perceive and respond to their world (Griffith, 1982). Nurses, as professionals, should constantly strive to improve the delivery of care to all people regardless of their gender orientation, socioeconomic background, ethnic origin, creed, or nationality (Holtz & Bairan, 1990). There is much more for nurses to know about how these three factors of gender, socioeconomics, and culture affect the teaching-learning process before we can competently, confidently, and sensitively deliver care to satisfy the needs of our socially, intellectually, and culturally diverse clientele.

REVIEW QUESTIONS

1. What are five gender-related characteristics in cognitive functioning and personality that affect learning?
2. How does the environment versus heredity influence gender-specific approaches to learning?
3. In what ways does SES negatively affect a person's health and, conversely, how does illness impact an individual's socioeconomic well-being?
4. How does the SES of individuals influence the teaching-learning process?
5. What is meant by the term *poverty circle*?
6. What is the definition of each of the following terms: *acculturation*, *assimilation*, *culture*, and *ethnocentrism*?
7. How can the concept of transcultural nursing be applied to the assessment and teaching of clients from culturally diverse backgrounds?
8. What are the six cultural phenomena that should be taken into account when conducting a nursing assessment?
9. Which four components are included in the Culturally Competent Model of Care?
10. What are the four major cultural groups in the United States?
11. What are the salient characteristics of each of the four major cultural groups?
12. Which teaching strategies are most appropriate to meet the needs of individuals from each of the four major cultural groups?
13. What can the nurse do to avoid cultural stereotyping?

REFERENCES

Anderson, J. M. (1987). The cultural context of caring. *Canadian Critical Care Nursing Journal*, December, 7–13.

Anderson, J. M. (1990). Health care across cultures. *Nursing Outlook, 38*(3), 136–139.

Andrews, M. M. (1992). Cultural perspectives on nursing in the 21st century. *Journal of Professional Nursing, 8*(1), 7–15.

Andrews, M. M. & Boyle, J. S. (1995). Transcultural nursing care. In M. M. Andrews & J. S. Boyle (Eds.), *Transcultural Concepts in Nursing Care* (2nd ed., pp. 49–95). Philadelphia: Lippincott.

Baker, D. W., Parker, R. M., Williams, M. V., Coates, W. C., & Pitkin, K. (1996). Use and effectiveness of interpreters in an emergency department. *Journal of the American Medical Association, 275*(10), 783–788.

Baron-Cohen, S. (2005). The essential difference: The male and female brain. *Phi Kappa Phi Forum, 85*(1), 23–26.

Baydar, N., Brooks-Gunn, J., & Furstenberg, F. F. (1993). Early warning signs of functional illiteracy: Predictors in childhood and adolescence. *Child Development, 64*, 815–829.

Begley, S. (February 19, 1996). Your child's brain. *Newsweek*, 55–62.

Begley, S., Murr, A., & Rogers, A. (March 27, 1995). Gray matters. *Newsweek*, 48–54.

Campinha-Bacote, J. (1995). The quest for cultural competence in nursing care. *Nursing Forum, 30*(4), 19–25.

Cantore, J. A. (2001). Earth, wind, fire and water. *Minority Nurse*, Winter, 24–29.

Carol, R. (2001). Taking the initiative. *Minority Nurse*, Fall, 24–27.

Caudle, P. (1993). Providing culturally sensitive health care to Hispanic clients. *Nurse Practitioner, 18*(12), 40, 43–44, 46, 50–51.

Chachkes, E. & Christ, G. (1996). Cross cultural issues in patient education. *Patient Education & Counseling, 27*, 13–21.

Chao, R. K. (1994). Beyond parental control and authoritarian parenting style: Understanding Chinese parenting through the cultural notion of training. *Child Development, 65*, 1111–1119.

Chideya, F. (1999). *The color of our future*. New York: William Morrow.

Cohen, D. (ed.). (1991). *The circle of life: Rituals from the human family album*. New York: Harper-Collins.

Corley, M. C. & Goren, S. (1998). The dark side of nursing: Impact of stigmatizing responses on patients. *Scholarly Inquiry for Nursing Practice: An International Journal, 12*(2), 99–118.

Crimmins, E. M. & Saito, Y. (2001). Trends in healthy life expectancy in the United States, 1970–1990: Gender, race, and educational differences. *Social Science & Medicine, 52*, 1629–1641.

Denboba, D. L., Bragdon, J. L., Epstein, L. G., Garthright, K., & Goldman, T. M. (1998). Reducing health disparities through cultural competence. *Journal of Health Education, 29*(5), 47–53.

Dreher, M. C. (1996). Nursing: A cultural phenomenon. *Reflections*, 4th Quarter, 4.

Duffy, M. M. & Snyder, K. (1999). Can ED patients read your education materials? *Journal of Emergency Nursing, 25*(4), 294–297.

Gage, N. L. & Berliner, D. C. (1992). *Educational psychology* (5th ed.). Boston: Houghton Mifflin.

Gage, N. L. & Berliner, D. C. (1998). *Educational psychology* (6th ed.). Boston: Houghton Mifflin.

Galanti, G. A. (1991). *Caring for patients from different cultures*. Philadelphia: University of Pennsylvania Press.

Giger, J. N. & Davidhizar, R. E. (1995). *Transcultural nursing: Assessment and intervention* (2nd ed.). St. Louis: Mosby-Year Book.

Gollop, C. J. (1997). Health information-seeking behavior and older African American women. *Bulletin of the Medical Library Association, 85*(2), 141–146.

Gorman, C. (January 20, 1992). Sizing up the sexes. *Time*, 42–51.

Griffith, S. (1982). Childbearing and the concept of culture. *Journal of Obstetrics, Gynecological, and Neonatal Nursing, 11*(3), 181–184.

Guralnik, J. M., Land, K. C., Blazer, D., Fillenbaum, G. G., & Branch, L. C. (1993). Educational status and active life expectancy among older Blacks and whites. *New England Journal of Medicine, 329*(2), 110–116.

Hahn, M. (1995). Providing health care in a culturally complex world. *Advance for Nurse Practitioners*, November, 43–45.

Hancock, L. (February 19, 1996). Why do schools flunk biology? *Newsweek*, 59.

Hirsch, E. D. (2001). Overcoming the language gap. *American Educator*, Summer, 5–7.

Holtz, C. & Bairan, A. (1990). Personal contact: A method of teaching cultural empathy. *Nurse Educator, 15*(3), 13, 23, 28.

Horton, M. & Freire, P. (1990). *We make the road by walking*. Philadelphia: Temple University Press.

Hosey, G. M. & Stracqualursi, F. (1990). Designing and evaluating diabetes education material for American Indians. *Diabetes Educator, 16*(5), 407–414.

Jackson, L. E. (1993). Understanding, eliciting, and negotiating clients' multicultural health beliefs. *Nurse Practitioner, 18*(4), 30–43.

Jezewski, M. A. (1993). Culture brokering as a model for advocacy. *Nursing & Health Care, 14*(2), 78–85.

Kawamura, M., Midorikawa, A., & Kezuka, M. (2000). Cerebral localization of the center for reading and writing music. *NeuroReport, 11*(14), 3299–3303.

Kelley, M. L. & Fitzsimmons, V. M. (2000). *Understanding cultural diversity: Culture, curriculum, and community in nursing*. Boston: Jones and Bartlett.

Kniep-Hardy, M. & Burkhardt, M. A. (1977). Nursing the Navajo. *American Journal of Nursing, 77*(1), 95–96.

Kubota, J. & Matsuda, K. J. (1982). Family planning services for southeast Asian refugees. *Family & Community Health, 5*(1), 19–25.

Leininger, M. (1978). *Transcultural nursing: Concepts, theories and practices*. New York: Wiley.

Leininger, M. (1994). Transcultural nursing education: A worldwide imperative. *Nursing & Health Care, 15*(5), 254–257.

Lipman, E. L., Offord, D. R., & Boyle, M. H. (1994). Relation between economic disadvantage and psychosocial morbidity in children. *Canadian Medical Association Journal, 151*(4), 431–437.

Lowe, J. & Struthers, R. (2001). A conceptual framework of nursing in Native American culture. *Journal of Nursing Scholarship*, 3rd Quarter, 279–283.

Luster, T. & McAdoo, H. P. (1994). Factors related to the achievement and adjustment of young African American children. *Child Development, 65*, 1080–1094.

Mail, P. D., McKay, R. B., & Katz, M. (1989). Expanding practice horizons: Learning from American Indian patients. *Patient Education & Counseling, 13*, 91–102.

Markides, K. S. & Coreil, J. (1986). The health of Hispanics in southwestern U.S.: An epidemiological paradox. *Public Health Reports, 101*(3), 253–265.

Marquand, B. (2001). On the front lines of diversity. *Minority Nurse*, Fall, 46–49.

Massett, H. A. (1996). Appropriateness of Hispanic print materials: A content analysis. *Health Education Research*, *11*(2), 231–242.

McGoldrick, M. (1995). *You can go home again*. New York: W. W. Norton.

Monastersky, R. (November 2, 2001). Land mines in the world of mental maps. *Chronicle of Higher Education*, A20–A21.

Morra, M. E. (1991). Future trends in patient education. *Seminars in Oncology Nursing*, 7(2), 143–145.

Nagoshi, C. T., Johnson, R. C., & Honbo, K. A. (1993). Family background, cognitive abilities, and personality as predictors of education and occupational attainment across two generations. *Journal of Biosocial Science*, *25*(2), 259–276.

Nash, J. M. (1997). Fertile minds. *Time*, *149*(5), 48–56.

Ormrod, J. E. (1995). *Educational psychology: Principles and applications*. Englewood Cliffs, NJ: Prentice-Hall.

Pappas, G., Queen, S., Hadden, W., & Fisher, G. (1993). The increasing disparity in mortality between socioeconomic groups in the United States, 1960 and 1986. *New England Journal of Medicine*, *329*(2), 103–109.

Parker, M. & Kiatoukaysy, L. N. (1999). Culturally responsive health care: The example of the Hmong in America. *Journal of the American Academy of Nurse Practitioners*, *11*(12), 511–518.

Perry, D. S. (1982). The umbilical cord: Transcultural care and customs. *Journal of Nurse-Midwifery*, *27*(4), 25–30.

Poss, J. E. & Rangel, R. (1995). Working effectively with interpreters in the primary care setting. *Nurse Practitioner*, *20*(12), 43–44, 46–47.

Price, J. L. & Cordell, B. (1994). Cultural diversity and patient teaching. *Journal of Continuing Education in Nursing*, *25*(4), 163–166.

Price, K. M. & Cortis, J. D. (2000). The way forward for transcultural nursing. *Nurse Education Today*, *20*, 233–243.

Primeaux, M. (1977). Caring for the American Indian patient. *American Journal of Nursing*, 77(1), 91–94.

Purnell, L. D. & Paulanka, B. J. (1998). *Transcultural health care: A culturally competent approach*. Philadelphia: F.A. Davis.

Rhem, J. (1998). Social class and student learning. *National Teaching & Learning Forum*, 7(5), 1–4.

Robinson, J. H. (2000). Increasing students' cultural sensitivity. *Nurse Educator*, *25*(3), 131–135.

Rooda, L. & Gay, G. (1993). Staff development for culturally sensitive nursing care. *Journal of Nursing Staff Development*, *9*(6), 262–265.

Schultz, S. L. (1982). How Southeast-Asian refugees in California adapt to unfamiliar health care practices. *Health & Social Work*, 7(2), 148–156.

Shomaker, D. M. (1981). Navajo nursing homes: Conflict of philosophies. *Journal of Gerontological Nursing*, 7(9), 531–536.

Sims, G. P. & Baldwin, D. (1995). Race, class, and gender considerations in nursing education. *Nursing & Health Care*, *16*(6), 316–321.

Smolan, R., Moffitt, P., & Naythons, M. (1990). *The power to heal: Ancient arts and modern medicine*. New York: Prentice Hall Press.

Speck, O., Ernst, T., Braun, J., Koch, C., Miller, E., & Chang, L. (2000). Gender differences in the functional organization of the brain for working memory. *NeuroReport*, *11*(11), 2581–2585.

Spector, R. E. (1991). *Cultural diversity in health and illness* (3rd ed.). Norwalk, CT: Appleton & Lange.

Spicer, J. G., Ripple, H. B., Louie, E., Baj, P., & Keating, S. (1994). Supporting ethnic and cultural diversity in nursing staff. *Nursing Management, 25*(1), 38–40.

Tear, J. (November 20, 1995). They just don't understand gender dynamics. *Wall Street Journal*, A14.

Thomas, D. A. & Ely, R. J. (1996). Making differences matter: A new paradigm for managing diversity. *Harvard Business Review, 74*(5), 79–90.

Torres, S. (1994). A challenge to nursing education: Meeting the health care needs of the Hispanic community. *Deans Notes: A Communication Service to Nursing School Deans, Administrators, and Faculty, 15*(5).

Tripp-Reimer, T. & Afifi, L. A. (1989). Cross-cultural perspectives on patient teaching. *Nursing Clinics of North America, 24*(3), 613–619.

U.S. Census Bureau. (2000). *Population estimates program*. Washington, DC: Author.

Westberg, J. (1989). Patient education for Hispanic Americans. *Patient Education & Counseling, 13*, 143–160.

Winkleby, M. A., Jatulis, D. E., Frank, E., & Fortmann, S. P. (1992). Socioeconomic status and health: How education, income, and occupation contribute to risk factors for cardiovascular disease. *American Journal of Public Health, 82*(6), 816–820.

Woolfolk, A. E. (1998). *Educational psychology* (7th ed.). Boston: Allyn and Bacon.

Yee, S-H., Liu, H-L., Hou, J., Pu, Y., Fox, P. T., & Gao, J-H. (2000). Detection of the brain response during a cognitive task using perfusion-based event-related functional MRI. *NeuroReport, 11*(11), 2533–2536.

CHAPTER 9

Special Populations

Kay Viggiani

CHAPTER HIGHLIGHTS

The Nurse's Role in Assessment
Types of Disabilities
Sensory Deficits
   Hearing Impairments
   Visual Impairments
Learning Disabilities
   Input Disabilities
   Output Disabilities
   Attention Deficit Disorder
Physical Disabilities
   Brain Injury

Communication Disorders
   Expressive Aphasia
   Receptive Aphasia
   Dysarthria
Chronic Illness
   The Family's Role in Chronic Illness or Disability
Adaptive Computing
   Types of Computer Adaptations

KEY TERMS

adaptive computing
attention deficit disorder
brain injury
chronic illness
disability
dysarthria
expressive aphasia
habilitation

hearing impairment
input and output disabilities
learning disability
receptive aphasia
rehabilitation
sensory deficits
visual impairment

OBJECTIVES

After completing this chapter, the reader will be able to

1. Describe how visual and hearing deficits require adaptive intervention.
2. Identify the various teaching strategies that are effective with learning disabilities.
3. Describe the appropriate adaptation of the teaching-learning plan for patients with a brain injury.

4. Enhance the teaching-learning process for someone with a communication disorder.
5. Discuss the teaching-learning process with patients and their families who are living with a chronic illness.
6. Describe adaptive computing and its application for people with disabilities.

Teaching others to be independent in self-management of their lives is a critical and challenging role for the nurse in any setting and with any population of individuals. However, the teaching-learning process is especially challenging when dealing with patients who have altered functional status due to a disabling condition affecting their physical, cognitive, or sensory capacities. The nurse's efforts must be directed toward assisting individuals with a disability and their significant others to maintain already established patterns of living or to develop new ones to accommodate changes in functional ability.

The terms *habilitation* and *rehabilitation* are frequently used to differentiate approaches for managing developmental and acquired types of disabilities. "Habilitation includes all the activities and interactions that enable an individual with a disability to develop new abilities to achieve his or her maximum potential, whereas rehabilitation is the relearning of previous skills, which often requires an adjustment to altered functional abilities and altered lifestyle" (Burkett, 1989, p. 239).

Unfortunately, an increasing number of individuals are faced with having to deal with a disability caused by an injury, a disease, or a birth defect that is permanent and has long-term consequences on their mode of living. Nurses need to be prepared to use teaching strategies that will meet the demands of a broad range of clients whose problems and situations are the result of a disability. The teaching-learning process is an essential part of habilitation and rehabilitation in assisting disabled clients to make the transition from being dependent to becoming independent in self-care. Appropriate patient education can help clients and their family members learn new information, develop new skills, and make changes in their lifestyles that will aid in recovery, add to their quality of life, prevent future disability, and allow them to adapt to future situations (Diehl, 1989; Weeks, 1995).

People with special needs may look like the average person, but then again, they may not. Some will have obvious physical disabilities, whereas others may have a limitation that on the surface may not make them appear different from anyone else. The one thing that they will have in common is a problem that makes learning more difficult for them. For the purpose of this chapter, the term *disability* is defined as "the inability to perform some key life functions" (Dittmar, 1989, p. 7).

On July 26, 1990, President George H. W. Bush signed into law the Americans with Disabilities Act (ADA). The definition of disability under the ADA is "a physical or mental impairment which substantially limits one or more of the major life activities of the individual." A "major life activity" includes functions such as caring for oneself, standing, lifting, reaching, seeing, hearing, speaking, breathing, learning, and walking. This significant legislation extends civil rights protection to an estimated 43 million Americans with disabilities (Merrow & Corbett, 1994). The ADA protects those who are disabled from being discriminated against. Therefore, people with disabilities are found in every setting in which nurses practice, such as schools, clinics, hospitals, nursing homes, occupational health, and home care. Persons who have special needs as a result of a disability will expect nurses and other health professionals to provide appropriate instruction adapted to meet their particular circumstances.

The role of the nurse in teaching the disabled client continues to evolve, as more than ever before clients are assuming greater responsibility as self-care agents. The focus of the nurse's teaching efforts should be on the strengths—not limitations—of the individual. In addition, the family should be encouraged to become involved in the habilitation and rehabilitation process. The family and significant others are the disabled person's support system in the community. They must be invited right from the beginning to take an active part in learning information as it applies to assisting with self-care activities for their loved ones. Thus, it is important for nurses to design and promote an environment conducive to learning (Diehl, 1989). We must become aware of the barriers that exist as well as the interventions and technologies that are available to help special populations overcome those barriers (Cunningham, 2001).

The nurse as teacher of special populations is a unique aspect of this book. Few other publications address the subject or suggest nursing interventions that involve teaching self-care measures to individuals with a wide range of disabilities. This chapter provides an overview of some of the more common disabilities. It addresses the learning problems of population groups with various types of deficits and highlights the role of the nurse in designing and implementing specific teaching strategies to accommodate the needs of disabled patients and their families. A resource list is provided in Appendix B as a further reference to the reader who seeks additional information about a specific disability.

THE NURSE'S ROLE IN ASSESSMENT

Prior to teaching, assessment is always the first step in determining the nature of the client's problems, the short- and long-term consequences of a disability, the effectiveness of the client's coping mechanisms, and the type and extent of the deficits being experienced. The nurse must determine the client's knowledge with respect to the disability, the amount and type of new information needed to change behavior, and the client's readiness to learn. At this initial stage, it is important that the nurse obtain information about the client and family by using the assessment skills of observation, testing, and interviewing. Also, information from other members of the healthcare team about their perceptions of the client's needs should be taken into account.

Diehl (1989) outlines the following questions to be asked when determining the client's readiness to learn:

1. Do the patient and family members demonstrate an interest in learning by requesting information or asking questions?
2. Are there obstacles to learning such as low literacy, vision problems, or hearing impairments? If so, is the client willing and able to use supportive devices?
3. What learning style best suits the client to process information?
4. Are the goals of the client and family the same?
5. Is the environment appropriate for learning?
6. Does the client value the learning of new information and skills as a means to achieve an optimal level of functioning?

TYPES OF DISABILITIES

The disabilities affecting millions of Americans can be categorized into two major types: mental and physical. These disabilities may result from injury, disease, heredity, or congenital defect. The following five categories have been chosen for discussion: sensory deficits, learning disabilities, physical disabilities, communication disorders, and chronic illness. Included within the section discussing each category are the specific teaching strategies that should be used to meet the needs of the learner who has a particular disability.

SENSORY DEFICITS

Hearing Impairments

People with impaired hearing have a complete loss (deafness) or a reduction in their sensitivity to sounds (hard of hearing). *Hearing impairment* is a term used to describe any type of hearing loss, the etiology of which may be related to either conductive or sensorineural problems resulting from congenital defect, trauma, or disease (Strong, 1996).

Currently about 10% of Americans (approximately 26 million people) have some degree of hearing loss, ranging from mild to severe (McCafferty, 2002). Approximately 1.8 million people in this country are deaf. A recent national health survey estimates that hearing loss among 18–44-year-olds increased by 17% between 1971 and 1990 (Stock, 2002). Regardless of the degree of hearing loss, any person with a hearing impairment faces communication barriers that interfere with efforts at patient teaching. Hearing loss poses a very real communication problem because deaf and hearing-impaired individuals may also have limited verbal abilities. This is especially true for adults who have been deaf since early childhood.

It is clear that individuals who are deaf will have different skills and needs depending on how long they have been without a sense of hearing. For those persons who have been deaf since birth, most likely they rely on American Sign Language (ASL) and lip-reading to communicate. If deafness has occurred early in life but after language has been acquired, they may speak quite understandably and have some lip-reading abilities. If deafness has occurred in later life, often caused by the process of aging, affected individuals will probably have poor lip-reading ability, but their reading and writing skills should be within average range, depending on their educational and experiential background. If aging is the cause of hearing loss, visual impairments may also be a complicating factor. Because vision and hearing are two common sensory losses in later adulthood, these deficits pose major communication problems when teaching older clients.

Deaf and hearing-impaired persons, like other individuals, will require health care and health education information at various periods during their life. Although nurses will encounter many differences among people who are deaf, there is one common denominator—they will always rely on their other senses for information input, especially their sense of sight. For patient education to be effective, then, communication must be visible.

Because there are several different ways to communicate with a person who is deaf, one of the first things you need to do is ask your client to identify how they prefer to communicate. Sign language, written information, lip-reading, and visual aids are some of the common choices. It is true that one of the simplest ways to transfer information is through visible communication signals such as hand gestures and facial expressions. However, these methods will not be adequate for any lengthy teaching sessions. The following modes of communication are suggested as ways to decrease the barriers to communication and facilitate teaching and learning for hearing-impaired patients in any setting in which nurses practice.

Sign Language

For most deaf people whose native language is ASL, this is often the primary mode of communication. If you do not know ASL, you need to obtain the services of a professional interpreter. Sometimes a family member or friend of the patient skilled in signing is willing and available to act as a translator during teaching sessions. However, before seeking the assistance of an interpreter, always be certain to ask for the patient's permission, because information communicated about health issues may be considered personal and private. If the information to be taught is confidential, it is advised that family or friends should not be asked to serve as an interpreter. Hiring a certified language interpreter is often the best strategy.

When considering the services of an interpreter, be certain that the deaf individual is the one who has made the choice. If a professional interpreter is requested by a deaf patient in a health facility receiving federal funds, it is required by federal law that one be secured (Section 504 of the Rehabilitation Act of 1973, PL 93-112). If the patient cannot provide the names of interpreters, contact the Registry of Interpreters of the Deaf (RID) in your state. This registry can provide an up-to-date list of qualified sign language interpreters.

When working with an interpreter, be sure to stand or sit next to the interpreter. Talk at a normal pace, and look and talk directly to the deaf person when speaking.

Lip-reading

One common misconception among hearing persons is that all people who are deaf can read lips. This assumption is potentially dangerous. Only about 40% of English sounds are visible on the lips. Therefore, only a skilled lip-reader will obtain any real benefit from this form of communication (DiPietro, 1979).

If the individual can lip-read, do not exaggerate your lip movements, because this action will distort the movements of the lips and interfere with interpretation of your words. If lip-reading is preferred, you must be sure to provide sufficient lighting on your face and remove all barriers from around your face so that your mouth can be clearly seen. Beards and mustaches also present a challenge to the lip-reader. Because less than half of the English language is visible on the lips, this form of communication should be supplemented with signing or written materials.

Written Materials

Written information is probably the most reliable way to communicate, especially when understanding is critical. In fact, always write down the important information to reinforce the spoken word even when the person is versed in lip-reading.

Be certain to provide printed patient education materials that match the readability level of your audience. When putting information in writing for your client who is deaf, keep the message as simple and specific as possible. For instance, instead of writing, "When running a fever, take two aspirin," revise your message to read, "For a fever of 100.5°F or more, take two aspirin." Remember that a person with low reading skills often interprets words literally; therefore, the word *running* could be confusing because it is often used in the context of someone who is "running to the store," for example (see the guidelines for writing or revising educational materials in Chapter 7). Visual aids such as simple pictures, drawings, diagrams, and models are useful tools to increase understanding of the message contained in written materials.

Verbalization by the Client

Sometimes clients who are deaf will choose to communicate through speaking, especially if you have established a rapport and a trusting relationship with them. Often the tone and inflection of the patient's voice will be different than normal speech, so you must give yourself time to listen carefully to what is being said. Listen without interruptions until you become accustomed to the person's particular tone of voice and speech rhythms. If you still have trouble understanding what a client is saying, try writing down what you hear, which may help you to get the gist of the message.

Sound Augmentation

For those patients who have a hearing loss but are not completely deaf, hearing aids are often a useful device. Clients who have already been fitted for a hearing aid should be encouraged to use it, and you should be sure it is readily available, fitted properly, turned on, and with the batteries in working order. If the client does not have a hearing aid, with permission of the patient and family you should make a referral to an auditory specialist, who can determine whether such a device is appropriate for your patient. Another means by which sounds can be amplified is by cupping your hands around the client's ear or using a stethoscope in reverse. That is, the patient puts the stethoscope in his or her ears, and you talk into the bell of the instrument (Babcock & Miller, 1994).

If the patient can hear better out of one ear than the other, always stand or sit nearest to the side of the "good" ear. Be sure to slow your speech, provide adequate time for the patient to process your message and to respond, and avoid shouting.

Telecommunications

Telecommunication devices for the deaf (TDD) are important resources for patient education. Television decoders for closed-caption programs are useful tools for further enhancing communication. Caption films for patient education are also available free of charge through Modern Talking Pictures and Services. Under the federal ADA law, these devices are considered to be "reasonable accommodations" for deaf and hearing-impaired persons.

In summary, the following guidelines should be applied when using any of the modes of communication mentioned above (Navarro & Lacour, 1980):

- Be natural:
    - Don't be rigid and stiff or attempt to over-articulate your speech.
    - Use simple sentences.
    - Be sure to get the person's attention by a light touch on the arm before you start to talk.
    - Face the patient and stand no more than 6 feet from the patient when trying to communicate.

- Be considerate and avoid:
    - Talking and walking at the same time.
    - Bobbing your head a lot.
    - Talking with your mouth full or while chewing gum.
    - Turning your face away from the deaf person when speaking.
    - Standing directly in front of a bright light, which may glare directly into the patient's eyes or cast a shadow across your face.
    - Placing an IV in either hand, because the patient will need to use both hands for communicating by sign language.

No matter what methods of communication for teaching you and your client choose, it is important to confirm that your health messages have been received and understood. It is essential that patient comprehension is validated in a nonthreatening manner. In attempts to avoid embarrassing or offending one another, patients as well as nurses will often smile or nod in response to what either one is trying to communicate when, in fact, the message is not understood at all. To ensure that the health education requirements of deaf or hearing-impaired patients are being met, nurses must find effective strategies to communicate the intended message clearly and precisely while at the same time demonstrating acceptance of individuals by making accommodations to suit their needs (Harrison, 1990). Patients who have lived with a hearing impairment for a while usually can tell you the ways to communicate that work best for them.

Visual Impairments

In the United States, a person is considered legally blind if vision is 20/200 or less in the better eye with correction or if visual field limits in both eyes are within 20 degrees diameter. People lose their vision and may become legally blind for a variety of reasons: infections, accidents, aging, disease, poisoning, or congenital degeneration such as retinitis pigmentosa. Most recently, blindness in AIDS patients as a result of infection has been associated with the end stages of this disease.

Visual impairment is especially common among older persons. According to the 2000 census, more than 2.5 million individuals older than age 65 are severely visually impaired (U.S. Census Bureau, 2000). The four leading eye diseases associated with the aging process are macular degeneration, cataracts, glaucoma, and diabetic retinopathy (Figure 9-1). Severe visual impairment after correction with glasses is defined as the inability to read newspaper print. Using this standard, studies of nursing home residents indicate that about 30% to 50% are considered to be significantly visually impaired (Nelson, 1991).

If you suspect that patients are legally blind but have not been evaluated by a low-vision specialist, you should put them in contact with the local Commission for the Blind and Visually Handicapped. Fortunately, many devices are available to help legally blind persons maximize their remaining vision. Patients who are without sight most likely have had services from a local agency for the blind and are familiar with which adaptations work best for them. However, you may want to further investigate their needs to assure yourself that you are using the most appropriate format and tools for teaching visually impaired clients.

Diabetes education, for example, consumes a great deal of a nurse's teaching time because of the high incidence of this disease in the American population. Diabetic retinopathy is a major cause of blindness, so it is likely that you will be teaching visually impaired patients who are also in need of diabetes education. This situation presents a unique challenge to the nurse. In 1993, a task force consisting of representatives from groups of diabetes educators and rehabilitation teachers for the blind developed a document entitled Adaptive Diabetes Education for Visually Impaired Persons (ADEVIP). ADEVIP provides consistent practice guidelines for the care of diabetics who are visually handicapped.

The following are some tips you might find helpful in caring for patients who are blind or visually impaired:

- Obtain the services of a low-vision specialist, who can prescribe optical devices such as a magnifying lens (with or without a light), a telescope, a closed-circuit

Major diseases causing serious vision impairment that cannot be corrected with conventional spectacles or lenses are cataract, macular degeneration, glaucoma, and diabetic retinopathy. People who have advanced stages of these diseases have difficulty performing ordinary visual tasks, like reading.

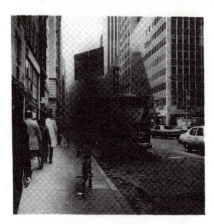

MACULAR DEGENERATION—The deterioration of the macula, the central area of the retina, results in an area of decreased central vision. Peripheral, or side, vision remains unaffected. This is the most prevalent eye disease.

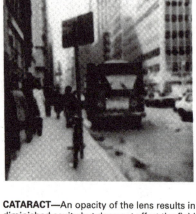

CATARACT—An opacity of the lens results in diminished acuity but does not affect the field of vision. There are no blind spots, but the person's vision is hazy overall, particularly in glaring light.

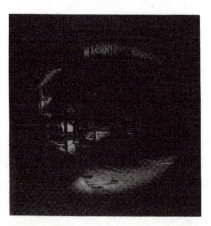

GLAUCOMA—Chronic elevated eye pressure in susceptible individuals may cause atrophy of the optic nerve and loss of peripheral vision. Early detection and close medical monitoring can help reduce complications.

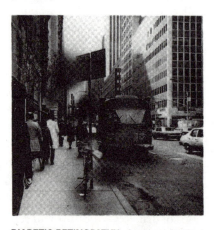

DIABETIC RETINOPATHY—Leaking of retinal blood vessels in advanced or long-term diabetes can affect the macula or the entire retina and vitreous, producing blinding areas.

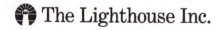

The Lighthouse Inc.

Figure 9-1   Photo Essay on Partial Sight (Low Vision)
Source: Reprinted courtesy of The Lighthouse Inc., New York, New York.

TV, or a pair of sun shields, any of which will enable you to adapt your teaching material to meet the needs of your particular client.

- Persons who have long-standing blindness have learned to use their other senses of hearing, taste, touch, and smell. Usually their listening skills are particularly acute, so avoid the tendency to shout. Just because they have impaired vision does not mean they cannot hear you well. Unlike a sighted person, the blind cannot see nonverbal cues such as hand gestures, facial expressions, and other body language. Before approaching a visually impaired person, always announce your presence, identify yourself, and explain clearly why you are there and what you are doing. Because their memory and recall also are better than the abilities of most sighted persons, you can use this talent to maximize learning (Babcock & Miller, 1994). When conveying messages, rely on their auditory and tactile senses as a means to help them learn information.

- When explaining procedures, be as clear as possible. Describe what you are doing, and explain any noises associated with treatments or the use of equipment. Allow the patient to touch, handle, and manipulate equipment. Use the patient's sense of touch when you are in the process of teaching psychomotor skills as well as when the client is learning to return demonstrate.

- Because persons who are blind are unable to see shapes, sizes, and the placement of objects, using their sense of touch is an important technique when teaching. For example, such patients can identify their medications by feeling the shape, size, and texture of tablets and capsules. Gluing pills to the tops of bottle caps and putting medications in different-sized or -shaped containers will aid in blind persons' ability to identify various medications (Boyd, Gleit, Graham, & Whitman, 1998). Keeping items in the same place at all times will help them independently locate their belongings. Arrange things in front of them in a regular clockwise fashion to help them perform a task that must be accomplished in an orderly, step-by-step manner (McConnel, 1996).

- When using written materials, enlarging the print (font) size is typically an important first step for those who have diminished sight.

- Color is a key factor in whether a visually impaired person can distinguish objects. Be sure to assess on which medium your client sees better—black ink on white paper or white ink on black paper. Bold colors are much better to use than pastels, which are more difficult to discriminate by the older person with vision problems.

- Proper lighting is most important when assisting the legally blind person to read the printed word. Regardless of the print size and the color of the type and paper used, if the light is insufficient, the visually impaired person will have a great deal of difficulty reading print or working with objects.

- Providing contrast is a very helpful technique. For example, using a dark placemat with white dishes or serving black coffee in a white cup will allow persons with visual problems to better see items in front of them.
- Large-print watches and clocks with either black or white backgrounds are available through the local chapter for the blind.
- Audiotapes and cassette recorders are very useful tools. Today, many health education texts as well as other printed health information materials are available as "talking books" and can be obtained through the Library of Congress in Washington, D.C., or through your state library for the blind and visually handicapped. Oral instruction can be audiotaped so that blind patients can listen to the information as often as they wish at another time and place. Repetition allows the opportunity for memorization to reinforce learning.
- The computer is a popular and useful tool for this population of learners. Although they are costly, some computers have synthetic speech as well as Braille keyboards.
- Most blind associations either have a Braille library or can direct you to appropriate resources for information written in Braille. If your client can read Braille and you have a large amount of printed material for patient education, local blind associations may Braille the materials so they can be used by the visually impaired learner.
- When assisting a person who is blind to ambulate, always use the "sighted guide" technique. That is, allow the person to grasp your forearm while you walk about one-half step ahead of them.
- Adaptive equipment, with large display screens or voice instructions, is available for self-monitoring blood glucose levels and for measuring insulin.

It is evident that a variety of useful mechanisms allow blind patients the opportunity to care for themselves and achieve a successful medical and rehabilitation outcome (Baker, 1993).

LEARNING DISABILITIES

The term *learning disability* is defined as "a heterogeneous group of disorders manifested by significant difficulties in acquisition and use of listening, speaking, reading, writing, reasoning or mathematical abilities" (Hammill, Leigh, McNutt, & Larsen, 1981, p. 336). Twenty-five years later, this still stands as the accepted working defini-

TABLE 9-1   Myths and Facts

Myth: Children are labeled "learning disabled" because they can't learn.
Fact: They can learn, but their preferred learning modality must be identified.

Myth: Children who have a learning disability must be spoken to more slowly.
Fact: Those who learn auditorily may become impatient with slower speech and stop listening; those who learn visually would benefit more from seeing the information.

Myth: Children who are learning disabled just have to try harder.
Fact: Telling these children to try harder is a turn off. They already do try hard.

Myth: Children outgrow their disabilities.
Fact: Children do not outgrow their disabilities. They develop strategies to compensate for and minimize their disabilities.

Myth: Children with learning disabilities should be treated like everyone else.
Fact: That treatment would be unfair; they would not get what they need.

Myth: Nearly all children with a learning disability are boys.
Fact: Boys are more often referred for proper identification of learning disabilities because they are more overt in acting out their frustrations.

Source: Copyright 1991, The American Journal of Nursing Company. Reprinted from *MCN: American Journal of Maternal Child Nursing*, Sept/Oct 1991, vol. 16, no. 5. Used with permission.

tion for purposes of assessing, diagnosing, and categorizing an array of perceptual processing deficits. Learning disabilities are disorders intrinsic to the individual and presumed to be due to central nervous dysfunction (Kirk & Kirk, 1983). Other general terms for a learning disability are *minimal brain dysfunction*, *attention deficit disorder (ADD)*, *dyslexia*, and *hyperactivity*.

An estimated 10% to 15% of the overall U.S. population is considered to be learning disabled. Approximately 6% to 10% of school-aged children are diagnosed with a learning disability, and an additional 20% have some degree of learning disability (Greenberg, 1991). In the past, a learning disability was thought to be a problem involving only children. Now, however, evidence supports the belief that most individuals do not "outgrow" the problem. Indeed, the percentage of adults with a learning disability is probably similar to that found in children. The American Council on Education reported that the proportion of full-time college students with learning disabilities has more than tripled in the last two decades—from less than 3% in 1978 to 9% in 1998 (Zirkel, 2000). The majority of people with learning disabilities have language and/or memory deficits.

Individuals with learning disabilities usually do not show any outward signs of having a problem and are often of at least average, if not superior (gifted), intelligence. Some very famous and successful people in world history are thought to have had some type of learning disability—Leonardo daVinci, Woodrow Wilson, George Patton, Winston Churchill, Nelson Rockefeller, and Albert Einstein. Table 9-1 lists common myths and facts about learning disabilities in children. Learning disabilities are not caused by retardation, emotional disturbances, physical impairments (blindness or deafness), or environmental deprivation such as lack of educational opportunity (Greenberg, 1991).

A person who is learning disabled may experience difficulty with one or more of the following:

- Memory
- Language
- Motor functioning
- Information processing

These difficulties fall under two general headings: "input" and "output" disabilities. *Input disabilities* refer to the process of receiving and recording information in the brain. They include visual perceptual, auditory perceptual, integrative processing, and memory disorders. *Output disabilities* refer to the process of orally responding and performing physical tasks. They include language and motor disorders. Although these problems are frequently identified in children, many of them can be found in people who have not been diagnosed as learning disabled until later in adulthood. It is important to remember that a learning disabled individual can experience one type of learning disability or a combination of different types. Greenberg (1991) outlines the characteristics of these learning disability problems and the teaching strategies useful in assisting the learning disabled to acquire the behaviors required for independent functioning.

Input Disabilities

Visual Perceptual Disorders

This type of disability results in an inability to read or difficulty with reading (dyslexia). Letters of the alphabet may be seen in reverse or rotated order—for example, d is b and p is q or g. Letters also may be confused with one another, such as the word *was* being perceived as the word *saw*. In addition, the individual may have trouble focusing on a particular word or group of words. There also may be a "figure ground" problem, such that the person is unable to identify a specific object within a group of objects, such as finding a cup of juice on a food tray. Furthermore, judging distances or positions in space or dealing with spatial relationships may prove difficult, resulting in the person's bumping into things, being confused about left hand-right hand or up and down, or being unable to throw a ball or do a puzzle.

People with visual perceptual deficits tend to be auditory learners. With these individuals, visual stimulation should be kept to a minimum. Visual materials such as pamphlets or books are ineffective unless the content is explained orally or the information is read aloud. If visual items are used, only one item should be given at a time with a sufficient period in between times to allow for the information to be focused on and mastered. Because persons with visual perceptual deficits usually learn best through hearing, using CDs and audiotapes (with or without earphones) and verbal instruction are keys in helping them learn. Recall and retention of information can be assessed by oral questioning, allowing learners to verbally express back to you what they understand and remember about the content that has been presented.

Auditory Perceptual Disorders

This type of disability is characterized by the inability to distinguish subtle differences in sounds—for example, "blue" and "blow" or "ball" and "bell." There also may be a problem with auditory "figure ground," such that the sound of someone speaking cannot be identified clearly when others are speaking in the same room. Auditory "lags" may occur, whereby sound input cannot be processed at a normal rate. Parts of conversations may be missed unless one speaks at a speed that allows the disabled person enough time to process the information. During instruction, it is important to limit the noise level and eliminate distractions in the background. Using as few words as possible and repeating them when necessary (using the same words to avoid confusion) are useful strategies. Direct eye contact helps keep the learner focused on the task at hand.

Visual teaching methods such as demonstration-return demonstration, gaming, and role playing, as well as using visual instructional tools such as pictures, charts, films, books, printed handouts, and the computer, are the best ways to communicate information. Pointing to objects that represent key words when giving verbal instructions, allowing the learner to have hands-on experiences, and providing opportunities for observation are useful techniques for learning. Directions for learning using these methods and tools should be in written form. Visual learners may intently watch your face for the formation of words, expressions, eye movements, and hand gestures. These are strategies they have developed to aid them in comprehending what you are saying. If the learner does not understand something being taught, he or she may show frustration by becoming irritable and inattentive.

Individuals with either visual or auditory perceptual problems often rely on tactile learning. They prefer to do things with their hands, like to use touch to explore things, enjoy writing and drawing, and choose to engage in physical activities.

Integrative Processing Disorders

Recording information in the brain requires that the information be organized to process it correctly. An inability to sequence visual, auditory, or tactile stimuli or understand abstract messages is characteristic of this type of disability. A child who has difficulty sequencing information may read and understand the word *dog* as *god* because the letters *d*, *o*, and *g* are processed in the wrong order. Thinking also may progress from the middle to the end rather than taking in information by starting at the beginning. The inability to grasp the meaning of words or phrases leads to misunderstandings. For example, abstract expressions, such as "window shopping" or "blowing smoke," are interpreted literally rather than figuratively.

Those with an integrative processing disability need specific explanations. You should avoid using confusing phrases, puns, or sarcasm with such patients. Frequently ask the person to repeat or demonstrate what was learned to immediately clear up any misconceptions.

Short-Term or Long-Term Memory Disorders

Once information is recorded and processed in the brain, it must be stored and remembered. Normally, most people can retrieve information fairly quickly and without much effort from either their short-term or long-term memories. *Short-term memory* refers to information that is remembered as long as one is paying attention. For example, being able to remember what you have been told recently or taking a telephone order and then being able to write it down completely soon after you have hung up the phone is evidence of short-term memory ability. *Long-term memory* refers to information that has been stored and becomes available whenever one thinks about it, such as being able to remember someone's telephone number (or your own, for that matter) after a long period of time. Individuals with short-term memory deficits may be unable to recall what they learned an hour before, but they may be able to recall the information they learned a long time ago. People with both short- and long-term memory disabilities need brief, frequent, repetitive teaching sessions for constant reinforcement of information.

Output Disabilities

Language Disorders

There are two types of oral language—spontaneous (initiating and carrying on a conversation) and demand (asking a question). With spontaneous language, persons select a topic, organize their thoughts, and choose the correct words to verbally express themselves. Demand language occurs when someone else starts a conversation and poses questions for another person to answer. In response to demand language, the person with a language disability may panic and answer "Huh?" or "What?" or "I don't know." If you detect this response pattern, allow them sufficient time either to process the information they received or formulate a response. This approach will reduce barriers to communication due to anxiety and frustration. For persons with either type of language disability, the greatest gift you can give them is time—time to process their thoughts, to find words, and then to speak for the purpose of starting or participating in a conversation or responding with answers to your questions.

The following are some adaptive techniques that can be used to help an individual with a language disorder:

- Provide information on tape, or give a learner the option of responding to questions orally with a tape recorder.
- Use hand signs for key words when giving verbal directions.
- Use hands-on experience or observation.
- Highlight important information.
- Use a computer.
- Capitalize on teachable moments.
- Use puzzles.
- Appeal to all senses—auditory, visual, and tactile.
- Use an active reading strategy such as SQ3R (skim, question, read, rehearse, revise).

Motor Disorders

Learning psychomotor tasks will be difficult if the individual has problems performing gross and fine motor tasks. Often people with this type of disability will avoid such tasks. For example, they will shy away from using writing as a form of communication because it requires fine motor coordination. Instead of forcing them to handwrite, allow them to use a tape recorder or computer to communicate their knowledge of information. Depending on the disabled person's auditory and visual strengths, various print and nonprint materials may prove helpful for teaching and learning. Safety also is always a concern for those with gross motor difficulties because they are prone to clumsiness, stumbling, or falling. The environment should be kept as uncluttered as possible to avoid injury and embarrassment.

Attention Deficit Disorder

The ability to pay attention is important for success in school, work, and personal life activities. Any difficulty with attending skills can have an adverse effect on learning. Three major subtypes of attention deficit disorder (ADD) are: attention deficit disorder with hyperactivity (ADDH), attention deficit disorder without hyperactivity (ADDNOH), and attention deficit disorder, residual type.

The onset of ADD is before the age of 7 years. Estimates of the prevalence of ADD range from 1–2% of all school-aged children. The exact cause of ADD is unknown. Its primary characteristics are signs of having difficulty paying attention and being impulsive that are developmentally inappropriate. The child often fails to finish projects, seems not to listen, is easily distracted, and has difficulty concentrating. Other thoughts, sights, or sounds keep getting in their way, especially when the task is difficult or not interesting to them. The child acts before thinking, moves from one activity to another before finishing any task, requires much supervision, and has difficulty with staying on schedule and organizing their time, work, and belongings. Hyperactivity (ADDH) often goes hand in hand with the inattentiveness and impulsivity. The older child and adolescent may be extremely restless and fidgety. His or her behavior tends to be haphazard, poorly organized, and not goal directed. ADD, residual type, is sometimes used to identify older adolescents who were previously identified as ADDH at a younger age but who no longer exhibit hyperactivity.

ADD affects children with average ability as well as those who are gifted. This problem and other learning disabilities frequently occur together. Often, medication therapy is the treatment of choice for children with ADD. Before beginning any educational intervention with these children, have an open discussion with the child and the parents to determine what works best for them. Most older children have been involved in special programs at school that help them consistently use specific learning strategies, which is of primary importance.

Provide new information to such patients in a quiet environment, which may require using another place for the teaching session than the child's hospital room. When giving instructions or assigning a task, give directions one step at a time, and divide the work into small parts. Reward achievement, and ignore inappropriate behavior. Eliminate as much distraction as possible. Encourage the older child to keep a notebook and write instructions down.

In summary, it is important to stress that people who are learning disabled are not mentally retarded; they just learn differently. They may have one or more disabilities, ranging from mild to severe. The challenge is to determine how the client learns best and then to adapt your teaching strategies to meet their preferred style of learning—auditory, visual, or tactile. The most reliable way to determine what accommodations need to be made in your teaching approach is to ask people with learning disabilities about problems they encounter in processing information and what they find to be the most appropriate instructional methods and tools to help them with learning. In the case of children, questions should be directed to both the child and the parents. Someone's strengths and weaknesses with respect to learning can be identified through direct, individualized assessment. A teaching plan can then be developed to promote learning through use of strategies that compensate for or minimize the effect of a disability (Greenberg, 1991).

PHYSICAL DISABILITIES

Brain Injury

A fall, car accident, gunshot wound, or blow to the head are just a few potential causes of traumatic brain injury (TBI). It is estimated that 5.3 million people in the U.S. (2% of the population) are living with a disability as a result of a traumatic brain injury (National Center for Injury Prevention and Control, 1999).

Most members of this special population, ages 15–24 years, were previously healthy and active young people. Also, there is a growing number of older individuals surviving a closed head injury. Often, these persons suffer from behavior and personality changes, as well as an impairment in cognitive ability, following their TBI (Tate, Fenelon, Manning, & Hunter, 1991).

The amount and types of deficits usually depend on the severity and location of the injury. Cognitive impairments may include poor attention span, slowness in thinking, confusion, difficulty with short-term or long-term memory, impulsive and socially inappropriate behaviors, poor judgment, and difficulty with organization and problem solving. Skills with reading and writing also are likely to be impaired. In addition, the person may have acquired a hearing loss. As might be expected, communication will more than likely be an issue.

Changes in communication, cognitive-perceptual abilities, and behavior may be dramatic. "The combined effects of these multiple deficits following a TBI create tremendous psychosocial consequences for patients and their families. Especially in the early stages of the injury, patients are not able to handle normal routine social situations" (Grinspun, 1987, p. 63). In fact, personality changes present the biggest burden for the family. Studies have shown that the level of family stress is directly related to personality changes and the relative's own perception of the symptoms arising from the head injury (Grinspun, 1987).

Although most of the literature deals with the importance of including the family during the rehabilitation period, it is clear that brain-injured persons will always need the involvement of their family. The benefits of participation in family groups are immeasurable. Considerable strength is gained from group participation, and learning is accomplished through a friendly, informal approach. Of particular importance for brain-injured persons and their friends and family is the need for unconditional acceptance.

Learning needs for this population center on the issues of client safety and family coping. Safety issues are related to cognitive, perceptual, and behavioral capabilities. Families are faced with a life-changing event and will require ongoing support and encouragement to take care of themselves. Recovery may take several years, and most often the person is left with some form of impairment. The symptoms of personality change, slowness, and poor memory in head-injured patients affect about 70% of this population (Tate et al., 1991).

Table 9-2 lists some "dos" and "don'ts" for effective teaching of the person with a brain injury.

COMMUNICATION DISORDERS

"Communication is a universal process by which human beings exchange ideas, impart feelings and express needs" (Adkins, 1991, p. 74). Communication occurs in a variety of ways, including drama, music, literature, and art. It is verbal and nonverbal, and there are both sending and receiving components. Stroke, or cerebrovascular accident, is the most common cause of impaired communication. As is true with the other disabilities discussed in this chapter, a stroke is a major crisis for both the person and the family. Many of the strategies discussed for teaching other individuals with impairments are also applicable to an educational program for the person who has suffered a stroke. This discussion will cover some useful strategies appropriate for working with a person with impaired communication, such as aphasia.

Table 9-2   Guidelines for Effective Teaching of the Brain-Injured Patient

DO
Use simple rather than complex statements.
Use gestures to complement what you are saying.
Give step-by-step directions.
Allow time for responses.
Recognize and praise all efforts to communicate.
Ensure the use of listening devices.
Keep written instructions simple, with only a small amount of information on each page.

DON'T
Stop talking or trying to communicate.
Speak too fast.
Talk down to the person.
Talk in the person's presence as though he or she is not there.
Give up (instead, seek the assistance of a speech-language pathologist).

Each year, 150 to 200 per 100,000 Americans suffer a stroke (Edwards, 2000). Stroke is a more common occurrence in older adult men and in the African American population. Perceptual deficits such as neglect and denial as well as spatial disturbances may also affect a person's ability to communicate (Olson, 1991). One of the most common residual deficits of a stroke is a problem with language. Language involves not only speaking, but also comprehending thoughts and ideas, as well as understanding and using symbols (Boss, 1986).

Aphasia is a communication problem, either with speaking, writing, or understanding. It may be defined as a loss of language ability, usually caused by damage to the dominant hemisphere (Adkins, 1991). When you prepare to work with someone with aphasia, it is necessary to determine which type of aphasia—expressive or receptive—is present. If your involvement with the client occurs during the early stages of rehabilitation, the speech therapist would be a good teammate.

The function of language primarily resides in the left hemisphere of the brain. Most often when an injury affects the dominant cerebral hemisphere (usually the left), the result is *expressive aphasia*. About three-quarters of the overall population has a dominant left hemisphere. Expressive aphasia occurs when an injury damages the inferior frontal gyrus, just anterior to the facial and lingual areas of the motor cortex, known as Broca's area (Table 9-3). Because Broca's area is so near the left motor area, the stroke often leaves the person with right-sided paralysis as well.

Table 9-3   Clinical Features of Aphasia

Type	Involved Anatomy	Expression	Auditory Comprehension	Written Comprehension	Naming	Word/Phrase Repetition	Ability to Write
Broca's (motor, expressive)	Precentral gyrus, Broca's area	Nonfluent, tele-graphic, may be mute	Subtle deficits	Subtle deficits	Impaired	Impaired	Impaired
Wernicke's (recep-tive, sensory)	Superior temporal gyrus	Fluent but con-tent inappropriate	Impaired	Impaired	Severely impaired	Impaired	Impaired
Global (mixed)	Frontal-temporal area	Nonfluent	Severely impaired	Impaired	Severely impaired	Impaired	Severely impaired
Conductive (central)	Arcuate fasciculus	Fluent	Intact	Intact	Impaired	Severely impaired	Impaired
Anomic (amnesic)	Angular gyrus	Fluent	Intact	Intact	Severely impaired	Intact	Subtle deficits
Transcortical sensory (TCSA)	Periphery of Broca's and Wernicke's areas (watershed zone)	Fluent	Impaired	Impaired	Impaired	Intact	Severely impaired
Transcortical motor (TCMA)	Anterior, superior, or lateral to Broca's area	Nonfluent, speech initiation difficult	Intact	Subtle deficits	Impaired	Intact	Impaired

Source: Reprinted by permission from Bronstein, Popovich, & Stewart-Amidi, *Promoting Stroke Recovery: A Research-Based Approach for Nursing.* Table 11-1. St. Louis: Mosby-Year Book, 1991.

Wernicke's area of the brain (Table 9-3) is located in the temporal lobe and is needed for auditory and reading comprehension. When this area is affected, persons are left with *receptive aphasia*. Although their hearing is unimpaired, they are nevertheless unable to understand the significance of the spoken word.

It is important to remember that although persons with both types of aphasia are unable to communicate verbally, or have difficulty doing so, it does not mean they are intellectually impaired. The inability to communicate verbally is one of the most frustrating experiences. Speech therapy should be an early intervention, and the nurse will need to incorporate those strategies into the teaching-learning plan. Every effort must be made to establish communication at some level. Remember, regardless of how severe the communication deficit, it is almost always possible to have stroke patients communicate within their own environment in some manner and to some extent.

Expressive Aphasia

In the event structured speech therapy is not available, the nursing staff will need to develop their own plan of care. When working with expressive aphasia, you might try having the person recall word images, first by naming commonly used objects (e.g., spoons, knives, forks) and then those objects in the immediate environment (e.g., bed, table). Another strategy is having the person repeat words spoken by the nurse. It is wise to begin with simple terms and work progressively to the more complex.

These exercises may be carried out frequently during the day, keeping the sessions short. Most people tire easily when sessions are longer than 30 minutes. Often their speech will become slurred, and they will experience mental fatigue. In the last section of this chapter, some helpful information is offered regarding adaptive computing. People with expressive aphasia find computers a wonderful tool to assist in their efforts to communicate.

Receptive Aphasia

When working with someone with receptive aphasia, you need to establish a means for nonverbal communication. Usually the tone of voice, facial expressions, and gestures will be effective in conveying a message. Most often, these persons are unaware of their impairment and will speak in what sounds like a correct statement. However, their words often do not make sense. Speak more slowly and slightly louder to the person with receptive aphasia, as auditory stimulation seems to be effective. When comprehension and memory span increase, the person will begin to respond appropriately.

Aphasic persons also have trouble with retention and recall. It seems that personal memories of the past return first and recent events take longer to reappear. "It is a lonely, isolated world for those who cannot communicate with other human beings" (Jennings, 1981, p. 39). As we attempt to work with and engage in a teaching-learning intervention, we must be aware of our own attitudes. The effort to communicate with someone without our usual speech and language is one of the more frustrating experiences. Be sure to take time out and reflect on the rewards of assisting the client and family in overcoming this barrier.

Encouragement and explanation when teaching persons with aphasia will go a long way in ensuring client participation and recovery. Keep your teaching sessions filled with praise, and always acknowledge the client's frustration. Keep distractions to a minimum. Be sure the radio and television are turned off so you have the full attention of the client. Always have one person speak at a time. Speak slowly, and be sure to stand where the client is able to see your face (Norman & Baratz, 1979). In teaching people with aphasia, it is easy to overestimate their understanding of speech. Often they will smile and agree when they are actually understanding only half of the message. The challenge is to provide enough time for learning and to constantly check with them to be sure the message is fully understood without getting upset or impatient with the client.

Blanco (1982) suggests the following general guidelines:

- Don't use baby talk.
- Speak in normal tones.
- Speak in short, slow, simple sentences.
- Allow the person time to answer.

Be patient, slow the person's response down, and involve the family. While working with individuals with this type of language deficit, the nurse should also be aware that their ability to read may be affected. Little is known about this aspect of the disability or how many stroke patients suffer from the inability to read. In a study carried out by Loughrey (1992), a small group of patients with aphasia were able to improve their reading ability. Two methods of reteaching reading were used: a multi-sensory technique and a visual-verbal technique. Both were successful in improving the subjects' ability to recognize and use their newly acquired words. Although teaching reading is not a usual nursing responsibility, the nurse may choose to encourage the family to help their loved one relearn reading by using these promising techniques.

Dysarthria

Many people with degenerative disorders, such as Parkinson's disease, multiple sclerosis, and myasthenia gravis, also have dysarthria. Dysarthria is a problem with the voluntary muscle control of speech. It occurs as a consequence of damage to the central or peripheral nervous system. The degree of unintelligible speech is directly related to the severity of the dysarthria (Dreher, 1981).

Several types of dysarthria exist: flaccid, spastic, ataxic, hypokinetic, or mixed. The difference in symptoms for each type depends not on the underlying disease, but on the site in the nervous system that the disease strikes (Dreher, 1981). The incidence of this category of communication problems will certainly increase as the medical treatments for the various brain diseases improve and people live longer. Those who do survive neurological disorders will need help in overcoming all of the residual social and communication problems that occur as a result of their disease.

A useful tool in relating with a person who has dsyarthria is sign language, which may be used if the person's arm and hand muscles are unaffected. The nurse should work with the speech therapist to determine whether any other nonverbal aids would be appropriate, such as communication boards or a portable electronic voice synthesizer. With the invention of the adaptive computer, the possibilities are limitless. Also, the intervention of a physical therapist may help improve the function of various muscles used for speech.

To improve communication with the dysarthric person, Dreher (1981) makes the following suggestions:

- Be sure the environment is quiet, because you are listening to a person whose speech muscles are weak and uncoordinated. A careful listener may detect a consistent pattern in the sound errors.
- Ask the speaker to repeat unclear parts of the message. Concentration on their speech sounds will aid clarity.
- Do not simplify your message. Dysarthria does not affect comprehension.
- Ask questions that need only short answers to prevent exhausting the dysarthric patient who expends great effort to shape sounds.
- Encourage the person to use more oral movement to produce each syllable, to slow the overall rate of speaking, and to speak more loudly.
- Ask the patient who cannot verbalize well to gesture, write, or point to messages on a communication board.

CHRONIC ILLNESS

Lubkin (2002) states that *chronic illness* is the number one medical problem in the United States. It is impossible within this chapter to cover specific teaching strategies for each chronic illness. Unlike acute illnesses, which usually have a clearly defined beginning and end, chronic illness is permanent. It is never completely cured. It fully involves its victims. Every aspect of life is affected—physical, psychological, social, economic, and spiritual. Because successful management of a chronic illness is a life-long process, the development of good learning skills is a matter of survival (Lubkin, 2002).

The learning process for individuals with a chronic illness begins with rehabilitation at the moment of the disability. From the onset of the problem, patients and their families need to acquire knowledge about the disease and arrive at an early understanding of its effects on their lives. Families need information and education to deal with the limitations and changes in their loved one's lifestyle. There is often a conflict between feelings of dependence and the need to be independent. Sometimes the energy and focus of maintaining independence are overwhelming, both physically and emotionally. Often, living with a chronic illness includes a loss or change in roles. When people suffer from role loss (e.g., a father who is no longer able to keep his job), their self-esteem may also be affected.

Controlling the symptoms of chronic illness is a major time-consuming activity. The following are eight key problem areas experienced by chronically ill patients (Strauss et al., 1984):

1. Prevention of medical crisis and the management of problems once they occur
2. Control of symptoms
3. Carrying out prescribed regimens and the management of problems related to carrying out the regimens
4. Prevention of, or living with, social isolation
5. Adjustment to changes in the course of the disease, whether the symptoms worsen or the person goes into remission
6. Attempts at maintaining a normal lifestyle and interactions with others
7. Finding the necessary funds to pay for treatments and to survive despite partial or complete loss of employment
8. Facing the psychological, marital, and family problems that arise due to the stress experienced by the patient and the caregivers

When working with a person with a chronic illness who must manage a sometimes complex therapeutic regimen, it is easy to see how the label of "noncompliance" might enter the assessment. The truth is, the person with a chronic illness requires more than just teaching. Acquiring knowledge does not necessarily help people gain the new skills needed to deal with the problems of everyday life. They need assistance with applying their new knowledge to find solutions that will allow them to lead as normal a life as possible. Therefore, learning must be made meaningful and, most important, useful. Nurses can encourage people to work with their particular regimen and help individuals meet their needs.

The Family's Role in Chronic Illness or Disability

The family's reaction to and perception of a chronic illness or disability will determine their ability to adjust to the changes in relationships and lifestyles. Family members are usually the care providers and the support system for the person with a chronic illness or other disability. They need to be included in all the teaching-learning interactions. The literature has documented that family participation does have a major influence on the success of a client's rehabilitation program.

Assessment of the client's and family's learning needs provides the data necessary to develop an individualized teaching plan. When the client and family are assessed, it is important to note what the family considers high-priority learning needs. Most often their identified needs will be related to each family member's perceived lifestyle change (Will I be able to garden? Go for lunch with friends?). It is important that the nurse assist the client and family to identify problems and develop mutually agreed-upon goals. Adaptation is key. Communication between and among family members is crucial.

Before teaching the client and family, the nurse must take into account how the family is coping with their relative's disability. "Having a disabled individual within the family unit requires that all other members adapt to a new family structure" (Fraley, 1992, p. 108). A chronic illness or disability can either destroy or strengthen family unity. Spouses, siblings, and children of the disabled person may be at different stages of acceptance. Denial may be present during the initial diagnosis of a disability. Later, as the client and his or her family realize the permanence and consequence of the illness or disability, the nurse may witness periods of anger, guilt, depression, fear, and hostility. Depending on the family's stage of acceptance, adapt teaching lessons to fit the circumstances. Flexibility on the part of the nurse and the family is vital to achieving a successful outcome. Be sure to treat each family member as unique, and recognize that some family members may never adjust. Table 9-4 lists some of the most common sources of tension in client and family education (LaRocca, 1994).

Nurses need to value their teaching role when they work with the family having a disabled member. Unlike families dealing with an acutely ill member, families with permanently disabled members will have intermittent contact with the healthcare system throughout their lives. Therefore, whenever teaching sessions are required, the family's availability should be a primary consideration. Given adequate support and resources, families with a chronically ill family member can adapt, make adjustments, and live relatively happy, full lives.

ADAPTIVE COMPUTING

The growth of modern technology has affected all areas of our lives. Without a doubt, though, the personal computer has become the technology that has had the greatest impact. As Max Cleland states, "The real disabled people of the future are going to be those who don't have a computer to use" (Green & Brightman, 1990). Until recently, however, computers have been inaccessible to individuals with a disability. When adaptive computing has been made available, special populations have experienced dramatic changes in their lives. Computers with the appropriate adaptations have liberated people from social isolation and feelings of helplessness and instilled feelings of self-worth and independence. *Adaptive computing*, which is relatively new, refers to the technology (both hardware and software) and the professional services that make computing technology accessible for persons with disabilities (Merrow & Corbett, 1994).

Since the enactment of the ADA in 1990, the diversity of our client population has grown to include more individuals with disabilities in every practice setting. An understanding of adaptive computing will enhance the ability of nurses to advocate for and assist people to obtain the appropriate equipment and training needed for independence. Just about every type of disability mentioned in this chapter could benefit from the use of adaptive computers. Merrow and Corbett (1994) describe the use of computers with various populations, such as the older adult, the physically disabled in long-term rehabilitation, and the hearing and visually impaired.

The Internet now provides access to Web sites on adaptive computing for persons with disabilities and their families and for anyone interested in computer resources for teaching and learning (Burgstahler, 1997). Technology has the potential to improve the lives of people with disabilities by giving them the tools to become more self-sufficient, more productive, and better able to participate in a wide range of life experiences related to employment, education, and recreation.

Table 9-4 Relieving External Tensions in Client and Family Education

Problem	Response
FAMILY DYNAMICS	
Client or family member feels overwhelmed	Set goals. Help the family refocus on tasks at hand. Review goals that have been attained to boost morale.
Anxiety and fear of performing complex procedures	Establish an atmosphere of acceptance. Don't be in a hurry. Offer opportunities for talk and questions. Reassure client and family that they have made the right treatment choice.
Emotions associated with chronic or terminal conditions	Provide opportunities to express feelings. Offer referrals to community resources.
Caregiver burnout and illness	Simplify client management where possible (e.g., scheduling drug doses to reduce nighttime treatment). Remain accessible. Remember: When caregiver needs are not being met, resentments increase. Provide information on respite care.
Client fatigue, especially with chronic illness	Help the client identify individual tolerance for tiredness in planning for as much active participation in the family life as possible.
Young clients are frequently overwhelmed by complex emotions about their illness and therapy	Encourage both children and adolescents to use artwork to express their feelings. Suggest support groups. Offer support to parents and siblings who must alter their family lifestyle.
GERIATRIC CONSIDERATIONS	
An increase in the number of drugs taken daily (on average four or more per day) increases the potential for adverse reactions	Use only one pharmacy so that one source keeps track of medications. Continually evaluate all drugs taken for need, safety, compatibility, potential adverse reactions, and expiration dates.
Decreased visual acuity	Use teaching materials with large, bold type. Encourage the use of a magnifying glass.

Source: Adapted by permission from *Mosby's Home Health Nursing Pocket Consultant*. St. Louis: Mosby-Year Book, 1995.

Although the personal computer has the potential to change the life of a person with even the most severe disability, the fact remains that it is a very individualized process. Personalized computer solutions are those that respond to a particular person, not to the particular disability (Green & Brightman, 1990; Merrow & Corbett, 1994).

Types of Computer Adaptations

The type of adaptation needed depends on whether a person's impairment is a learning disability or a problem with mobility, hearing, seeing, or communicating. Head pointers, mouth sticks, voice recognition systems, joysticks, and trackballs are alternatives to using the traditional keyboard and mouse. These devices can be positioned in unique places and activated with different parts of the body for people who do not have a wide range of movement in their arms or hands.

For people with communication problems, especially those who are unable to speak or whose speech is difficult to understand, the computer adds a whole new dimension to their lives. Within the last 10 years, technology to assist those with impaired speech has become available. Several software packages are now on the market for patients with such problems (see Appendix B). For example, computer-based electronic augmentative communication helps people use a synthetic voice to speak out loud (Green & Brightman, 1990).

The visually and hearing impaired also can benefit from adaptive computing. As previously noted, there are many types of visual impairments, ranging from a person with low vision to a person who is blind. It is obvious that the problem with this population relates to output—in other words, the monitor and the printer. There are many types of adaptive devices that can enable individuals with vision impairment to use a personal computer—everything from large-size monitors to large-print software. For people who are unable to see the screen at all, a solution may be to have the computer "speak" the screen contents. Another solution for computer users who are blind is tactile output. The images on the screen are converted into Braille on a device known as Optacon, which gives the person an exact tactile representation of the letters and lines.

Learning disability problems can often be solved with a creative software package; for example, outliners, a type of thought processor, are programs that help people organize their ideas. They are very helpful in writing papers or reports. Sometimes the outliners software can be used in place of a word processor.

Every computer-based solution is the result of a carefully planned, individually determined approach. Individuals with a disability are the experts on what works best for them. However, some guidelines should be considered when selecting the most appropriate adaptive computer. The best computer solution for individuals with disabilities is that which allows for independent and effective use. Other criteria include affordability, portability, flexibility, and simplicity of learning. If these criteria are met, then the adaptive computer is probably in line with the ADA's recommendations for providing "reasonable accommodations."

SUMMARY

The shock of any disability, no matter when it occurs along the continuum of life, has a tremendous impact on individuals and their families. At the onset and all through the habilitation or rehabilitation process, patients and their families are met with new information to be learned. Successful habilitation or rehabilitation means acquiring knowledge and applying it to their situation. Inner strength and courage are attributes needed to face each new day, as the effort to live a "normal" life never ends. The physical, social, emotional, and vocational implications of living with a disability require the nurse in the role of teacher to be well prepared to meet any member of this special population right where they are in their struggle to live independently.

REVIEW QUESTIONS

1. How do the terms *habilitation* and *rehabilitation* differ from one another?
2. What are the major causes of disabilities?
3. Which six questions should be asked by the nurse when assessing a disabled person's readiness to learn?
4. What are the two major types of disabilities?
5. What are the five categories of disabilities addressed in this chapter?
6. When should the nurse enlist the help of a professional interpreter rather than a member of the family when teaching a hearing impaired person?
7. What are ten tips you might find helpful in teaching a blind or visually impaired person?
8. What are the four types of input disabilities and the two types of output disabilities?
9. What are the characteristic behaviors of persons with ADD, and what are the educational interventions that nurses should use when teaching people with ADD?

10. What are the guidelines for effective teaching of brain-injured patients?
11. What are the strategies that can be used to teach patients with the three types of communication disorders?
12. What are some effective approaches for teaching patients and their families who are dealing with a chronic illness?
13. What types of adaptive computing devices are available to allow people living with a disability to function independently?

REFERENCES

Adkins, E. R. H. (1991). Nursing care of the client with impaired communication. *Rehabilitation Nursing, 16*(2), 74–76.

Babcock, D. E. & Miller, M. A. (1994). *Client education: Theory and practice*. St. Louis: Mosby.

Baker, S. S. (1993). Teamwork between the healthcare community and the blind rehabilitation system. *Journal of Visual Impairment and Blindness, 87*(9), 349–352.

Blanco, K. M. (1982). The aphasic patient. *Journal of Neurosurgical Nursing, 14*, 34–37.

Boss, B. J. (1986). The neuroanatomical and neurophysiological basis for learning. *Journal of Neuroscience Nursing, 18*(5), 256–264.

Boyd, M. D., Gleit, C. J., Graham, B. A., & Whitman, N. I. (1998). *Health teaching in nursing practice* (3rd ed.). Stamford, CT: Appleton & Lange.

Bronstein, K. S., Popovich, J., & Stewart-Amidei, C. (1991). *Promoting stroke recovery: A research-based approach for nurses*. St. Louis: Mosby-Year Book.

Burgstahler, S. (April 1997). Teaching on the Net: What's the difference? *T.H.E. Journal*, 61–64.

Burkett, K. W. (1989). Trends in pediatric rehabilitation. *Nursing Clinics of North America, 24*(1), 239–255.

Cunningham, C. (February 2001). Breaking the barriers to math and science for students with disabilities. *Syllabus*, 41–42.

Diehl, L. N. (1989). Client and family learning in the rehabilitation setting. *Nursing Clinics of North America, 24*(1), 257–264.

DiPietro, L. (1979). *Deaf patients, special needs, special responses*. Washington, DC: National Academy of Gallaudet College.

Dittmar, S. (1989). *Rehabilitation nursing*. St. Louis: Mosby-Year Book.

Dreher, B. (1981). Overcoming speech and language disorders. *Geriatric Nursing, 2*, 345–349.

Edwards, P. A. (2000). *The specialty practice of rehabilitation: A core curriculum* (4th ed.). Glenville, IL: Association of Rehabilitation Nurses.

Fraley, A. M. (1992). *Nursing and the disabled: Across the life span*. Boston: Jones and Bartlett.

Green, P. & Brightman, A. J. (1990). *Independence day: Designing computer solutions for individuals with disability*. Allen, TX: DLM.

Greenberg, L. A. (1991). Teaching children who are learning disabled about illness and hospitalization. *MCN: American Journal of Maternal Child Nursing, 16*(5), 260–263.

Grinspun, D. (1987). Teaching families of traumatic brain-injured adults. *Critical Care Nursing Quarterly, 10*(3), 61–72.

Hammill, D. D., Leigh, J. E., McNutt, G., & Larsen, S. C. (1981). A new definition of learning disabilities. *Learning Disability Quarterly, 4*, 336–342.

Harrison, L. L. (1990). Minimizing barriers when teaching hearing-impaired clients. *MCN: American Journal of Maternal Child Nursing, 15*(2), 113.

Jennings, S. (1981). Communicating with your aphasic patients. *Journal of Practical Nursing, 31*, 22–23.

Kirk, S. A. & Kirk, W. D. (1983). On defining disabilities. *Journal of Learning Disabilities, 16*(1), 20–21.

LaRocca, J. C. (1994). *Handbook of home care IV therapy*. St. Louis: Mosby-Year Book.

Loughrey, L. (1992). The effects of two teaching techniques on recognition and use of function words by aphasic stroke patients. *Rehabilitation Nursing, 17*(3), 134–137.

Lubkin, I. M. (2002). *Chronic illness: Impact and interventions* (5th ed.). Boston: Jones and Bartlett.

McCafferty, L. A. E. (January 21, 2002). Sounds of understanding: Nurses can help spot and treat hearing loss. *Advance for Nurses*, 5.

McConnel, E. A. (1996). Clinical do's & don'ts: Caring for a patient with a vision impairment. *Nursing, 26*(5), 28.

Merrow, S. L. & Corbett, C. (1994). Adaptive computing for people with disabilities. *Computers in Nursing, 12*(4), 201–209.

National Center for Injury Prevention and Control. (December 1999). Traumatic brain injury in the United States: A report to Congress. Retrieved from http://www.CDC.gov/NCIPC/pub-res/pubs.htm.

Navarro, M. R. & Lacour, G. (1980). Helping hints for use with deaf patients. *Journal of Emergency Nursing, 6*(6), 26–28.

Nelson, K. (1991). *Projected increase in the prevalence of severe visual impairment among elderly Americans*. New York: American Foundation for the Blind.

Norman, S. & Baratz, R. (1979). The brain-damaged patient: Approaches to assessment, care, and rehabilitation. Understanding aphasia, Part 4. *American Journal of Nursing, 79*, 2135–2138.

Olson, E. (1991). Perceptual deficits affecting the stroke patient. *Rehabilitation Nursing, 16*(14), 212–213.

Stock, S. (January 21, 2002). When silence isn't golden. *Advance for Nurses*, 28–29.

Strauss, A. L., Corbin, J., Fagerhaugh, S., et al. (1984). *Chronic illness and quality of life* (2nd ed.). St. Louis: Mosby.

Strong, M. (1996). *Language learning and deafness*. New York: Cambridge University Press.

Tate, R. L., Fenelon, B., Manning, M. L., & Hunter, M. (1991). Patterns of neuropsychological impairment after severe blunt injury. *Journal of Nervous and Mental Disease, 179*(3), 117–126.

U.S. Census Bureau. (2000). *Population estimates program*. Washington, DC: Author.

Weeks, S. K. (1995). What are the educational needs of the prospective family caregiver of newly disabled adults? *Rehabilitation Nursing, 20*(5), 256–260.

Zirkel, P. A. (2000). Sorting out which students have learning disabilities. *The Chronicle of Higher Education, 47*(15), B15–B16.

PART III

Techniques and Strategies for Teaching and Learning

CHAPTER 10

Behavioral Objectives

Susan B. Bastable and Julie A. Doody

KEY TERMS

affective domain
behavioral objectives
cognitive domain
goal
intrinsic and augmented feedback

learning curve
psychomotor domain
taxonomy
teaching plans

OBJECTIVES

After completing this chapter, the reader will be able to

1. Identify the difference between goals and objectives.
2. Recognize the value of using behavioral objectives for teaching and learning.
3. Write behavioral objectives accurately using the three components of condition, performance, and criterion.
4. List the most frequent errors made in writing objectives.
5. Define the three domains of learning.
6. Select the instructional methods appropriate for teaching in the cognitive, affective, and psychomotor domains.
7. Develop teaching plans that reflect internal consistency between the elements.
8. Recognize the role of the nurse in writing objectives for the planning, implementation, and evaluation of teaching and learning.

With appreciation to Cynthia Sculco, EdD, RN for her contribution to the first edition of this chapter.

In previous chapters, the characteristics and attributes of the learner with respect to learning needs, readiness to learn, and learning styles have been addressed. Clearly, assessment of the learner is an essential first step in the teaching-learning process. Assessment determines what the learner needs to know, when and under what conditions the learner is most receptive to learning, and how the learner actually learns best. Before a decision can be made about selecting the content to be taught or choosing the teaching methods and materials to be used to change learner behavior, the teacher must first decide what the learner is expected to accomplish. Patient and family needs are determined by identifying the gaps in their knowledge, attitudes, or skills. Identification of needs is essential before writing behavioral objectives that guide the planning, implementation, and evaluation of teaching and learning.

Educators and educational psychologists have developed approaches to writing and classifying behavioral objectives that offer teachers assistance in organizing instructional content for learners functioning at various levels of ability. Mager (1997) has been the primary educator credited with developing a system for writing behavioral objectives. His system helps teachers make appropriate instructional decisions as well as assists learners in understanding what they need and are expected to know. The underlying principle has been, if one does not know where he or she is going, how will the person know when he or she has arrived? In addition, the taxonomic system devised by Bloom and associates (1956) for categorizing objectives according to a hierarchy of behaviors has been the cornerstone of teaching for one-half century.

The technique of writing behavioral objectives requires that behaviors be categorized according to their type and complexity. This skill is a necessary function of the nurse's role when teaching patients and their families. Understanding how to write and classify behavioral objectives ensures that learner outcomes are measurable and that teaching efforts are consistent.

This chapter examines the importance of behavioral objectives for effective teaching; describes how to write clear and precise behavioral objectives; explores the levels of achievement by the learners in the cognitive, affective, and psychomotor domains; and outlines the development of teaching plans. All of these elements provide a framework for the successful instruction of the learner.

CHARACTERISTICS OF GOALS AND OBJECTIVES

The terms *goal* and *objective* are often used interchangeably, but there is a real difference between the two terms. This difference must be clearly understood by all teachers. Time span and specificity are the two factors that differentiate goals from objectives (Haggard, 1989). Goals and objectives must be directed to what the learner is expected to be able to do, not what the teacher is expected to teach.

A *goal* is the final outcome of what is achieved at the end of the teaching-learning process. Goals are global and broad, and serve as long-term targets for both the learner and the teacher. Goals are the desired outcomes of learning that are realistically achievable in weeks or months. An *objective*, on the other hand, is a specific, single behavior. Objectives are short-term and should be achievable at the end of one teaching session or within a matter of a few days following a series of teaching sessions.

According to Mager (1997), an objective describes a performance that learners should be able to demonstrate before they are considered competent. Thus, objectives that describe learner behaviors are known as behavioral objectives. They are the intended result of instruction, not the process or means of instruction itself. Therefore, behavioral objectives are action-oriented rather than content-oriented and learner-centered rather than teacher-centered. Behavioral objectives describe what the learner will be able to do following a teaching experience.

Objectives are statements of specific or short-term behaviors that lead step by step to the more general, overall long-term goal. Objectives must be achieved before the goal can be reached. They must be observable and measurable to be able to determine whether they have been met by the learner. Objectives inform the learner what behaviors are expected in the cognitive, affective, or psychomotor domains to meet the intended outcome (Babcock & Miller, 1994). Objectives are derived from a goal and must be consistent with and related to that goal. As an analogy, a goal can be thought of as an entire pie and the objectives as individual pieces of the pie that make up the goal.

Objectives and goals form a map that provides directions (objectives) for how to arrive at a particular destination (goal). For example, a goal might be that a diabetic patient will learn to manage diabetes. To accomplish this goal, which has been agreed on by both the nurse and the patient, specific objectives must be outlined to address changes in behavior such as the need to learn diet therapy, insulin administration, exercise regimens, stress management, and glucose monitoring. The objectives to accomplish the goal become the blueprint for attaining the desired outcomes of learning. The successful achievement of predetermined objectives is, in part, the result of appropriate instruction.

If the teaching-learning process is to be successful, then determining which goals and objectives are to be achieved must be a mutual decision on the part of both the teacher and the learner. It is the responsibility of both parties to participate in the decision-making process and "buy into" the immediate objectives and ultimate goals. Involving the learner right from the start in creating goals and objectives is absolutely crucial. Otherwise, time and effort on the part of the teacher and the learner may be wasted. Blending what the learner wants to learn with what the teacher has determined that the learner needs to know into a common set of objectives and goals provides for an educational experience that is mutually accountable, respectful, developmental, and fulfilling (Reilly & Oermann, 1990).

Objectives and goals must also be clearly written, realistic, and learner-centered. If they do not precisely state what the learner is expected to do in the short and long term, then there are no clear guidelines to follow nor an obvious end result of the learning process. If goals and objectives are too difficult to achieve, the learner will become easily discouraged, which decreases motivation and interferes with compliance. For example, a goal that a patient will maintain a *salt-free* diet is likely to be impossible to accomplish or adhere to over an extended period of time. Establishing a goal of maintaining a *low-salt* diet, with the objective of learning to avoid eating and preparing high-sodium foods, is a much more realistic and achievable expectation of the learner.

THE IMPORTANCE OF USING BEHAVIORAL OBJECTIVES FOR TEACHING

Robert Mager (1997), a recognized authority on preparing behavioral objectives, points out three major advantages to writing explicit objective statements:

1. They provide a basis for the selection and design of instructional content, methods, and materials.
2. They provide learners with the means to organize their efforts and activities toward accomplishing the objectives.
3. They allow for a determination as to whether an objective has been accomplished.

As Mager (1997) states, "If you don't know where you're going, how will you know which road to take to get there?" (p. 14). Before the teacher prepares instruction, before materials and teaching methods are selected, before the means to evaluate learning are chosen, it is important to clearly state what the intended results of instruction are to be. To paraphrase Mager's thinking, mechanics do not select repair tools until they know what has to be fixed, surgeons do not choose instruments until they know what operation is to be performed, and builders do not buy construction materials before drafting a blueprint.

Haggard (1989) summarized the following questions that arise if objectives are not always written:

- How will anyone else know what objectives have been set?
- How will the educator evaluate and document success or failure?
- How will learners keep track of their progress?

The following considerations justify the need for writing behavioral objectives (Ferguson, 1998). Careful construction of objectives

- helps to keep teachers' thinking on target and learner-centered.
- communicates to both learners and healthcare team members what is planned for teaching and learning.
- helps learners understand what is expected of them so they can keep track of their progress.
- forces the teacher to organize educational materials so as not to get lost in content and forget the learner's role in the process.
- encourages nurses as teachers to question their own motives, to think deliberately about why they are doing things, and to analyze what positive results will be attained from accomplishing specific objectives.
- tailors teaching to the learner's particular circumstances and needs.
- creates guideposts for teacher evaluation and documentation of success or failure.
- focuses attention not on what is taught but on what the learner will come away with once the teaching-learning process is completed.
- orients both teacher and learner to the specific end result of instruction.
- makes it easier for the learner to visualize performing the required actions.

Developing behavioral objectives not only helps nurses explore their own knowledge, values, and beliefs about teaching and learning, but also encourages them to examine the experiences, values, motivations, and knowledge of the patients and family members they teach. The setting of objectives and goals is considered by many nurses to be the initial, most important consideration in the teaching/learning process (Haggard, 1989; Mager, 1997).

The teacher and learner must work together to compose objectives and goals that focus on what is to be accomplished both short and long term. This process provides direction that helps the nurse identify the time that will be needed for teaching, how the learner best learns, the teaching methods that will work most effectively, and the best ways to evaluate the learner's progress. The process of stating well-written objectives encourages the teacher to seriously contemplate what is worth teaching and what is worth spending time to accomplish.

WRITING BEHAVIORAL OBJECTIVES

Well-written behavioral objectives give learners very clear statements about what is expected of them and assist teachers in being able to measure learner progress toward achieving the objectives. Over the past three decades, Robert Mager's (1997) approach to writing behavioral objectives has been widely accepted. His message to teachers is that for objectives to be meaningful, they must precisely, clearly, and very specifically communicate the teacher's instructional intent (Arends, 1994).

According to Mager (1997), the format for writing concise and useful behavioral objectives includes the following three important characteristics:

1. **Performance:** Describes what the learner is expected to be able to do to demonstrate the kinds of behaviors the teacher will accept as evidence that objectives have been achieved. Activities performed by the learner may be quite visible, such as being able to "write" or "listen," or less visible, such as being able to "recognize" or "recall."
2. **Condition:** Describes the situation(s) under which the behavior will be observed or the performance is expected to occur.
3. **Criterion:** Describes how well or with what accuracy the learner must be able to perform the behavior to be considered competent.

These characteristics translate into the following questions: (1) What should the learner be able to do? (2) Under what condition(s) should the learner be able to do it? (3) How well must the learner be able to do it? A fourth component must also be included that describes the "who" to ensure that the behavioral objective is learner-centered. Behavioral objectives are statements that communicate *who* will *do what* under *what condition(s)* and *how well* (Cummings, 1994). To link together the parts of a behavioral objective, the following three steps are recommended:

1. Identify the testing situation (condition).
2. State the learner and the learner's behavior (performance).
3. State the performance level (criterion).

For example: "Following a 20-minute teaching session on hypoglycemia (*condition*), Mrs. Smith will be able to identify (*performance*) three out of four major symptoms of low blood sugar (*criterion*)."

Table 10-1 outlines the three-part method of objective writing. Table 10-2 gives samples of well-written and poorly written objectives.

Table 10-1 The Three-Part Method of Objective Writing		
Condition **(Testing Situation)**	**Performance** **(Learner Behavior)**	**Criterion** **(Quality of Accuracy)**
	The learner will be able to:	
Without using a calculator	solve	5 out of 6 problems
Using a model	demonstrate	the correct procedure
Following a group discussion	list	at least two reasons
After watching a video	select	with 100% accuracy

Table 10-2   Samples of Written Objectives
WELL-WRITTEN OBJECTIVES
After watching a demonstration on tube feeding, the patient's wife will be able to use the correct technique to provide her husband with nutrition three times per day.
Following a class on hypertension, the patient will be able to state three out of four causes of high blood pressure.
On completing the reading materials provided for the care of a newborn, the mother will be able to express any concerns she has about caring for her baby after discharge.
POORLY WRITTEN OBJECTIVES
The patient will be able to prepare a menu using low-salt foods (*condition and criterion missing*).
Given a list of exercises to relieve low back pain, the patient will understand how to control low back pain (*performance not stated in measurable terms, criterion missing*).
The nurse will demonstrate crutch walking postoperatively to the patient (*teacher-centered*).

Performance Words with Many or Few Interpretations

When writing behavioral objectives using the format suggested by Mager (1997), the recommendation is to use precise action words (verbs as labels, known as verbals) that describe a specific action.

An objective should clearly state what a learner must demonstrate for mastery in a knowledge, attitude, or skill area. A performance verb describes what the learner is expected to do. A performance may be visible or audible—for example, the learner is able to *list*, to *write*, to *state*, or to *walk*. These performances are directly observable. A performance also may be indirectly observed—for example, the learner is able to *identify*, to *solve*, to *recall*, or to *recognize*. Any performance, whether directly or indirectly observed, must be measurable. Verbs that describe what the patient is thinking, feeling, or believing, such as to *understand*, to *know*, to *enjoy*, or to *appreciate* should be avoided because they are difficult to measure (Mager, 1997).

It is impossible to identify all behavioral terms that may be used in objective writing. The important thing to remember in selecting verbs to describe performance is that they are specific, can be measured, and are action-oriented. The lists in Table 10-3 give examples of verbals that are not recommended because they are too broad, ambiguous, and hard to evaluate. It also lists those that are recommended because they are specific and relatively easy to measure (Gronlund, 1985).

COMMON MISTAKES WHEN WRITING OBJECTIVES

In formulating behavioral objectives, a number of common pitfalls can easily be made by the novice as well as by the seasoned teacher. The most frequent errors in writing objectives are

- to describe what the instructor rather than the learner is expected to do.
- to include more than one expected behavior in a single objective (avoid using the compound word *and* to connect two verbs—e.g., the learner will select *and* prepare).
- to forget to include all three components of condition, performance, and criterion.
- to use terms for performance that are not action oriented and are difficult to measure.
- to write an objective that is unattainable and unrealistic.
- to write objectives that do not relate to the goal.
- to clutter an objective by including unnecessary information.

TAXONOMY OF OBJECTIVES ACCORDING TO LEARNING DOMAINS

A *taxonomy* is an approach used to categorize things according to their relationships to one another. In science, for example, taxonomies are used to classify plants and animals in a systematic and logical fashion (Arends, 1994). In the late 1940s, psycholo-

Table 10-3 Verbals with Many or Few Interpretations

Terms with Many Interpretations (Not Recommended)	Terms with Few Interpretations (Recommended)	
to know	to apply	to explain
to understand	to choose	to identify
to appreciate	to classify	to list
to realize	to compare	to order
to be familiar with	to contrast	to predict
to enjoy	to construct	to recall
to value	to define	to recognize
to be interested in	to describe	to select
to feel	to demonstrate	to state
to think	to differentiate	to verbalize
to learn	to distinguish	to write

Source: Adapted from Gronlund, N. E. (1985). *Stating objectives for classroom instruction* (3rd ed.). New York: Macmillan.

gists and educators became concerned about the need to develop a way for defining and ordering levels of behavior according to their type and complexity (Reilly & Oermann, 1990). Bloom et al. (1956) and Krathwohl, Bloom, and Masia (1964) developed a very useful system, known as the *Taxonomy of Educational Objectives*, as a tool for classifying behaviors. This taxonomy divided behaviors into three broad categories or domains: cognitive, affective, and psychomotor. Although these three domains of behaviors are described as existing as separate entities, they are interdependent and can be experienced simultaneously. Humans do not possess thoughts, feelings, and actions in isolation of one another. For example, behaviors in the affective domain influence behaviors in the cognitive domain. Likewise, the processes of thinking and feeling influence psychomotor performance (Menix, 1996).

Behaviors in each domain are ordered in a taxonomic form of hierarchy and are classified into low, medium, and high levels, with simple behaviors listed first (designated by numbers 1.0 or 2.0) and the most complex behaviors listed last (designated by numbers 5.0 or 6.0). Learners must successfully achieve behaviors at the lower levels of the domains before they are able to adequately learn behaviors at the higher levels of the domains.

The Cognitive Domain

The *cognitive domain* is known as the "thinking" domain. Learning in this domain involves the acquiring of information and refers to the learner's intellectual abilities, mental capacities, and thinking processes. Objectives in this domain are divided into six levels, each specifying cognitive processes ranging from the simple (knowledge) to the more complex (evaluation), as listed and described in the following section (Bloom et al., 1956).

Levels of Cognitive Behavior

Knowledge (1.00): Ability of the learner to memorize, recall, define, recognize, or identify specific information, such as facts, rules, principles, conditions, and terms, presented during instruction.

Comprehension (2.00): Ability of the learner to demonstrate an understanding of information such as grasping an idea by defining it or summarizing it in his or her own words (knowledge is a prerequisite behavior).

Application (3.00): Ability of the learner to use ideas, principles, abstractions, or theories in particular and concrete situations, such as figuring, writing, reading, or handling equipment (knowledge and comprehension are prerequisite behaviors).

Analysis (4.00): Ability of the learner to recognize and structure information by breaking it down into smaller parts and specifying the relationship between the parts (knowledge, comprehension, and application are prerequisite behaviors).

Synthesis (5.00): Ability of the learner to put together parts and elements by creating a unique product that is written, oral, pictorial, and so on (knowledge, comprehension, application, and analysis are prerequisite behaviors).

Evaluation (6.00): Ability of the learner to judge the value of something, such as an essay, design, or action, by applying appropriate standards or criteria (knowledge, comprehension, application, analysis, and synthesis are prerequisite behaviors).

Table 10-4 lists verbs commonly used in writing cognitive-level behavioral objectives.

Examples of Behavioral Objectives in the Cognitive Domain

Analysis level: "After reading handouts provided by the nurse, the family member will calculate the correct number of total grams of protein included on average per day in the family diet."

Table 10-4   Commonly Used Verbs According to Domain Classification

COGNITIVE DOMAIN

Knowledge: choose, circle, define, identify, label, list, match, name, outline, recall, report, select, state

Comprehension: describe, discuss, distinguish, estimate, explain, generalize, give an example, locate, recognize, summarize

Application: apply, demonstrate, illustrate, implement, interpret, modify, order, revise, solve, use

Analysis: analyze, arrange, calculate, classify, compare, conclude, contrast, determine, differentiate, discriminate

Synthesis: categorize, combine, compile, correlate, design, devise, generate, integrate, reorganize, revise, summarize

Evaluation: appraise, assess, conclude, criticize, debate, defend, judge, justify

AFFECTIVE DOMAIN

Receiving: accept, admit, ask, attend, focus, listen, observe, pay attention

Responding: agree, answer, conform, discuss, express, participate, recall, relate, report, state willingness, try, verbalize

Valuing: assert, assist, attempt, choose, complete, disagree, follow, help, initiate, join, propose, volunteer

Organization: adhere, alter, arrange, combine, defend, explain, express, generalize, integrate, resolve

Characterization: assert, commit, discriminate, display, influence, propose, qualify, solve, verify

PSYCHOMOTOR DOMAIN

Perception: attend, choose, describe, detect, differentiate, distinguish, identify, isolate, perceive, relate, select, separate

Set: attempt, begin, develop, display, position, prepare, proceed, reach, respond, show, start, try

Guided response, mechanism, and complex overt response: align, arrange, assemble, attach, build, change, choose, clean, compile, complete, construct, demonstrate, discriminate, dismantle, dissect, examine, find, grasp, hold, insert, lift, locate, maintain, manipulate, measure, mix, open, operate, organize, perform, pour, practice, reassemble, remove, repair, replace, separate, shake, suction, turn, transfer, walk, wash, wipe

Adaptation: adapt, alter, change, convert, correct, rearrange, reorganize, replace, revise, shift, substitute, switch

Origination: arrange, combine, compose, construct, create, design, exchange, reformulate

Source: Adapted from Gronlund, N. E. (1985). *Stating objectives for classroom instruction* (3rd ed.). New York: Macmillan.

Synthesis level: "Given a sample list of foods, the patient will write a menu to include foods from the four food groups (dairy, meat, vegetables and fruits, and grains) in the recommended amounts for daily intake."

Teaching in the Cognitive Domain

A variety of teaching methods and tools exist for the purpose of developing cognitive abilities. The methods most often used to stimulate learning in the cognitive domain include lecture, one-to-one instruction, and gaming (see Chapter 11). Verbal, written, and visual tools also are useful in supplementing the teaching methods to help learners master cognitive skills.

Cognitive domain learning is the traditional focus of most teaching. In education of patients and their family members (as well as nursing staff and nursing students), emphasis remains on the sharing of facts, ideas, and concepts. Perhaps this emphasis has occurred because nurses in the role of teacher typically feel more confident and more skilled in being the "giver of information" rather than being the facilitator and coordinator of learning. Lecture and one-to-one instruction are the most often used teaching methods. Both of these instructional approaches, when taught in a typical fashion, are directed almost exclusively at teaching cognitive behaviors.

The Affective Domain

The *affective domain* is known as the "feeling" domain. Learning in this domain involves influencing feelings expressed as emotions, interests, attitudes, values, and appreciations. The affective domain is divided into categories that specify the degree of a person's depth of emotional responses to tasks. It represents the extent to which feelings or attitudes are incorporated into one's personality or value system (Arends, 1994; Reilly & Oermann, 1990).

Although nurses recognize the need for individuals to learn in the affective domain, the learner's attitudes, beliefs, and values cannot be directly observed, but can only be inferred from words and actions (Maier-Lorentz, 1999). Teachers tend to be less confident and more challenged in writing behavioral objectives for the affective domain because it is difficult to develop easily measurable objectives for the evaluation of learning outcomes.

Behavior in the affective domain is guided by notions held by individuals and society as to what is considered good and right, which involves moral reasoning and ethical decision making. For staff nurses, competency in the affective domain is measured to determine if care is given to patients in a humanistic and sensitive manner.

Reilly and Oermann (1990) differentiate between the terms *beliefs*, *attitudes*, and *values*. *Beliefs* are what an individual perceives as reality; *attitudes* represent feelings about an object, person, or event; and *values* are beliefs that guide actions and ways of living.

Objectives in the affective domain are divided into five categories, each specifying the associated level of affective responses as listed and described in the following section (Bloom et al., 1956; Krathwohl et al., 1964).

Levels of Affective Behavior

Receiving (1.00): Ability of the learner to show awareness of an idea or fact or a consciousness of a situation or event in the environment.

Responding (2.00): Ability of the learner to respond to an experience, at first obediently and later willingly and with satisfaction (receiving is a prerequisite behavior).

Valuing (3.00): Ability of the learner to accept the worth of a theory, idea, or event, demonstrating commitment to an experience believed as having value (receiving and responding are prerequisite behaviors).

Organization (4.00): Ability of the learner to organize, classify, and prioritize values by integrating a new value into a general set of values (receiving, responding, and valuing are prerequisite behaviors).

Characterization (5.00): Ability of the learner to integrate values into a total philosophy or world view (receiving, responding, valuing, and organization are prerequisite behaviors).

Table 10-4 lists verbs commonly used in writing affective-level behavioral objectives.

Examples of Behavioral Objectives in the Affective Domain

Receiving level: "During a group discussion session, the patient will admit to any fears he may have about needing to undergo a repeat angioplasty."

Responding level: "At the end of one-to-one instruction, the child will verbalize feelings of confidence in managing her asthma using the Peak Flow Tracking Chart."

Characterization level: "Following a series of in-service education sessions, the staff nurse will display consistent interest in maintaining strict hand-washing technique to control the spread of nosocomial infections to patients in the hospital."

Teaching in the Affective Domain

A variety of teaching methods have been found to be reliable in helping the learner acquire affective behaviors. Questioning, case study, role playing, gaming, and group discussion sessions are examples of instructional methods that can be used to help patients and their families develop values and explore attitudes, interests, and feelings. Another powerful tool for affective teaching is role modeling by the nurse to instill desired behaviors into the learner.

Unfortunately, adequate weight is not usually given to teaching in the affective domain. The nurse in the role of teacher more often emphasizes cognitive processing and psychomotor functioning with little time set aside for exploration and clarification of learner feelings, emotions, and attitudes (Ellis, 1993; Rinne, 1987).

Schoenly (1994) examined affective teaching strategies that can be used to assist learners in acquiring affective domain behaviors. Once appropriate objectives, an accepting climate, and a trusting relationship have been established, the following teaching techniques can be selected and implemented:

Questioning: The technique of careful questioning during the lecture process or one-to-one instruction can assist in meeting objectives in the affective domain. Affective questioning increases interest and motivation to learn about feelings, values, beliefs, and attitudes regarding a topic under study. *Low-level* affective questions are directed at stimulating learner awareness and responsiveness to a topic. *Midlevel* affective questioning assists in determining the strength of a belief or the internalization of a value. *High-level* affective questioning probes for information about the depth of integration of a value.

Case study: This method can assist the learner in developing problem solving and critical thinking skills through exploration of participant attitudes, beliefs, and values. Using learning groups, with the reader assuming the role of a key player in the situation (nurse, family member, patient) rather than being a neutral observer, will help develop affective behavioral responses.

Role playing: This method provides an excellent opportunity to practice new behaviors and explore feelings, attitudes, and values; to problem solve; and to resolve personal problems associated with human circumstances. Role playing allows the learner to "walk in someone else's shoes." Being an observer during role playing can sensitize the learner to the situation. Active participation in role playing energizes the learner to attend and respond to the circumstance being presented.

Gaming: Games that are controlled by the participants and that have flexible rules, rather than games that have structured roles and specific rules, are more appropriate for accomplishing affective behavioral objectives. Gaming promotes active involvement of the learner in goal-directed, although not necessarily competitive, activities. Debriefing following gaming is an important aspect of acquiring affective domain behaviors.

Group discussion: This method provides an opportunity for clarifying personal values and exploring social values and moral issues. Value clarification involves identifying and sharing personal values for the purpose of increasing self-awareness and self-discovery. Values inquiry involves investigating the value systems of various ethnic groups. Both approaches provide the chance for in-depth learning of affective behaviors.

The affective domain encompasses three levels that govern attitudes and feelings (Richards & Vicary, 1985):

- The intrapersonal level includes personal perceptions of one's own self, such as self-concept, self-awareness, and self-acceptance.
- The interpersonal level includes the perspective of self in relation to other individuals.
- The extrapersonal level involves the perception of others as established groups.

All three levels are important in affective skill development and can be taught through a variety of methods as described above.

The Psychomotor Domain

The *psychomotor domain* is known as the "skills" domain. Learning in this domain involves acquiring fine and gross motor abilities such as walking, handwriting, handling equipment, or carrying out a procedure. Psychomotor skill learning, according to Reilly and Oermann (1990) "is a complex process demanding far more knowledge than suggested by the simple mechanistic behavioral approach" (p. 81). For development of psychomotor skills to take place, there must be integration of the other two domains of learning as well. The affective component conveys recognition of the value or worth of the skill being learned. The cognitive component relates to knowing the principles, relationships, and processes in carrying out the physical movement. Although all three domains are involved in demonstrating a psychomotor competency, the psychomotor domain can be examined separately and requires different teaching approaches and evaluation strategies (Reilly & Oermann, 1990).

Psychomotor skills are easy to identify and measure because they include primarily movement-oriented activities that are relatively easy to observe.

Psychomotor learning, including perceptual-motor tasks, can be classified in a variety of ways (Dave, 1970; Harrow, 1972; Moore, 1970; Simpson, 1972). Simpson's system seems to be the most widely recognized as relevant to patient teaching. Objectives in this domain, according to Simpson, are divided into seven levels, as listed and described in the following section.

Levels of Psychomotor Behavior

Perception (1.00): Ability of the client to show sensory awareness of objects or cues associated with some task to be performed. This level involves reading directions or observing a process with attention to steps or techniques involved in doing a task.

Set (2.00): Ability of the learner to exhibit readiness to take a particular kind of action, such as following directions, through expressions of willingness, sensory attending, or body language favorable to performing a motor act (perception is a prerequisite behavior).

Guided response (3.00): Ability of the learner to exert effort under the guidance of an instructor to imitate an observed behavior with conscious awareness of effort (perception and set are prerequisite behaviors).

Mechanism (4.00): Ability of the learner to repeatedly perform steps of a desired skill with a certain degree of confidence, indicating mastery to the extent that some or all aspects of the process become habitual. The steps are blended into a meaningful whole and are performed smoothly with little conscious effort (perception, set, and guided response are prerequisite behaviors).

Complex overt response (5.00): Ability of the learner to automatically perform a complex motor act with independence and a high degree of skill, without hesitation and with minimum expenditure of time and energy (perception, set, guided response, and mechanism are prerequisite behaviors).

Adaptation (6.00): Ability of the learner to modify or adapt a motor skill to suit the individual or various situations, indicating mastery of highly developed movements that can be applied to a variety of conditions (perception, set, guided response, mechanism, and complex overt response are prerequisite behaviors).

Origination (7.00): Ability of the learner to create new motor acts, such as novel ways of manipulating objects or materials, as a result of an understanding and ability to perform skills (perception, set, guided response, mechanism, complex overt response, and adaptation are prerequisite behaviors).

Table 10-4 lists verbs commonly used in writing psychomotor-level behavioral objectives.

Examples of Behavioral Objectives in the Psychomotor Domain

Guided response level: "After watching a 15-minute video on the procedure for self-examination of the breast, the client will perform the exam on a model with 100% accuracy."

Set level: "Following demonstration of proper use of crutches, the patient will attempt to walk using the correct three-point gait technique."

Teaching of Psychomotor Skills

When teaching psychomotor skills, it is important for the teacher to remember to keep skill instruction separate from a discussion of principles underlying the skill (cognitive component) or a discussion of how the learner feels about carrying out the skill (affective component). Psychomotor skill development is very egocentric and usually requires a great deal of concentration as the learner works toward mastery of a skill. It is easy to interfere with psychomotor learning if the teacher asks a knowledge (cognitive) question while the learner is trying to focus on the performance (psychomotor response) of a skill. For example, while the patient is learning to self-administer parenteral medication, it's not unusual for the teacher to ask "What are the actions or side effects of this medication?" or "How do you feel about injecting yourself?" These questions demand cognitive and affective responses during psychomotor performance. Although a teacher frequently intervenes with questions in the midst of a learner's performance, it is definitely an inappropriate teaching technique. What the teacher is doing, in fact, is asking the learner to demonstrate at least two different behaviors at the same time. This technique can result in frustration and confusion, and ultimately it may result in a delay or failure to achieve any of the behaviors successfully. Questions related to the cognitive or affective domain should take place before or after, not during the learner's practicing of a psychomotor skill (Oermann, 1990).

In psychomotor skill development, the ability to perform a skill is not equivalent to learning a skill. Performance is a transitory action, whereas learning is a more permanent behavior that follows from repeated practice and experience (Oermann, 1990). The actual learning of a skill requires practice to allow the individual to repeat the performance with accuracy and coordination, and out of habit. Practice does make perfect, and so repetition leads to perfection and reinforcement of the behavior. The riding of a bicycle is a perfect example. When one first attempts to ride a bicycle, movements tend to be very jerky, and the act requires a great deal of concentration. Once the skill is learned, bicycle riding becomes a smooth, automatic operation that requires minimal attention to the details of fine and gross motor movements acting in concert to allow the learner to achieve the skill of riding a bicycle. Some behaviors that are learned do not require much reinforcement, even over a long period of disuse, whereas other behaviors, once learned, need to be rehearsed or relearned to perform them at the level of skill once achieved. The amount of practice required to learn any new skill varies with the individual, depending on many factors. Oermann (1990) and Bell (1991) have addressed some of the more important variables:

Readiness to learn: The motivation to learn affects the degree of perseverance exhibited by the learner in working toward mastery of a skill.

Past experience: If the learner is familiar with equipment or techniques similar to those needed to learn a new skill, then mastery of the new skill may be achieved at a faster rate. The effects of learning one skill on the subsequent performance of another related skill is known as *transfer of learning* (Gomez & Gomez, 1984). For example, if a family member already has experience with aseptic technique in changing a dressing, then learning to suction a tracheostomy tube using sterile technique should not require as much time to master.

Health status: Illness state or other physical or emotional impairments in the learner may affect the time it takes to acquire or successfully master a skill.

Environmental stimuli: Depending on the type and level of stimuli, distractions in the immediate surroundings may interfere with acquiring a skill.

Anxiety level: The ability to concentrate can be affected by how anxious someone feels. Nervousness about performing in front of someone is a key factor in psychomotor skill development. High anxiety levels interfere with coordination, steadiness, fine muscle movements, and concentration levels when performing complex psychomotor skills. It is important to reassure learners that they are not necessarily being "tested" during psychomotor skill performance. Reassurance and support reduce anxiety levels related to the fear of not meeting the expectations of themselves or of the teacher.

Developmental stage: Physical, cognitive, and psychosocial stages of development all influence an individual's ability to master a movement-oriented task. A young child's fine and gross motor skills as well as cognitive abilities are at a different level than those of an adult. The older adult will likely exhibit slower cognitive processing and increased response time (needing more time to perform an activity) than younger clients.

Practice session length: During the beginning stages of learning a motor skill, short and carefully planned practice sessions and frequent rest periods will help increase the rate and success of learning. These techniques can prevent physical fatigue and restore the learner's attention to the task at hand.

Another hallmark of psychomotor learning is the type and timing of the feedback given to learners. Psychomotor skill development allows for immediate feedback so learners have an idea on the spot about how they performed. During skill practice, learners receive *intrinsic feedback* that is generated from within the self, giving them a feel for how they have performed. They may sense either that they did quite well or that they felt awkward and need more practice. In addition, the teacher has the opportunity to provide *augmented feedback* by sharing with learners an opinion or conveying a message through body language about how well they performed (Oermann, 1990). The immediacy of the feedback, together with the self-generated and teacher-supplemented feedback, makes this a unique feature of psychomotor learning. Performance checklists, which can serve as guides for teaching and learning, are also effective tools for evaluating the level of skill performance.

An important point to remember is that it is all right to make mistakes in the process of teaching or learning a psychomotor skill. If the teacher makes an error when demonstrating a skill or the learner makes an error during return demonstration, this is the perfect teaching opportunity to offer anticipatory guidance: "Oops, I made a mistake. Now what do I do?" Unlike cognitive skill development, where errorless learning is the objective, in psychomotor skill development a mistake represents an opportunity to demonstrate how to correct an error and to learn from the not-so-perfect initial attempts at performance. The old saying, "You learn by your mistakes" is most applicable to psychomotor skill mastery.

Learning is a very complex phenomenon. It is clear that the cognitive, affective, and psychomotor domains, although representing separate behaviors, are to some extent interrelated. For example, the performance of a psychomotor skill often requires a certain degree of cognitive knowledge or understanding of information, such as the scientific principles underlying a practice or why a skill is important to carry out. Also, there may be an affective component of valuing the performance of a psychomotor behavior as part of the learner's overall experience.

DEVELOPMENT OF TEACHING PLANS

After mutually agreed-upon goals and objectives have been written, it should be clear what the learner is to learn and what the teacher is to teach. Predetermined goals and objectives serve as a basis for developing a teaching plan. Organizing and presenting information in the format of an internally consistent teaching plan requires skill by the nurse. Developing an action plan to achieve the goals and objectives should include the actual purpose, content, methods and tools, sequence, timing, and evaluation of instruction. The teaching plan should be clear and concise.

The three major reasons for constructing teaching plans are:

1. To force the teacher to examine the relationship among the steps of the teaching process and to ensure a logical approach to teaching.
2. To communicate in writing and in an outline format exactly what is being taught, how it is being taught and evaluated, and the time allotted for accomplishment of the behavioral objectives.
3. To legally document that an individual plan for each learner is in place and is being properly implemented.

A complete *teaching plan* consists of eight basic parts (Ryan & Marinelli, 1990):

1. The purpose
2. A statement of the overall goal
3. A list of objectives
4. An outline of the related content
5. The instructional method(s) used for teaching the related content
6. The time allotted for the teaching of each objective
7. The instructional resources (materials/tools) needed
8. The method(s) used to evaluate learning

The major criterion for judging a teaching plan is whether it facilitates a relationship between its parts. A sample teaching plan format is shown in Figure 10-1. This format is suggested because the use of columns allows the teacher, as well as anyone else who is using it, to see all the parts of the teaching plan at one time and provides the best structure for monitoring internal consistency of the plan.

When constructing a teaching plan, the teacher must be certain that internal consistency exists within the plan (Ryan & Marinelli, 1990). A teaching plan is said to be internally consistent when all eight parts of the plan are related to one another. Internal consistency requires that the domain of learning in any objective that is written is reflected across the elements of the teaching plan, from the purpose all the way through to the end process of evaluation. The following example is adapted from Ryan and Marinelli's (1990) self-study module on *Developing a Teaching Plan*:

For example: If the nurse has decided to teach to the psychomotor domain, then the goal, objectives, and related content should reflect the psychomotor domain.

Purpose: To provide the client with the information necessary for monitoring blood glucose.

Goal: The client will demonstrate the ability to test for blood glucose on a regular basis.

Objective: Following a 20-minute teaching session, the client will be able to use a reagent strip, Chemstrip bG, to determine blood glucose level with 100% accuracy.

The purpose, goal, and objective in this above example all relate to the psychomotor domain. Therefore, the content, instructional method(s), instructional resource(s), time allotment, and evaluation method(s) also should be appropriate to the domain. The decision about what domains(s) should be the focus of a teaching plan must be made prior to developing the plan and should remain consistent throughout the plan. If the purpose and goal are written with a focus on just the cognitive domain, then the objectives and the remaining five parts should be reflective of teaching to the cognitive domain. If the purpose and goal is written for the accomplishment of a skill set that includes more than one domain, then the teaching plan should reflect objectives, content, methods of teaching, and methods of evaluation in these different domains (see Figure 10-1). As identified below, the overall design of the teaching plan must match whatever domains of learning have been selected.

Domain	Teaching Design
Cognitive	Topic-Centered
Affective	Feeling-Centered
Psychomotor	Performance-Centered

What is included in the *content outline* depends on the complexity and detail of the material to be taught. This decision is based on assessment of the client's readiness to learn, learning needs, and learning style. The amount and depth of information included should depend on the learning level of the client. The focus for teaching a low-level learner would be to concentrate on the "need to know" information to ensure that a skill can be performed safely. By comparison, a high-level learner can handle (and may desire) additional "nice to know" information. Whoever the client may be, the content to be taught for each objective must be directly related to the objective.

The *method of instruction* chosen also should be appropriate for the information being taught. If, for example, the purpose is to teach a client to self-administer medication from an asthma inhaler (psychomotor domain), the primary methods of teaching should be demonstration and return demonstration. If the purpose of teaching is to impart knowledge of what is in a low-fat diet (cognitive domain), lecture and programmed instruction are appropriate teaching methods.

The *time allotted* for the teaching and learning of each objective must be specified. Each teaching session should be no more than 20 to 30 minutes in length. In this period of time, one or more objectives may be accomplished or partially accomplished. Additional teaching sessions may be required for the learner to attain expected outcomes.

The *resources* used should appropriately match the content and teaching method(s). If the purpose is to teach breast self-examination, then written and audiovisual materials or an anatomical model of the breast would be useful instructional tools. A variety of resources may be necessary to maintain the learner's attention and to serve as reinforcers of information. An important consideration is the literacy level of the learner. Giving a low-literate person difficult reading materials may frustrate and confuse the learner and defeat the plan for teaching.

Finally, the *method of evaluation* should match the domain in which learning is to take place. If the behavioral objective is for the learner to be able to identify (cognitive) three major symptoms of an impending heart attack, then the evaluation method to test that knowledge could be obtained by giving a written post-test, or by using an oral question and answer approach. Evaluation methods must measure the desired learning outcomes to determine if and to what extent the learner actually learned.

In summary, just as with a nursing care plan, all elements of a teaching plan need to "hang together." The goal must be reflective of the purpose. The objectives depend on and must derive from the goal. The instructional content depends on and must be derived from the objectives. The teaching method depends on and must be related to the content, and so forth. If content outlined in the plan is not related to any of the objectives, then the content is either unnecessary or another objective must be written as a basis for including the extra content. If a teaching plan has no content relative to a particular stated objective, then additional content must be included or the objective should be eliminated. Whether a plan is adhered to or revised, it must, above all else, reflect internal consistency. (See Figure 10-1 for a sample teaching plan.)

PURPOSE: To provide patient with information necessary for self-administration of insulin as prescribed

GOAL: The patient will be able to perform insulin injections independently according to treatment regimen

Objectives	Content Outline	Method of Instruction	Time Allotted (in min.)	Resources	Method of Evaluation
Following a 20-minute teaching session, the patient will be able to:					
Identify the five sites for insulin injection with 100% accuracy (cognitive)	Location of five anatomical sites Rotation of sites	1:1 instruction	2	Anatomical chart	Post-testing
Demonstrate proper techniques according to procedure for drawing up insulin from a multidose vial (psycho-motor)	Accepted technique according to procedure

Reading syringe unit dose markings | Demonstration Return demonstration | 5 | Alcohol sponges Sterile SQ needles and insulin syringes Multidose vial of sterile water | Observation of return demonstration |
| Give insulin to self in thigh area with 100% accuracy (psychomotor) | Procedure for injecting insulin SQ at 90-degree angle using aseptic technique | Demonstration Return demonstration | 10 | Human model SQ needle and syringe Multidose vial of sterile water Alcohol sponges | Observation of return demonstration |
| Express any concerns about self-administration of insulin (affective) | Summarize common concerns Exploration of feelings | Discussion | 3 | Video Written handouts | Question and answer |

Figure 10-1   Completed Teaching Plan for Self-Administration of Insulin

THE CONCEPT OF LEARNING CURVE

Learning curve is a term commonly used to determine how long it takes for a learner to acquire a knowledge, attitude, or motor skill. To understand the learning curve concept as it relates to the process of teaching and learning, one must refer to educational psychology literature. The learning curve has been described as basically nothing more than a graphic depiction of changes in performance or output during a specified time period (McCray & Blakemore, 1985). A learning curve shows the relationship between practice and performance of some type of a skill. It provides a concrete measure of the rate at which a person learns a task. Cronbach (1963) defined a learning curve specifically as it relates to psychomotor skill development as "a record of an individual's improvement made by measuring his ability at different stages of practice and plotting his scores" (p. 297).

According to Cronbach (1963), the learning curve theory is divided into six stages (see Figure 10-2):

1. **Negligible progress:** This "pre-readiness" period is when the learner is not ready to perform the entire task, but learning is taking place, such as developing attention, manipulation, and perceptual skills. This period can be relatively long in young children who are developing physical and cognitive abilities and in older adults who may have difficulty in making key discriminations.

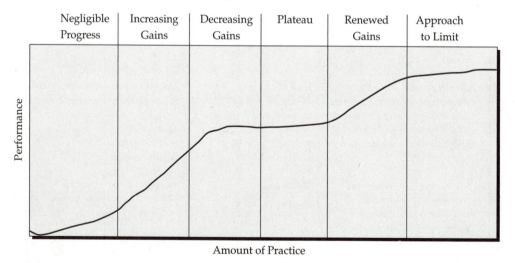

Figure 10-2 A Schematic Learning Curve
Source: Adapted from Cronbach. (1963). *Educational Psychology* (2nd ed.). New York: Harcourt, Brace & World, p. 299.

2. **Increasing gains:** Rapid gains in learning occur as the learner grasps the essentials of the task. Scores rise rapidly as the learner becomes aware of cues to attend to, goals to attain, or ways to effectively organize responses. Motivation to perform a skill increases when the learner has interest in the task, receives approval from others, or experiences a sense of pride in discovering the ability to perform.

3. **Decreasing gains:** In this period the rate of improvement in mastering a task slows down and additional practice does not produce much, if any, gains. Learning occurs in smaller increments as the learner incorporates changes by using cues to smooth out performance.

4. **Plateau:** No substantial gains are made. This "leveling off" period is characterized by a small rate of progress in performance. During this stage, the learner is making minor adjustments in mastering a skill. However, the belief that this is a "period of no progress" is considered false. Gains in skills can occur even though overall performance scores remain stable.

5. **Renewed gains:** During this period, additional progress can be made after the plateau period has ended. If gains occur, they are usually due to growth in physical development, renewed interest in the task, a response to a challenge, or the drive for perfection.

6. **Approach to limit:** Progress at this point becomes negligible. The ability to perform has reached its potential. The "limit" is a hypothetical stage only because there is never certainty that a learner cannot improve further.

Individual learning curves are characterized by irregularity (see Figure 10-3) and are often unlike the smooth theoretical curve. Fluctuations in performance can be attributed to changes in the learner, such as focus, interest, energy, and ability, or in the environment, such as situational circumstances or favorable/unfavorable conditions for learning (Barker, 1994; Cronbach, 1963; Gage & Berliner, 1998).

The concept of learning curve has been primarily applied to business and industry to measure employee productivity, which, in turn, has a direct effect on cost of labor, the time it takes to manufacture a product or deliver a service, the quality of the product or service, and the pricing of goods and services. Nursing research must be conducted on application of the learning curve concept to the teaching and learning of patients (or any other audience of learners whom the nurse may teach). Research could answer such questions in patient and staff education as the following:

- Can a learning curve be shortened given the characteristics of the learner, the situation, or the task at hand?

- Why is the learning curve steeper, more drawn out, or more irregular for some learners than for others?
- Can we predict the learning curves of our patients or nursing staff depending on their educational or experiential backgrounds?
- What can we do from an educational standpoint to influence the pace and pattern of learning for earlier or more complete achievement of expected outcomes?
- How can the learning curve concept be applied to improve staff performance, thereby increasing work satisfaction and productivity, decreasing costs of care, and improving the quality of care?

The answers to these questions could lead to changes in the nurse's approach to teaching and learning.

The advantages of applying the learning curve concept to patient teaching and learning are many. Perhaps one key benefit to understanding this concept is to realize that the pattern and pace of learning are irregular. The learning of any task is often rapid after an initial slow start, inevitably decreases, reaches a plateau, and then increases again, until a limit is reached where no more significant improvement in mastery of a skill is likely to be achieved. Understanding this concept will help

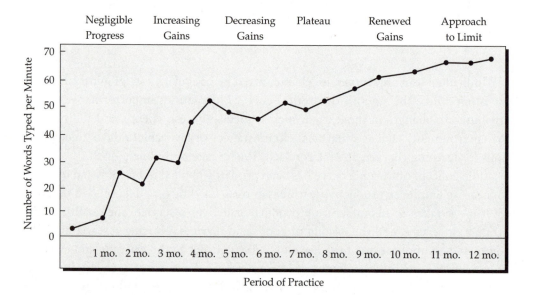

Figure 10-3   Learning Curve During One Year of Typing Practice
Source: Adapted from Cronbach. (1963). *Educational Psychology* (2nd ed.). New York: Harcourt, Brace & World, p. 303.

teachers adjust their expectations when different paces and patterns of learning occur in individuals as they attempt to master any psychomotor skill.

Awareness that learning does not occur in a straight upward fashion, and that the amount of practice needed to improve performance is variable, should also be shared with learners to reduce their expectations and frustrations when mastering a skill. For example, a patient who is undergoing rehabilitation to learn how to walk again may easily become discouraged with the progress he or she is making. Gains in learning may slow down or the patient may experience a time at the beginning or in the middle of the curve when he or she does not seem to be making any improvement toward goal achievement. Teachers can realistically support the learner if they understand the pace and pattern of skill development.

SUMMARY

The major portion of this chapter focused on differentiating goals from objectives, preparing accurate and concise objectives, classifying objectives according to the three domains of learning, and the teaching of cognitive, affective, and psychomotor skills using appropriate instructional interventions. The writing of behavioral objectives is fundamental to the education process. Goals and objectives serve as a guide to the teacher in the planning, implementation, and evaluation of teaching and learning.

Assessment of the learner is a prerequisite to writing objectives. Prior to selecting the content to be taught and the methods and materials to be used for instruction, there must be a clear understanding of what the learner is expected to be able to do. Appraisal should be based on a mutual determination between the teacher and the learner as to what needs to be learned, under what conditions learning can best occur, and the teaching and evaluation methods most preferred. Objectives setting must be a partnership effort by the learner and the teacher for any learning experience to be successful and rewarding in the achievement of expected outcomes. The communication of desired behavioral outcomes and the mechanisms for accomplishing behavioral changes in the learner are essential elements of both teaching and learning.

This chapter also outlined the development of teaching plans, which provide the blueprint for organizing and presenting information in a coherent manner. A teaching plan must reflect internal consistency of its parts. Active involvement and accountability on the part of the learner must be encouraged. In addition, the concept of learning curve is relevant to the process of teaching and learning and must be explored from a nursing practice perspective.

REVIEW QUESTIONS

1. What are the two major differences between goals and objectives?
2. What are the definitions of the terms *goal* and *objective*?
3. What five reasons justify the need for writing objectives?
4. What are the three major characteristics that should be included in every written behavioral objective?
5. What mistakes are commonly made when writing behavioral objectives?
6. What are the three domains of learning?
7. Which levels of behavior, according to the taxonomic form of hierarchy, are considered the most simple and the most complex in the cognitive, affective, and psychomotor domains?
8. Why is it important for the teacher to remember to keep psychomotor skill instruction separate from the cognitive and affective components of skill development?
9. What five factors or variables influence the amount of practice required to learn any new skill?
10. What are the eight basic components of a teaching plan?
11. Why is the concept of learning curve an important consideration in teaching and learning for nursing practice?

REFERENCES

Arends, R. I. (1994). *Learning to teach* (3rd ed.). New York: McGraw-Hill.

Babcock, D. E. & Miller, M. A. (1994). *Client education: Theory and practice*. St. Louis: Mosby YearBook.

Barker, L. M. (1994). *Learning and behavior: A psychobiological perspective*. New York: Macmillan.

Bell, M. L. (1991). Learning a complex nursing skill: Student anxiety and the effect of preclinical skill evaluation. *Journal of Nursing Education, 30*(5), 222–226.

Bloom, B. J., Englehart, M. S., Furst, E. J., Hill, W. H., & Krathwohl, D. R. (1956). *Taxonomy of educational objectives: The classification of educational goals, Handbook 1: Cognitive domain*. New York: David McKay.

Cronbach, L. J. (1963). *Educational Psychology* (2nd ed.). New York: Harcourt, Brace, & World.

Cummings, C. (1994). Tips for writing behavioral objectives. *Nursing Staff Development Insider, 3*(4), 6, 8.

Dave, R. (1970). *Psychomotor levels in developing and writing objectives*. Tucson, AZ: Educational Innovators Press.

Ellis, C. (1993). Incorporating the affective domain into staff development programs. *Journal of Nursing Staff Development, 9*(3), 127–130.

Ferguson, L. M. (1998). Writing learning objectives. *Journal of Nursing Staff Development, 14*(2), 87–94.

Gage, N. L. & Berliner, D. C. (1998). *Educational Psychology* (6th ed.). Boston: Houghton Mifflin.

Gomez, G. E. & Gomez, E. A. (1984). The teaching of psychomotor skills in nursing. *Nurse Educator, 9*(4), 35–39.

Gomez, G. E. & Gomez, E. A. (1987). Learning of psychomotor skills: Laboratory versus patient care setting. *Journal of Nursing Education, 26*(1), 20–24.

Gronlund, N. E. (1985). *Stating objectives for classroom instruction* (3rd ed.). New York: Macmillan.

Haggard, A. (1989). *Handbook of patient education.* Rockville, MD: Aspen.

Harrow, A. J. (1972). *A taxonomy of the psychomotor domain: A guide for developing behavioral objectives.* New York: David McKay.

Krathwohl, D. R., Bloom, B. J., & Masia, B. B. (1964). *Taxonomy of educational objectives: The classification of educational goals. Handbook II: The affective domain.* New York: David McKay.

Mager, R. F. (1997). *Preparing instructional objectives* (3rd ed.). Atlanta, GA: Center for Effective Performance.

Maier-Lorentz, M. M. (1999). Writing objectives and evaluating learning in the affective domain. *Journal for Nurses in Staff Development, 15*(4), 167–171.

McCray, P. & Blakemore, T. (1985). *A guide to learning curve technology to enhance performance prediction in vocational evaluation.* Menomonie, WI: Research and Training Center, Stout Vocational and Rehabilitation Institute, School of Education and Human Services, University of Wisconsin-Stout.

Menix, K. D. (1996). Domains of learning: Interdependent components of achievable learning outcomes. *Journal of Continuing Education in Nursing, 27*(5), 200–208.

Moore, M. R. (1970). The perceptual-motor domain and a proposed taxonomy of perception. *Audio Communications Review, 18*, 379–413.

Oermann, M. H. (1990). Psychomotor skill development. *Journal of Continuing Education in Nursing, 21*(5), 202–204.

Reilly, D. E. & Oermann, M. H. (1990). *Behavioral objectives: Evaluation in nursing* (3rd ed.). Pub. No. 15-2367. New York: National League for Nursing.

Richards, B. & Vicary, J. R. (1985). The affective domain in health occupations education. *Nursing Management, 16*(7), 52–54.

Rinne, C. (1987). The affective domain: Equal opportunity in nursing education. *Journal of Continuing Education in Nursing, 18*(2), 40–43.

Ryan, M. & Marinelli, T. (1990). *Developing a teaching plan.* Unpublished Self-Study Module, College of Nursing, State University of New York Health Science Center at Syracuse.

Schoenly, L. (1994). Teaching in the affective domain. *Journal of Continuing Education in Nursing, 25*(5), 209–212.

Simpson, E. J. (1972). The classification of educational objectives in the psychomotor domain. In M. T. Rainier (ed.), *Contributions of behavioral science to instructional technology: The psychomotor domain* (3rd ed., pp. 43–56). Englewood Cliffs, NJ: Gryphon Press, Prentice-Hall.

CHAPTER 11

Teaching Methods and Instructional Settings

Kathleen Fitzgerald

CHAPTER HIGHLIGHTS

Teaching Methods
   Lecture
   Group Discussion
   One-to-One Teaching
   Demonstration and Return
     Demonstration
   Gaming
   Simulation

Selection of Teaching Methods
Evaluation of Teaching Methods
Increasing the Effectiveness of Teaching
   Techniques to Enhance the Effectiveness
     of Verbal Presentations
   General Principles for All Teachers
Instructional Settings
   Sharing Resources among Settings

KEY TERMS

demonstration
gaming
group discussion
healthcare-related setting
healthcare setting
instructional setting

lecture
nonhealthcare setting
one-to-one teaching
return demonstration
simulation
teaching method

OBJECTIVES

After completing this chapter, the reader will be able to
1. Define the term *teaching method*.
2. Explain the various types of teaching methods.
3. Describe how to use each method effectively.
4. Identify the strengths and limitations of each method.
5. Identify the variables that influence the selection of a method.
6. Recognize strategies to enhance teaching effectiveness.
7. Explain how to evaluate the method(s) used.
8. Classify the instructional setting in which the role of the nurse as teacher is played out.

With appreciation to Virginia E. O'Halloran, EdD, RN for her contribution to information on instructional settings in this chapter.

After an excellent presentation, have you ever heard someone comment, "Now, there is a born teacher!"? This comment makes it seem that teaching well comes automatically. In reality, teaching is a learned skill. Development of this skill requires knowledge of the teaching methods available and ways to use them effectively. Stimulating and effective learning experiences are designed, not accidental. *Teaching methods* are the techniques or approaches the teacher uses to bring the learner into contact with the content to be learned. Methods are a way, an approach, or a process to communicate information, whereas instructional materials or tools (see Chapter 12) are the actual vehicles by which information is shared with the learner. Some examples of methods are lecture, group discussion, one-to-one teaching, demonstration and return demonstration, gaming, and simulation. Books, videos, and posters are examples of materials and tools.

This chapter will review the types of teaching methods available and consider how to use them efficiently and effectively. It will also identify the strengths and limitations of each method. Throughout this chapter, examples will be presented to highlight various methods of teaching for patient education, such as assisting a client in a wellness program to stop smoking or instructing patients on how to self-manage their diabetes. The nurse is expected to be able to choose and use the most appropriate approaches when teaching a variety of patients and families in a variety of instructional settings.

TEACHING METHODS

Teaching is a vital role for nurses. When teaching, the importance of selecting the most appropriate methods to meet the needs of the learners should not be underestimated. There is no one perfect method for all learners and learning experiences. Whatever the method chosen, it will usually be most effective if it is used in combination with other instructional approaches to enhance learning. For example, the lecture may be used as a primary method, with opportunities for question and answer periods and short discussion sessions being interspersed throughout the lecture period.

Decisions about which methods to use will be based on such variables as audience size, diversity (e.g., age, educational background, culture), preferred learning style, and the setting for teaching. Methods that help patients become active participants in the learning process are also an important consideration. Passive learning leads to boredom and inattention.

Lecture

Lecture is a highly structured method by which the teacher verbally transmits information directly to groups of learners for the purpose of instruction. It is one of the oldest and most often used methods of teaching. In its purest form, the lecture format allows for only minimal exchange between the teacher and the learner, but it can be an effective method of teaching in the lower-level cognitive domain to impart content knowledge. Lecture is an efficient and cost-effective method for getting large amounts of information across to a large number of people at the same time and within a reasonable time frame. For example, the lecture might be used to explain diabetes mellitus to a group of laypeople. It is the nurse's expertise that can substantially contribute to the patient's understanding of a subject. Lecture is also useful for providing background information as a basis for group discussions and for summarizing data and presenting the latest research findings on a particular topic (Boyd, Gleit, Graham, & Whitman, 1998). In addition, the lecture can be easily supplemented with handout materials and other audiovisual aids.

With respect to its limitations, the lecture method is ineffective in teaching affective and psychomotor behaviors, it does not provide for much stimulation of learners, and there is limited opportunity for learner involvement. Rather, learners are passive recipients of the information being presented. Also, because the lecture does not account for individual differences in background, attention span, or learning style, all learners are exposed to the same information regardless of their ability or need. This is particularly evident in patient groups, where cognitive abilities and stages of coping with some topics vary widely. This diversity within groups makes it difficult and challenging for the nurse to effectively meet the needs of all patients in the group.

Although the lecture method is considered cost-effective, cost should not be determined just by calculating the nurse–patient ratio of contact hours. Teacher preparation time, the number of times the material needs to be presented, and the follow-up time used to individualize learning and evaluate outcomes must also be taken into account.

Using Lecture Effectively

Each lecture should include an introduction, body, and conclusion. During the introduction, learners should be presented with an overview of the behavioral objectives pertinent to the lecture topic, along with an explanation of why these objectives are significant. Engage learners' attention by conducting an informal survey or stating the objectives as questions that will be answered during the body of the lecture. Use humor and your personality to help establish rapport with your audience.

The next portion of the lecture is the body, or the actual delivery of the content. Careful preparation is needed so that the important aspects are covered in an accurate, logical, cohesive, and interesting manner. Examples should be used throughout to enhance the important points you wish to make, but avoid including too much information that can reduce the impact of your message. Because the lecture format tends to be very passive for learners, you can enhance the effectiveness of your presentation by mixing it with other teaching methods, such as discussion or question and answer sessions.

Use of audiovisual materials, such as a video, overhead projections, or PowerPoint slides, can also add variety to your presentation. Some general guidelines for these materials are as follows (Evans, 2000):

- Do not put all your content on slides. Instead, focus on the key concepts to supplement your presentation.
- Use the largest font possible, and include fewer than 25 words per slide.
- Use color and graphics when appropriate.
- Bold colors provide contrast between background and text, which is especially necessary if you plan to lecture in a large room with bright lights.
- Tables and charts are very useful when you are presenting large amounts of data

Make sure that all audiovisual equipment is functional and that you know how to use it before beginning the lecture. A technical malfunction can easily embarrass you as well as distract your audience.

If you are nervous or inexperienced in presenting before groups, practice ahead of time before a mirror or in front of a colleague. Outline key points of your presentation on index cards, overhead projections, or slides. Avoid reading the entire printed copy of your presentation. Vary your tone of voice, move around the room, be enthusiastic, show interest in the topic, and stay within the planned amount of time to capture and hold the group's attention.

The final section of the lecture format is the summary or conclusion. Review the major concepts presented. It is very important that your lecture not exceed the prescribed time so that you do not have to end abruptly because time has run out. Try to leave some opportunity for questions and summary information. If you are using a microphone with a large group, be sure to repeat the questions so the rest of the audience can hear them. If time runs short, state that you will be able to answer only a few questions, but invite immediate follow-up by meeting with interested individuals alone.

Group Discussion

Group discussion is a method of teaching in which learners get together to exchange information, feelings, and opinions with one another and with the nurse as teacher. Discussion is one of the most common teaching techniques. Group size can vary, but the group discussion technique can be used with as few as 3 people and with as many as 15 to 20 people. Group discussion is a good method for teaching in both the affective and cognitive domains.

Using Group Discussion Effectively

The discussion should focus on the behavioral objectives for learning that have been established before the session begins. Objectives should be presented at the beginning of the session. These objectives should be carefully followed to prevent the discussion from going off in directions different than you intended. The nurse's role in this teaching method is to act as a facilitator to keep the discussion on track and to tie points together. The nurse must be well versed in the subject matter to answer questions, to move the discussion along in the right direction, and to give appropriate feedback.

Group discussion requires the teacher to be able to tolerate less structure and organization than other methods, such as lecture or one-to-one teaching. The group must have some knowledge of the content before this method can be used. Otherwise, the discussion will be based on what is known as "pooled ignorance"; that is, people will offer opinions and ideas that are not based on facts. An experienced support group may need little input while they work out a complex self-care problem. A new group of patients or family members with little understanding or experience with a chronic illness, for example, will need information and guidance from the nurse before they can knowledgeably participate in problem solving.

It is also the teacher's responsibility to make sure that every member of the group understands what is being said, or else they may jump to conclusions based on incorrect information or may not be able to deal with what is being discussed. For this reason, patients need to be assessed before being assigned to groups. Although diversity within a group is beneficial, a large range in literacy skills, states of anxiety, and experiences with acute and chronic conditions may lead to difficulty in meeting one or more members' needs.

It is important for the nurse to maintain the trust of the group. Everyone must feel safe and comfortable enough to express his or her point of view. Respect and tolerance toward others should be modeled by the teacher and required of all group members. Of course, this consideration does not preclude correcting errors or disagreements. A clear message must be given that although personal opinions can be debatable and errors in thinking can be corrected, what each member has to say is valued and the member's right to participate is guaranteed.

The major advantage of group discussion is that it stimulates learners to actively think about issues and problems and to exchange their own experiences. It provides opportunities for sharing of ideas, receiving peer support, fostering a feeling of belonging, giving guidance, and reinforcing previous learning. Discussion is effective in assisting learners to identify resources and to reflect on the personal meaning of the topic being discussed (Brookfield & Preskill, 1999). It is well recognized that active learning leads to greater retention of information.

Working with people in groups rather than individually allows the teacher to reach a number of learners at the same time. With healthcare costs rising, this method should be considered as an efficient and effective method to teach groups with similar objectives, such as preparation for childbirth or cardiac bypass surgery. For other groups of patients, these programs may be economically valuable in preventing frequent hospitalization or in reducing time in acute care.

Through group work, members share common concerns and receive reinforcement from one another. Support from peers fosters the belief that "we're all in the same boat" or "if you can do it, I can do it," which serves to stimulate motivation for learning.

Group size, a major consideration in this method of teaching, should be determined by the purpose or task to be accomplished (Boyd et al., 1998). Although a large group has the potential for greater diversity because members will have different knowledge and experience, there will be less chance for everyone to participate and for individual needs to be met (Anderson, 1990). Arnold and Boggs (1989) suggest that a group size of six to eight members is ideal to achieve diversity of ideas and yet allow for balanced interaction among members. Larger groups can be broken down into smaller units to promote greater interaction by all members and to better develop the skills in knowledge and attitudes of each individual.

Group discussion has proved particularly helpful to patients and families dealing with chronic illness. It offers them a chance to share information, learn new coping skills, and receive ongoing support to maintain independence in self-care. The process also helps people learn how to respond to situations and explore ways to make needed changes in their lives. This approach increases patients' and families' confidence in their ability to handle an illness (Lorig & Gonzalez, 1993). Group discussion is most effective during the accommodation stage of psychological adjustment to chronic illness, because the interactions help reduce isolation and foster identification with others who are in similar circumstances (Fredette, 1990).

The opportunity for all members to be active participants is the major benefit of group discussion. But this method can also lead to difficulties if one or two members dominate the discussion or lose focus on the objectives for learning. Those who dominate or get off track may need to be redirected in a tactful manner that decreases their influence on the group but does not damage their self-esteem or the trust among the group members. Shy patients or family members, on the other hand, may refuse to become involved or may need a great deal of encouragement to participate. One helpful approach to encourage equal participation is to tell the group at the beginning of the session that the goal is to hear from all members. Let them know that everyone's input and points of view are welcomed, but everyone should have the chance to speak. Members who have additional questions that are important but unique to their circumstances can ask them after the discussion has ended. The discussion method is challenging for the novice teacher when faced with a group whose members do not easily interact.

One-to-One Teaching

In *one-to-one teaching*, the nurse delivers individual instruction designed specifically to meet a particular patient's needs. It is an opportunity to openly communicate ideas and feelings as well as receive nonverbal messages. This method should never be a lecture delivered to an audience of one to satisfy the nurse's goals for teaching. Instead, the experience should actively involve the patient and be based on his or her unique objectives for learning.

Using One-to-One Teaching Effectively

One-to-one teaching begins with an assessment of the learner and the mutual setting of objectives and goals to be accomplished. Establishing mutual objectives and goals by the teacher and learner is very important. It has been proven that patient education and counseling in chronic illness lead to better outcomes when the patient plays an active role in discussing alternatives and in setting the objectives and goals for learning (Kaplan, Greenfield, & Ware, 1989).

One-to-one teaching can be tailored to meet objectives in all three domains of learning. For example, teaching a patient to give insulin would address both the cognitive and psychomotor domains. Coaching an expectant mother so she feels she has enough control in using the techniques learned in birth preparation classes is an example of teaching primarily in the affective domain.

It is also important to determine at which stage of change the person is regarding a problem behavior such as smoking, and then to tailor the interventions to that stage (Saarmann, Daugherty, & Riegel, 2000). (See Chapter 6 for the Stages of Change model that explains motivation and compliance for behavioral change.)

Whenever teaching is done on a one-to-one basis, instructions should be specific and followed by immediate response from the learner and feedback from the teacher. Allowing learners the opportunity to state their understanding of information gives the teacher an opportunity to evaluate the extent of learning. Also, communicating to learners what further information is forthcoming allows them to connect what they have just learned with what they will be learning. For example, the nurse teaching a patient about hypoglycemia might say, "Now that you understand what causes low blood sugar, we will talk about how to tell when you have it and what to do if you experience it after discharge."

The process of one-to-one teaching involves moving patients from repeating the information to applying what they have learned. In the preceding example regarding hypoglycemia, you might give the person a hypothetical situation as close to the patient's lifestyle as possible and let the person work through how to respond to it. In this type of simulation, a potentially threatening situation can be presented in a non-threatening manner (Boyd et al., 1998). For instance, you might ask a busy executive who has diabetes how he would respond to feeling shaky and sweaty at 2:00 p.m. on a day when a meeting runs late and he misses lunch. Be sure to clearly state that this scenario is not a test but rather a "dress rehearsal" for life situations. You can change the scenarios with further questioning to help learners plan how they could prevent such situations in the future. This technique gives learners a chance to use the information at a higher cognitive level. It also gives the nurse a chance to evaluate learning in a nonthreatening way.

Questioning is an excellent technique for the one-to-one method of teaching. It can be used to involve patients as active participants in the learning process. The responses the patient gives to the questions you ask can also allow the nurse to provide feedback on his or her progress. Questions can be matched to the cognitive objectives. For example, for the knowledge level, you might ask "What is the next step?" in a procedure.

For the higher level of thinking, you might ask a patient to plan a meal with a new diet that has been prescribed. Questioning should be done in such a way that the learner does not feel like their knowledge is being tested, but rather in a way that exchanges information and stimulates thinking. Two problems can occur with questioning. Questions may be confusing and unclear such that the learner does not know what you are asking, or they can contain too many facts for the person to process them effectively (House, Chassie, & Spohn, 1990). Watch your learner's nonverbal reactions, and rephrase the question if you detect either of these problems. If the learner seems confused, it is helpful to take the responsibility that perhaps you did not ask the question in a clear manner. This technique will guard against the learner feeling guilty or becoming discouraged if a question was incorrectly answered. It is important to give learners time to process information and respond to your questions. Sometimes nurses are uncomfortable waiting in silence for an answer or are impatient and attempt to correct an answer before learners complete their responses. Interrupting patients may further interfere with their thinking process and create a tense atmosphere.

One-to-one teaching has many advantages. The major benefit is the ability to individualize teaching. This method is an ideal approach for both initial assessment of the learner and ongoing evaluation of the learner in all three domains of learning. It is especially suitable for teaching those who are educationally disadvantaged or who have been diagnosed with low-level literacy skills or learning disabilities. The teaching can be paced, the content can be tailored to meet individual patient needs, and immediate feedback from the teacher on progress toward achieving objectives and goals can be provided.

The major drawback of one-to-one teaching is the isolation of the learner from others who may have similar needs or concerns. Learners are deprived of the opportunity for identification with others through the sharing of ideas, thoughts, and feelings with those who may be in like circumstances. For example, patients recently diagnosed with cancer can benefit from group interaction that allows them to explore mutual concerns and find support in relating with others.

Exercise caution when using the one-to-one method to avoid having patients feel "put on the spot" because they are the only ones who are the object of teaching—the sole focus of attention. The nurse must also be careful in the use of questioning because learners may interpret this technique as a "test" of their knowledge and skills. In addition, it is not unusual for the teacher to make the mistake of cramming too much information into each session, which can result in the learner feeling overwhelmed and anxious. Also, one-to-one teaching of patients and families can be an inefficient approach because the nurse is reaching only one person at a time. Since this method is very labor-intensive, it must be well tailored to make the expense worthwhile in terms of achievement of learner outcomes and improved patient satisfaction rates.

Demonstration and Return Demonstration

Demonstration is a method by which the patient is shown by the nurse how to perform a particular skill. *Return demonstration* is a method by which the patient attempts to perform the skill with cues from the nurse as needed. These two methods require different abilities by both the nurse and the patient. Each is effective in teaching psychomotor domain skills. Both may also enhance cognitive and affective learning.

Using Demonstration and Return Demonstration Effectively

Prior to giving a demonstration, patients should be informed of the purpose of the procedure, the sequential steps involved, the equipment being used, and the actions expected of them. Equipment should be tested beforehand to ensure that it is complete and in working order. For the demonstration method to be employed effectively, the patient and family must be able to clearly see and hear the steps being taught. Therefore, the demonstration method is best suited to teaching individuals or small groups.

Watching a demonstration can be a passive activity for patients, whose role is to observe the teacher presenting an exact performance of the required skill. In the process of demonstrating a skill, it is important to explain why each step needs to be carried out in a certain manner. The performance should be flawless, but the teacher should take advantage of a mistake to show how errors can be handled. Used correctly, an error may increase rapport with patients. However, too many mistakes disrupt the mental image that the patient is forming.

When demonstrating a psychomotor skill, if possible, work with the exact equipment that the learner will be expected to use. For instance, a patient or family member who is learning to administer tube feedings at home will be anxious and frustrated if taught how to use one pump in the hospital when a different type is used in the home after discharge. Often the learner is too inexperienced to see the skill pattern and will have difficulty transferring learning of the task from one piece of equipment to another.

Return demonstration should be planned to occur close to when the demonstration was given. The nurse may need to give reassurance to reduce anxiety prior to the beginning of the patient's performance because the opportunity to return demonstrate may be viewed by the patient as a test. Often patients believe that they are expected to perform perfectly the first time around. Once a patient recognizes that the nurse is a coach and not an evaluator, the climate will be less stressful. Explaining that the initial performance likely will not be perfect and allowing the patient to manipulate the equipment before using it will help the learner to feel more comfortable in attempting to practice a new skill.

When the patient is giving a return demonstration, the nurse should remain silent except for offering cues when necessary or briefly answering questions. Learners may be prompted by a series of pictures or a checklist. Casual conversation or asking questions should be avoided because they interrupt the learner's thought processes and interfere with efforts to actually perform the task.

Breaking the steps of the procedure into small increments will give the learner the opportunity to master one sequence before attempting the next. Praising the patient along the way for each step correctly performed will reinforce behavior and give the learner confidence in being able to successfully accomplish the task in its entirety (Haggard, 1989). Emphasis should be on what to do, rather than on what not to do. Practice should be supervised until the patient is competent enough to independently perform all steps accurately.

Learners will need a varying amount of practice to become competent. Once a skill has been acquired, doing a task repeatedly increases speed and proficiency of performance.

Return demonstration sessions should be planned close enough together that the learner does not lose the benefit of the last practice session. As with demonstration, the equipment for return demonstration needs to exactly match that which will be used by the patient at home. Learners may also require help in compensating for individual differences. For example, if you are right-handed and the learner is left-handed, perhaps sitting across from each other during the demonstration would be more helpful than sitting next to one another. The patient with difficulty seeing the increments on an insulin syringe may need a magnifying device or an insulin pen to accurately perform the skill of self-administering the medication.

These methods actively engage the learner through stimulation of multiple visual, auditory, and tactile senses. The opportunity afforded for mental rehearsal of procedures being demonstrated prior to actual return demonstration has been associated with increased performance levels (Haggard, 1989). Repetition of movement and constant reinforcement through practice are the mainstays of successful learning in the psychomotor domain. Overlearning by extended practice instills confidence in the learner that the skill will be competently performed and will be retained for a longer period of time.

Although the cliché "practice makes perfect" is quite true, demonstration and return demonstration sessions are very time-consuming and require plenty of time to be set aside for teaching as well as for learning. These methods are expensive because of the need to keep the group size small, to provide individual supervision during follow-up practices, and to make available the equipment for practice.

Gaming

Gaming is a teaching method in which the learner participates in a competitive activity with preset rules. Although these activities do not have to reflect reality, they are designed to accomplish educational objectives. The goal is for the learners to win a game by applying knowledge and skills just learned or previously rehearsed. Gaming is fun with a purpose. It promotes retention of information by stimulating learner enthusiasm and increasing learner involvement. Games can be created or modified for individual or group learning. More complex games require the learner to use problem solving and critical thinking. This method adds variety to the learning experience and is excellent for dull or repetitive content.

Using Gaming Effectively

Games can be placed anywhere in the sequence of a learning activity—as a way to introduce a topic, check learner progress, or summarize information (Joos, 1984). This teaching method is primarily effective for objectives in the cognitive domain, but can also be used to enhance skills in the psychomotor domain and to influence affective behavior through increased social interaction (Robinson, Lewis, & Robinson, 1990).

In gaming, the teacher's role is that of a facilitator. At the beginning of a game, the group of patients should be told the objectives and the rules. Any materials needed to play a game are distributed, and various teams are assigned. Once the game starts, the nurse keeps the flow going and interprets the rules. The game should be interrupted as seldom or as briefly as possible so as not to disturb the pace (Joos, 1984). When the game is completed, winners should be rewarded. Prizes do not have to be expensive because their main purpose is to acknowledge achievement of learners in a public manner (Robinson et al., 1990). At the end of the game, the teacher should conduct a debriefing session with the learners to give them a chance to discuss what they learned, ask questions, and receive feedback regarding the outcome of the game.

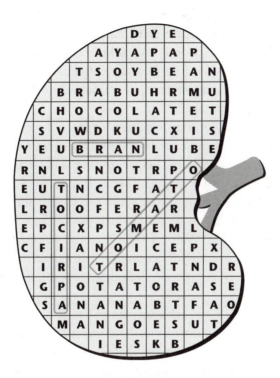

Figure 11-1 Sample Word Search Game for Patients
Source: Reprinted with permission of the American Nephrology Nurses Association, publisher, *ANNA Journal*, Volume 17/Number 4 (August 1990), page 307.

Games may be either purchased or designed. Well-known commercial games, such as Trivial Pursuit, Bingo, Monopoly, or Jeopardy, are useful because their formats can be modified to include content related to the objectives for patient education, the equipment is reusable, and many players already are familiar with the rules of play. Word searches, crossword puzzles, treasure hunts, and card and other board games are also flexible in format and can be developed inexpensively and with relative ease. See Figure 11-1 for an example of a word search game that helps patients with end-stage renal disease learn about foods that are known to elevate serum potassium (Robinson et al., 1990).

Computer games, although more expensive, are becoming increasingly available and are a popular option for many learners. Gaming is also a particularly attractive method for children, who enjoy the challenge of learning through playlike activity.

For example, an interactive video game was used with young people from ages 8 to 16 with Type I diabetes to learn about the daily challenges of self-care. Participants were told to play this simulation game as much or as little as they wished. By the end of the 6-month trial, there was a 77% drop in diabetes-related urgent care as well as an increase in diabetes-related self-efficacy, in communication with parents about diabetes, and in self-care (Lieberman, 2001).

Be sure to pilot games prior to using them for teaching and learning. To participate, learners must have sufficient ability and background knowledge to play the game. Remember, games that challenge reading skills likely will not be useful with patients who have literacy problems. Games should be exciting, fun, and challenging enough to stimulate learner interest but not so difficult or competitive as to result in frustration or inability to succeed, which would cause learners to avoid this type of learning opportunity (Walts, 1982). Games, whether purchased or self-developed, must serve the purpose of helping the learner accomplish the behavioral objectives. The question is: Are people learning something useful while they are having fun?

Along with its advantages, the gaming method has some limitations. Gaming can create a competitive environment that may be threatening to some learners. In addition, the group size must be kept small so that all members can participate, and the room must be more flexible than a traditional setting for teaching to allow for clusters of teams and higher noise level. Also, because gaming tends to be more physically demanding than many other methods, some learners may be excluded from playing due to age or a disability. Finally, the cost of purchasing games or the time taken by the nurse to design, pilot, and update the content of the games needs to be considered. Figure 11-2 is a game suitability checklist to determine if gaming is a good method to meet the objectives for learning.

Simulation

Simulation is a method that uses an artificial or hypothetical experience to engage patients in an activity reflecting real-life conditions but without the risk-taking consequences of an actual situation (Rystedt & Lindström, 2001). A variety of activities can be presented to help patients learn problem-solving skills. Simulations are effective for teaching in the cognitive, affective, and psychomotor domains. Actually, games and simulations are a lot alike because both methods require learners to actively participate in dealing with concrete, realistic situations. Experiential learning occurs when a learner must choose an action and handle the consequences.

GAME SUITABILITY CHECKLIST		
Criteria	Yes	No
• Does the game meet the program objectives?	_____	_____
• Can the game be completed within the time allotted?	_____	_____
• Is the size and layout of the room conducive to the game?	_____	_____
• Will the available participants meet the minimum number required for the game?	_____	_____
• Do staff members have the time and interest to design or adapt games? If not, are funds available to purchase games?	_____	_____
• If the game requires equipment or supplies, are they readily available?	_____	_____
a. Are resources or funds available to design or purchase needed materials?	_____	_____
b. Does the game require replacement of materials following each use?	_____	_____
• Does the game require preparation or cleanup time?	_____	_____

Figure 11-2 Game Suitability Checklist

Source: Lewis et al. (1989). Reprinted with permission from *The Journal of Continuing Education in Nursing*.

Simulations are effective in helping someone find solutions to problems, change attitudes, or prepare for possible events they may encounter (Rorden, 1987).

Using Simulation Effectively

When planning a simulation, it is most effective if the learning experience is made to resemble real life as much as possible, but in a nonthreatening way. The activity should challenge the decision-making abilities of the patients and family members by imposing time limits, creating levels of tension, using actual equipment, or subjecting them to stimuli in the environment to observe and evaluate. For example, a scenario could be developed to help parents of a baby with sudden infant death syndrome work through how they would handle a situation when the monitor signals respiratory difficulty in their infant. Another example would be to provide the patients in a diabetes self-management education program the opportunity to select foods from a restaurant menu and set their insulin pumps for the correct bolus of insulin to learn how to master these skills. Models can also be used in simulation to teach patients. An example would be how to change the dressing on a venous access device using a torso model.

The learning laboratory is a setting where patients and family members can easily use models, computers, videotapes, and actual equipment, with the nurse in the role of facilitator, to practice various skills such as transfer techniques, sterile procedures, and other care-giving activities. Even though the equipment for simulation remains permanently assigned to the learning center, it is ideal if the equipment is portable so that it may be used on hospital units, in outpatient clinics, or in home settings.

Simulated learning experiences should be followed with the actual experience as soon as possible. The simulation is never exactly the same as the real experience, and therefore the patient or family member will need help with the transfer of skills to the actual situation.

Limitations of this teaching method are few, but significant. They include cost of equipment and time needed for teaching and learning.

Table 11-1 summarizes the general characteristics of each of the teaching methods described above.

SELECTION OF TEACHING METHODS

Selecting a teaching method requires the nurse to conduct an assessment of each learner's needs, readiness to learn, and learning style as well as to determine with the client the behavioral objectives to be accomplished. There is no one right method, because the best approach depends on many variables, such as the audience, the content to be taught, and the setting in which teaching and learning are to take place. Also, consideration must be given to available resources such as time, money, space, and materials, to support the teaching and learning activities. The teacher's expertise is also an important variable in the selection process.

Nurses as teachers are at different levels on the novice-to-expert continuum. A nurse may be an expert clinician but have only limited experience and effectiveness in the teaching role. Nevertheless, the ideal method for any given situation is the one that best suits the learner's needs, not your own. If you are a novice, begin instruction with very familiar content so that you can focus on the teaching process itself and feel more confident trying out different techniques and instructional materials.

Periodically examining your role as a teacher gives you the opportunity to assess the personal factors of energy, attitudes, knowledge, and skills that can influence the priority you assign to your teaching responsibilities, your ability to teach effectively, and the amount of satisfaction you derive from teaching others.

Table 11-1   General Characteristics of Teaching Methods

Methods	Domain	Learner Role	Teacher Role	Advantages	Limitations
Lecture	Cognitive	Passive	Presents information	Cost-effective Targets large groups	Not individualized
Group discussion	Affective Cognitive	Active—if learner participates	Guides and focuses discussion	Stimulates sharing ideas and emotions	Shy or dominant member
One-to-one teaching	Cognitive Affective Psychomotor	Active	Presents information and facilitates individualized learning	Tailored to individual's needs and goals	High levels of diversity Labor-intensive Isolates learner
Demonstration	Cognitive	Passive	Models skill or behavior	Preview of "exact" skill/behavior	Individual or small groups needed to facilitate visualization
Return demonstration	Psychomotor	Active	Individualizes feedback to refine skill	Immediate individual guidance	Labor-intensive to view individual performance
Gaming	Cognitive Affective	Active—if learner participates	Oversees pacing Referees Debriefs	Captures learner enthusiasm	Environment too competitive for some learners
Simulation	Cognitive Psychomotor	Active	Designs environment Facilitates process Debriefs	Practice "reality" in safe setting	Labor-intensive Equipment costs

Elements to consider (Narrow, 1979):

- At any given point in time, your energy level will be affected by both psychological and physical factors, such as the demands of your professional and personal life, the state of your health, and the support you get from colleagues.
- Your relationship with the learners can influence the enthusiasm you bring to the teaching-learning situation. If you feel drawn to the patient and family members because you find them interesting or you are concerned or anxious about their situation, then teaching will most likely be a satisfying experience. If, on the other hand, they are demanding or display inappropriate behavior, you may feel negatively toward them and find the teaching-learning encounter more difficult and less fulfilling. You can develop the ability to accept individuals without necessarily approving of their behavior.
- Your confidence in the nature of the subject matter to be taught affects your overall performance. If you find certain content to be stressful to teach because you lack relevant knowledge or skills, then additional study and practice to increase your understanding of the subject will likely relieve your discomfort and apprehension, which allows you to function more effectively in the teaching role.
- Your comfort level will depend on how difficult it is for you to communicate with others about what you may consider sensitive material, such as sexual behavior, mental illness, abortion, birth defects, disfigurement, or terminal illness. It is important for you to examine your own feelings, seek support from colleagues, and locate resources to help you discover effective approaches in addressing these topics.

If the teaching-learning process is to be a partnership, it is crucial not only to assess the learner, but also to assess yourself as the teacher.

EVALUATION OF TEACHING METHODS

Evaluating any instructional approach requires you to make a judgment as to the effectiveness and efficiency of the method you used. The following four questions should be asked to help you decide if the method chosen was appropriate.

1. Did the method help the learners to achieve the stated objectives? This question is the most important criterion for evaluation. The method must help accomplish the objectives or else all the other criteria for selection are unimportant. Examine how well matched the method is to the learning domain of the objec-

tives. Did the method expose learners to the necessary information and training to learn the desired behaviors?

2. Did the resources available adequately support the method? This requires you to consider such factors as the size of the audience, the characteristics of the space, and the equipment at your disposal.

3. To what extent did the method allow for active participation to accommodate the needs, abilities, and style of the learner? Active participation has been well documented as a way to increase interest in learning and the retention of information.

4. Did the method match the preferences of the learner(s)? No one approach will satisfy all learners, but adhering to one method exclusively addresses the preferred style of only a segment of your audience.

INCREASING THE EFFECTIVENESS OF TEACHING

Excellent teachers have one thing in common—a passion to keep improving their abilities. One does not "arrive" at being an expert teacher. The drive toward excellence is an ongoing process that continues throughout the nurse's entire professional life. The following are techniques to improve your teaching.

Techniques to Enhance the Effectiveness of Verbal Presentations

Present information enthusiastically. No matter how well a lesson is planned or how clearly it is presented, if it is delivered in a dry and dull monotone, it will likely fall on deaf ears (Cunningham & Baker, 1986). Try to vary the quality and pitch of your voice, use a variety of gestures and facial expressions, change position if necessary to make direct and frequent eye contact with patients and families, and demonstrate a true interest in the topic to attract and hold an audience's attention. Be careful not to overuse body language and movements because excessive mannerisms can be distracting.

Include humor. Use humor as a technique to grab and maintain the attention of the learner. Appropriate humor can help establish a rapport with learners by humanizing the nurse. Humor does not necessarily require the teacher to tell jokes, and joke telling should not be attempted if this is not a skill one possesses. Furthermore, the teacher should avoid making someone the object of humor if it results in a "put-down." Humor establishes an atmosphere that allows for human error without embarrassment and encourages freedom and comfort to explore alternatives in the learning situations. Humor is a means to reduce anxiety when dealing with sensitive material, to provide unforgettable examples of everyday life experiences, and to reinforce traditional teaching methods (Freitas et al., 1991).

Choose problem-solving activities. Learners need to be exposed to activities that help them develop problem-solving skills. Patients, especially those with chronic conditions, need problem-solving skills to know how to respond to changes demanded by their condition. What should they do differently on a "sick day," or what constitutes an "emergency"? Patients and families need more than just low-level cognitive information to make adjustments in their lives. The nurse must therefore devise opportunities that help patients and families to critically analyze situations as well as support the learner in exploring possible alternatives.

Use anecdotes and examples. Use stories and examples to illustrate points. Anecdotes are valuable in driving a point home, clarifying a topic under discussion, or helping someone better relate to an issue. Use examples to reinforce the learning principle that simple illustrations can help with understanding complex ideas. Using examples related to past experiences and the knowledge base of patients helps them identify and connect in a concrete way with the material being taught.

General Principles for All Teachers

The following are some general principles that should be used by all nurses in their role as teachers.

Give positive reinforcement. It is well known that giving praise to someone or using words of approval for the ideas, actions, and opinions of others by making statements such as "That's a good answer," "I agree with you," and "You have a very good point," or using nonverbal expressions of acceptance such as smiling or nodding, will encourage patients to participate more readily or to try harder. Rewarding even a small success can instill satisfaction in the learner. Disapproval or criticism, on the other hand, will dampen motivation and cause learners to withdraw. However, what works as positive reinforcement for one individual may not be effective for another, as rewards are closely tied to value systems. The amount of reinforcement needed also varies from one individual to another. For example, a small amount of praise can have a strong effect on the learner who is not used to succeeding.

Project an attitude of acceptance and sensitivity. If you come across as believable, trustworthy, caring, and competent, you help to put your patients at ease, which serves as an invitation for them to learn. When you demonstrate patience and sensitivity with respect to age, race, culture, and gender, people feel accepted for who they are. Establishing rapport with your patients and family members opens up the avenues of communication for the sharing of ideas and concerns. People learn better in a comfortable and supportive environment. Not only is it important that the physical environment be conducive to learning, but the psychological climate should also be respectful of their needs and circumstances. Nurses must have a clear view of their roles as expert coaches and as partners in the teaching and learning situation, rather than as only givers of information.

Be organized and give direction. Excellent group discussions, interesting lectures, and successful attempts at using simulation are examples of teaching that do not happen by accident. They are the result of hours of preparation, careful planning, and organization, which allow the patient to stay focused on the objectives. Material should be logically organized, objectives should be clearly defined, and directions should be given in a straightforward, specific, and easily understood manner. Teaching sessions should be relatively brief so as not to overload the patient with too much detail and unnecessary content. "Need to know" information should take precedence over the "nice to know" information to be sure that enough time is set aside to cover the essentials. Regardless of the method of teaching used, the attention span of the learner waxes and wanes over time, and what is learned first and last is usually retained the most (Ley, 1972).

Elicit and give feedback. Feedback should be a two-way process. It is a strategy to give information to the learner about their performance as well as to receive information from learners about your teaching. Feedback can take the form of either verbal or nonverbal responses to a situation. It should be encouraged during and at the end of each teaching-learning encounter. Learners are often able to judge their own performance by comparing it to what they expect of themselves or what they think others expect of them. To get feedback, the learner might ask, "How well did I do?", "Am I on track?", "Did I do all right?", or "What do you think?" Feedback about your teaching is equally important because it helps you to decide if you should proceed with teaching or modify your approach to teaching, take time to review or explain, or stop altogether for the moment. For example the teacher should ask, "What questions do you have?", "Is this clear?", "What more do you want to know?", or "What else can I help you with?" Also, the teacher should be sensitive to nonverbal expressions such as a nod, a smile, a look of bewilderment, or a frown indicating either an understanding or a lack thereof.

Use questions. Questioning is one of the means for both the nurse and the patient to get information about performance. If the nurse is skillful in the use of questioning, it serves multiple purposes in the teaching-learning process. Questions help to clarify concepts, assess what the patient already knows about the topic, stimulate interest in a new subject, or evaluate the patient's mastery of the objectives.

Babcock and Miller (1994) identified three types of questions that can be used to elicit different types of answers:

1. The first type, known as a factual or descriptive question, begins with words such as *who, what, where, which,* or *when* and asks for recall-type responses from the learner. Answers to questions such as "Which foods are high in fat?" or "Whom should you call if you run out of medication?" reveal the facts that were learned. Descriptive questions take a more open-ended approach, such as "What kinds of exercise do you get daily?", "What problems do you have with activities of daily living?", or "What are the signs and symptoms of infection?", and require a more detailed response from the learner.

2. The second type involves clarifying questions that ask for more information and help the learner to convey thoughts and feelings. Such questions might include "What do you mean when you say . . . ?" or "I'm not sure I understand exactly what you are expressing."

3. The third type, known as a high-order question, requires more than memory or perception to answer. It requires the learner to establish cause and effect, or compare and contrast concepts. Examples include "Why does a low-salt diet help to control blood pressure?", "What do you think will happen if you don't take your medication?", or "What do you see as the advantages and disadvantages in following the treatment plan?"

After asking questions, a period of silence may occur, which can be uncomfortable for both the nurse and the patient. Encouraging the patient to think about the answer before responding may reduce anxiety over the silence. In a group, this strategy also allows all participants to have a chance to think through their responses to the questions, which gives them the opportunity to make more thoughtful and deliberate responses. Questioning helps the teacher pace the material being presented and judge the progress the learner is making in the achievement of the behavioral objectives.

Know your audience. It is important to know what patients and families need and want to learn. The effectiveness of teaching will be severely limited when the choice of teaching method is based on the interest and comfort level of the teacher and not on the assessed needs of the learner (Freitas et al., 1991). Use methods that match the topic rather than the teacher's personality. Most teachers have a preferred style of teaching and tend to rely on that approach regardless of the content to be taught. Skilled nurses, however, adapt themselves to a teaching style appropriate to the subject matter, setting, and various styles of the learners. Flexibility is their hallmark in tailoring the instruction to the unique needs of learners. Be willing to use a variety of teaching methods to provide the best possible experience for achievement of objectives.

Use repetition and pacing. Repetition, if used appropriately, is a technique that strengthens learning. It reinforces learning by helping people retain information. If overused, repetition can lead to boredom and frustration because you are repeating what is already understood and remembered. If used correctly, it can assist the patient in focusing on important points and keeping the learner on track. Repetition is especially important when presenting new or difficult information. The opportunity for repeated practice of behavioral tasks is called *skill inoculation*. Repetition can take the form of a simple reminder, a review of previously learned material, or the continued practice of a skill. Assessing the learner's understanding will help you to use repetition effectively. Pacing refers to the speed at which information is presented. Constantly assessing will help you to pace your teaching so that it is slow enough for information to be absorbed, yet fast enough to maintain interest and enthusiasm (Narrow, 1979).

Summarize important points. Summing up information at the end of the teaching-learning encounter gives a perspective on what has been covered, how it relates to the objectives, and what you expect the learner to have achieved. Summarizing also reviews key ideas to instill information in the mind and helps the learner to see the parts of a whole. Summary reinforces retention of information. It provides feedback as to the progress made, which leaves the learner with a feeling of satisfaction with what has been accomplished.

INSTRUCTIONAL SETTINGS

Traditionally, the primary focus of nursing practice has been on the delivery of acute care in hospital settings. In recent years, however, the practice of nursing in community-based settings has experienced tremendous growth. The reasons for the shift in orientation of nursing practice from inpatient care sites to outpatient sites relate to the trends affecting the nation's healthcare system as a whole. These trends include public and private reimbursement policies, changing population demographics, advances in healthcare technology, an emphasis on wellness care, and increased consumer interest in health. In response to these trends, the domains of nursing practice have broadened to include a greater emphasis on the delivery of care in community settings such as homes, clinics, health maintenance organizations (HMOs), physicians' offices, public schools, and the workplace.

With the increased focus on prevention, promotion, and independence in self-care activities, today's newly emerging healthcare system mandates the education of consumers to a greater extent than ever before. Opportunities for client teaching have become increasingly more varied in terms of the types of clients encountered, their particular learning needs, and the settings in which healthcare teaching occurs. Because health education has become an increasingly important responsibility of nurses in all practice environments, it is important to acknowledge the various settings where clients, well or ill, are consumers of health care.

Instructional settings are classified according to the relationship health education has to the primary purpose of the organization or agency that provides or sponsors health instruction. An *instructional setting* is defined as any place where nurses engage in teaching for disease prevention, health promotion, and health maintenance and rehabilitation. Three types of settings for the education of clients are classified as follows:

1. A *healthcare setting* is one in which the delivery of health care is the primary or sole function of the institution, organization, or agency. Hospitals, visiting nurse associations, public health departments, outpatient clinics, extended-care facilities, health maintenance organizations, physician offices, and nurse-managed centers are examples of organizations whose primary purpose is to deliver health care. Health education is an integral aspect of the overall care delivered within these settings. Nurses provide direct patient care, and their role encompasses the teaching of clients.

2. A *healthcare-related setting* is one in which health-related services are offered as a complementary function of the agency. Examples of this type of setting include the American Heart Association, the American Cancer Society, and the Muscular Dystrophy Association. These organizations provide client advocacy, conduct health screenings and self-help groups, distribute health education information and materials, and support research on disease and lifestyle issues for the benefit of consumers within the community. Education on health promotion, disease prevention, and improving the quality of life for those who live with a particular illness is the key function of nurses within these agencies.

3. A *nonhealthcare setting* is one in which health care is an incidental or supportive function of an organization. Examples of this type of setting include businesses, industries, schools, and military and penal institutions. The primary purpose of these organizations is to produce a manufactured product or offer a nonhealth-related service to the public. Industries, for example, are involved in health care

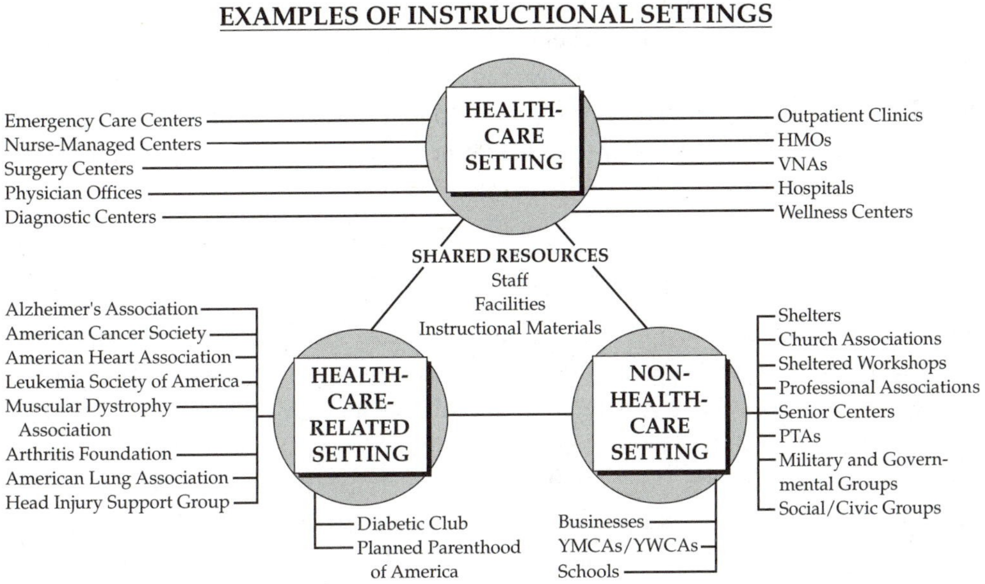

EXAMPLES OF INSTRUCTIONAL SETTINGS

FIGURE 11-3   Instructional Settings and Their Relationships

only to the extent of providing health screenings and nonemergent health coverage to their employees through a health office within their place of employment. Such services make instruction available on job-related health and safety issues to meet Occupational Safety and Health Administration (OSHA) regulations, or providing opportunities for health education through wellness programs to reduce absenteeism or improve employee morale.

Classifying instructional settings in which the nurse functions as teacher provides a frame of reference through which to better understand the interrelationship among the components of the organizational climate, the target audience, and the resources within the environment influencing the educational tasks to be accomplished. The role and functioning of the nurse is affected differently by these components in each of the identified settings.

An instructional setting, then, is any environment in which health education takes place to provide individuals with learning experiences for the purpose of improving their health or reducing their risk for illness and injury. Nurses must recognize the numerous opportunities available for the teaching of those who are currently or potentially consumers of health care. Given that teaching is an important aspect of healthcare delivery and given the fact that nurses are functioning as teachers in a multitude of settings, they encounter clients of differing ages and at various stages along the wellness-illness continuum. Wherever and whenever teaching takes place, nurses need to recognize the importance of consciously applying the principles of teaching and learning to these encounters for maximum effectiveness in helping clients to attain and maintain optimal health.

Sharing Resources Among Settings

Professional nurses involved in client health education should use available opportunities to share resources among the three identified settings (Figure 11-3). Many already perform this service as printed or audiovisual materials are borrowed, rented, or purchased for small fees from area institutions, organizations, or agencies. Nurses from healthcare or healthcare-related settings are contracted for or voluntarily provide health education programs to small and large groups in other healthcare, healthcare-related, or nonhealthcare settings. And, nurses from each category of setting collaborate on individual client situations or on major community health projects. The nurses from each of these settings can establish a health education committee in their community to coordinate health education programming, ensure effective use of all resources, and reduce duplication of efforts. The members of this committee can develop standardized health education content, clarify roles and services for each of the instructional settings, and share resources to provide a well-planned, comprehensive community program of health education for a wide spectrum of clients.

Classification of instructional settings for the education of consumers offers a method for analyzing the role of the nurse as teacher and for selecting teaching strategies that best fit the organizational climate, the resources available, and the clientele served. Instructional settings are classified according to the purpose of the organization, institution, or agency that provides or sponsors health instruction. Healthcare settings exist for the primary purpose of providing direct patient care, with education occurring as an integral part of healthcare delivery services within the setting. Healthcare-related settings consist of voluntary agencies whose purposes are advocacy, research, and educating the general public as well as professionals regarding specific healthcare problems affecting society. Nonhealthcare settings include institutions engaged in anything other than health care as their operational purpose, though they may choose to provide health education or healthcare services as benefits to their membership or employees.

Even where organizational and environmental resources are limited, creative thinking and resourcefulness on the part of the nurse in the role of teacher can expand the opportunities possible in any instructional setting to provide cost-effective client education that is well planned and comprehensive.

SUMMARY

This chapter presented an in-depth review of various teaching methods, highlighted how to use them effectively to address the specific domains for learning, and compared the strengths and limitations of each approach. Emphasis was given to the importance of taking into account the learner characteristics, behavioral objectives, teacher characteristics, and available resources prior to selecting any method. In many instances, guidelines were suggested to assist nurses in planning and developing their own teaching activities. Also, the major questions to be considered when evaluating the effectiveness of teaching methods were discussed. In addition, tips to enhance verbal presentations as well as the general principles all nurse teachers should use to effectively communicate with patients were reviewed. Nurses in the role of teachers are urged to use a combination of teaching methods to accomplish the objectives and to meet the different needs and styles of each patient. Multisensory stimulation is best for increasing the acquisition of skills and the retention of information. Finally, an overview of how instructional settings can be classified was presented. It is the responsibility of nurses in all practice environments to teach clients, well or ill, the information needed to independently maintain or improve their quality of life.

REVIEW QUESTIONS

1. How is the term *teaching method* defined?
2. What are the strengths and limitations of each teaching method?
3. Which teaching methods encourage active participation by the learner?
4. Which teaching methods are best for learning cognitive skills? Psychomotor skills? Affective skills?
5. What teaching method isolates the learner from others who may have similar needs/concerns?
6. What is meant by the term *pooled ignorance* and in which method does this likely occur?
7. What are the variables that influence the selection of any method of instruction?

8. What questions should you ask yourself when evaluating the effectiveness of any teaching method?

9. What is the difference between factual/descriptive questions, clarifying questions, and high-order questions?

10. What are the techniques that teachers can use to enhance the effectiveness of teaching?

11. What are the three classifications of instructional settings?

REFERENCES

Anderson, J. M. (1990). Health care across cultures. *Nursing Outlook, 38*, 136–139.

Arnold, E. & Boggs, K. (1989). *Interpersonal relationships*. Philadelphia: Saunders.

Babcock, D. E. & Miller, M. A. (1994). *Client education: Theory and practice*. St. Louis: Mosby-Year Book.

Boyd, M. D., Gleit, C. J., Graham, B. A., & Whitman, N. I. (1998). *Health teaching in nursing practice: A professional model* (3rd ed.). Stamford, CT: Appleton and Lange.

Brookfield, S. D. & Preskill, S. (1999). *Discussion as a way of teaching: Tools and techniques for democratic classrooms*. San Francisco: Jossey-Bass.

Cunningham, M. A. & Baker, D. (1986). How to teach patients better and faster. *RN, 49*(9), 50–52.

Evans, M. (2000). Polished, professional presentation: Unlocking the design elements. *Journal of Continuing Education in Nursing, 31*(5), 213–218.

Fredette, S. L. (1990). A model for improving cancer patient education. *Cancer Nursing, 13*, 207–215.

Freitas, L., Lantz, J., & Reed, R. (1991). The creative teacher. *Nurse Educator, 16*(1), 5–7.

Haggard, A. (1989). *Handbook of patient education*. Rockville, MD: Aspen.

House, B. M., Chassie, M. B., & Spohn, B. B. (1990). Questioning: An essential ingredient in effective teaching. *Journal of Continuing Education in Nursing, 21*, 196–201.

Joos, I. R. M. (1984). A teacher's guide for using games and simulation. *Nurse Educator, 9*(3), 25–29.

Kaplan, S. H., Greenfield, S., & Ware, J. E. Jr. (1989). Assessing the effects of physician-patient interactions on the outcomes of chronic disease. *Medical Care, 27*(Suppl. 3), S110–S127.

Lewis, D. J., Saydak, S. J., Mierzwa, I. P., & Robinson, J. A. (1989). Gaming: A teaching strategy for adult learners. *Journal of Continuing Education in Nursing, 20*, 80–84.

Ley, P. (1972). Primacy, rated importance, and recall of medical statements. *Journal of Health and Social Behavior, 13*, 311–317.

Lieberman, D. (2001). Management of chronic pediatric diseases with interactive health games: Theory and research findings. *Journal of Ambulatory Care Management, 24*(1), 26–38.

Lorig, K. & Gonzalez, V. M. (1993). Using self-efficacy theory in patient education. In B. Gilroth (ed.), *Managing hospital-based patient education* (pp. 327–337). Chicago, IL: American Hospital Publishing.

Narrow, B. (1979). *Patient teaching in nursing practice: A patient and family centered approach*. New York: Wiley.

Robinson, K. J., Lewis, D. J., & Robinson, J. A. (1990). Games: A way to give laboratory values meaning. *American Nephrology Nurses Association Journal, 17*, 306–308.

Rorden, J. W. (1987). *Nurses as health teachers: A practical guide*. Philadelphia: Saunders.

Rystedt, H. & Lindström, B. (2001). Introducing simulation technologies in nurse education: A nursing practice perspective. *Nurse Education in Practice, 1*(3), 134–141.

Saarmann, L., Daugherty, J., & Riegel, B. (2000). Patient teaching to promote behavior change. *Nursing Outlook, 48*(6), 281–287.

Walts, N. S. (1982). Games and simulations. *Nursing Management, 13*(2), 28–29.

CHAPTER 12

Instructional Materials

Diane S. Hainsworth

KEY TERMS

analogue
delivery system
illusionary representations
instructional materials
learner, media, and task characteristics

realia
replica
symbol
symbolic representations
tailoring

OBJECTIVES

After completing this chapter, the reader will be able to

1. Differentiate between instructional materials and teaching methods.
2. Identify the three major variables (learner, task, and media characteristics) to be considered when selecting, developing, and evaluating instructional materials.
3. Cite the three components of instructional materials required to effectively communicate educational messages.
4. Discuss general principles applicable to all types of media.
5. Identify the multitude of audiovisual tools—both print and nonprint materials—available for education of patients and their families.
6. Compare the advantages and disadvantages specific to each type of instructional medium.
7. Determine the type of media suitable for use depending on the characteristics of the learner, the behavioral objectives to be achieved, the setting for teaching, and the resources available.
8. Describe what should be considered when evaluating print and nonprint tools.
9. Recognize the supplemental nature of media's role in patient education.

Whereas teaching methods are the *approaches* used for instructor–client communications, instructional materials are the *vehicles* that help to convey information. Often, educators also use the terms *instructional strategies* and *teaching techniques*, which include both the methods and the materials used in teaching. To be exact, instructional materials are the audio and visual tools that aid learning. They stimulate a learner's senses and help the teacher simplify complex messages (Babcock & Miller, 1994).

In this chapter, the term *instructional materials*, also referred to as tools and aids, include both print and nonprint media. They are intended to supplement, rather than replace, actual teaching. It is up to the teacher to select and/or develop materials that are best suited to the methods chosen for teaching.

The purpose of instructional materials is to assist the nurse to deliver messages creatively and clearly during patient education. A multimedia approach for teaching helps learners to retain more effectively what they learn (Rankin & Stallings, 2001), helps clarify abstract or complex concepts, adds variety to the teaching-learning experience (Babcock & Miller, 1994), reinforces learning, and potentially brings realism to the experience. It is well documented that the use of audiovisual aids facilitates learning. Therefore, nurses must look for ways to supplement their teaching with methods that help the learner to more easily acquire knowledge, attitudes, and skills.

This chapter provides guidance in selecting, developing, using, and evaluating instructional materials. The advantages and disadvantages of the different types of media will be discussed. Although the choice of which instructional materials to use often depends on availability or cost, whatever materials are selected should enhance the client's learning. This chapter is intended to inform nurses about various media options and allow them to make informed choices regarding appropriate instructional materials that fit the learner, that will accomplish the learning task, and that will positively affect the motivation of the learner. Whether nurses educate patients and families or other healthcare professionals, the same principles apply in making decisions about the type of instructional materials to use for teaching.

GENERAL PRINCIPLES

Before selecting or developing media for teaching, you should be aware of the following general principles about the effectiveness of audiovisual tools:

- The teacher must be familiar with media content before a tool is used.
- Print and nonprint materials do change learner behavior by influencing a gain in cognitive, affective, or psychomotor skills.

- No one tool is better than another in enhancing learning.
- The tools should complement the teaching methods.
- The choice of media should be consistent with subject content and match the tasks to be learned.
- The instructional materials should reinforce and supplement—not substitute for—the nurse's teaching efforts.
- Media should match the available financial resources.
- Instructional aids should be appropriate for the learning environment, such as the size and seating of the audience, acoustics, space, and lighting.
- Media should be appropriate for the sensory abilities, developmental stages, and educational level of the intended audience.
- Instructional materials must be accurate, up-to-date, and free of any unintended messages.
- The media should contribute to learning by adding diversity and additional information.

CHOOSING INSTRUCTIONAL MATERIALS

Many important variables must be considered when choosing instructional materials. The role of the nurse as teacher goes beyond the giving of information only; it also involves skill in effectively designing and planning instruction. Learning can be made more enjoyable for both the learner and the teacher if the nurse knows how to select and use instructional tools to enhance the teaching-learning experience. Making appropriate choices of instructional materials depends on an understanding of three factors: (1) characteristics of the learner, (2) characteristics of the media, and (3) characteristics of the task to be achieved (Frantz, 1980). A useful way to remember these factors is LMAT: Learner, Media, and Task.

1. **Characteristics of the learner:** It is important to "know your audience" so media can be chosen that best suit the learners' perceptual abilities, physical abilities, reading abilities, motivational levels, developmental stages, and learning styles.
2. **Characteristics of the media:** A wide variety of media, print and nonprint, are available to enhance your teaching. The tools selected are the form through which the information will be communicated. No single medium is most effective. Therefore, using a multimedia approach is suggested.
3. **Characteristics of the task:** The task to be accomplished depends on identifying the complexity of the behavior and the domains for learning—what the learner needs to know, value, or be able to do.

THE THREE MAJOR COMPONENTS OF INSTRUCTIONAL MATERIALS _____

Three major components of media should be kept in mind when choosing print and nonprint materials for instruction: delivery system, content, and presentation.

Delivery System

The delivery system is both the physical form of the materials and the hardware used to present the materials. For example, overhead transparencies or slides are the physical form, and a projector is the hardware. Likewise, computer programs are the physical form and the computer is the hardware. The choice of the delivery system depends on the size of the audience, how quickly or slowly the information needs to be presented, and the sensory abilities of the clients (Weston & Cranston, 1986).

Content

The content, or message, is the actual information that is shared with the learner. When selecting media for teaching, the nurse must consider several things:

- Does the tool give accurate information? For example, it is important to question the qualifications of the author(s) who produced the printed material you are thinking of using.
- Is the tool appropriate for the particular content being taught? For example, audiotapes can be a very appropriate tool for teaching knowledge but not a good tool for teaching a psychomotor skill, which might be better taught by showing a current video or using real equipment to demonstrate the skill.
- Is the tool up-to-date? For example, a videotape may be outdated and therefore the information it contains does not include the latest research findings and most recent treatment protocols.
- Can printed materials be read and understood by the audience? It is important that instructions are written at a level suitable to the reader. Including illustrations in printed materials or rewriting instructions in simple language makes information more understandable to a poor reader (see Chapter 7 on literacy).

Presentation

The form of a message is most important when selecting or developing instructional materials. The form of the message can occur along a continuum from concrete (real objects) to abstract (symbols) (Weston & Cranston, 1986).

Realia

Realia, that which is or represents the real thing, is the most concrete form of stimulus that can be used to deliver information. For example, an actual woman demonstrating breast self-examination is the most concrete way to teach this skill. Because this form of presentation is not appropriate for teaching in front of a large number of people, the next best choice would be a model. Models have many characteristics of reality because they are three-dimensional. The message is less concrete, yet using a model allows for an accurate presentation. Further along the continuum of realia is a video presentation of a woman performing breast self-examination. The learner could still learn accurate breast self-examination this way, but because the aspect of dimensionality is absent, the message is less concrete and more abstract.

Illusionary Representations

Many realistic cues, including dimensionality, are missing from this category of instructional materials. Moving or still photographs, audiotapes, and drawings and graphs are good examples of illusionary representations (Weston & Cranston, 1986). They are less concrete and more abstract, but the instructional advantages of illusionary media are that these forms can offer learners experiences to which they might otherwise not have access due to factors such as size, location, or expense. For instance, pictures of different stages of decubitus ulcers or diagrams showing the steps of how to draw up and give insulin are more abstract in form, but do, to some degree, resemble realia.

Symbolic Representations

Numbers and words are symbols that are written and spoken to convey ideas or represent objects. They are the most common form of instruction, yet are the most abstract types of message. Audiotaped presentations, written texts and handouts, and the use of blackboards are just a few examples of messages delivered in symbolic form. The chief disadvantage of symbolic representations stems from their lack of concreteness. For that reason, their use should be limited with young children, learners from different cultures, learners with low literacy skills, and cognitively and sensory impaired patients.

When making decisions about how to best accomplish teaching objectives, the nurse must carefully consider these three components of instructional materials. The various delivery systems available, the content or message to be conveyed, and the form in which information will be presented are all important choices. Remember, no one medium provides a clear advantage over another in helping learners gain knowledge and skills. In other words, nurses must know how to select the tools that will best complement and support their teaching efforts for a particular audience.

TYPES OF INSTRUCTIONAL MATERIALS

Written Materials

Handouts, leaflets, books, pamphlets, brochures, and instruction sheets are the most widely used and most accessible type of media for teaching. Printed teaching materials have been described as "frozen language" (Redman, 2001). Nonetheless, written materials are the most common form of teaching tool even though they are the most abstract.

The use of printed materials offers some distinct advantages. They are:

- available to the learner as a reference for information when the nurse is not immediately present to answer questions or clarify information.
- widely acceptable and familiar to the public.
- available through commercial sources and, thus, are easily obtainable.
- usually relatively low in cost.
- portable and convenient to use.
- published in a variety of languages, such as Spanish.
- becoming more widely available.
- especially useful for learners who prefer reading rather than receiving messages in other formats.
- able to be altered to target specific audiences.

The disadvantages of printed materials include that:

- they are the most abstract form of reality.
- possibilities for immediate feedback are limited.
- a large percentage of materials are written at too high a level for comprehension by learners with low literacy skills.
- those persons who are visually or cognitively impaired may not be able to take full advantage of them (Doak, Doak, Friedell, & Meade, 1998).

Commercially Prepared Materials

Brochures, posters, pamphlets, and instruction sheets are examples of materials that are commercially prepared in bulk. Several questions must be asked when reviewing commercial materials for possible use (Foster, 1987):

- Who produced the item?
- Did healthcare professionals have input in the preparation of the tool?
- Can the material be previewed for accuracy and appropriateness of content before it is used for teaching?
- Is the price of the teaching tool reasonable?
- Can the tool be used with large numbers of learners?
- How quickly will the information become outdated?

The advantages of using commercial materials are that they are:

- easily available.
- often cheaper than designing new instructional materials, often costing 50 cents or less when bought in large quantities.
- a real time saver when compared with the hours it would take nurses to research, write, and copy materials to create information packets of equal quality.

The disadvantages of using commercial materials may include:

- issues of cost, because some educational booklets are expensive to purchase and give away in large quantities to learners.
- level of readability, which often is a problem for patients with low literacy skills.
- the content, which might not completely and accurately cover all the information the learner needs to know.

Self-Composed Materials

Nurses may choose to write their own instructional materials to save costs or include content needed by specific audiences. Advantages to composing your own materials are many (Brownson, 1998). By writing your own materials, you can:

- include the information to fit your own institution's policies, procedures, and equipment.
- build in answers to those questions asked most frequently by your patients.
- tailor your written materials to reinforce specific oral instructions.

Rice and Johnson (1984) found that groups of patients receiving specific instructions were more likely to follow directions and required less oral teaching time than groups of patients receiving general or nonspecific instructions.

Tailoring personalizes the message to fit an individual patient's learning needs. Doak et al. (1998) outlined specific suggestions for tailoring information to help patients want to read and remember the message and to act on it. It has been found that tailoring instruction improves reading, recall, and follow-through in health teaching (Campbell et al., 1994; Skinner, Strecher, & Hospers, 1994).

The disadvantages to composing your own materials include:

- Needing time to prepare materials that are well written and laid out effectively
- The tendency to write information that is too detailed and written at too high a level for the intended learner

Format and appearance are equally important factors in encouraging learners to read the printed word. Pay attention to illustrations. If the format and appearance are too detailed, learners will feel overwhelmed, and may become easily discouraged and abandon attempts at learning. Figures 12-1 and 12-2 illustrate the importance of keeping written directions and pictures simple so as to convey clear, uncluttered messages that attract and keep the learner's attention.

Nurses are expected to enhance their methods of teaching with audiovisual materials, but few have ever had formal training in the development and application of written materials. Specific guidelines for writing patient education materials with clarity and completeness can be found in Chapter 7.

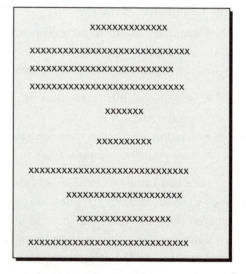

FIGURE 12-1   Inadequate versus Adequate Appearance and Formatting

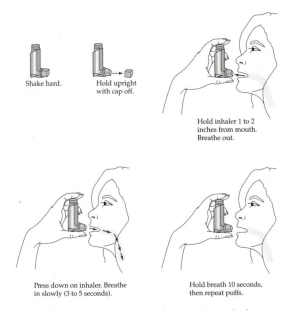

Shake hard.

Hold upright with cap off.

Hold inhaler 1 to 2 inches from mouth. Breathe out.

Press down on inhaler. Breathe in slowly (3 to 5 seconds).

Hold breath 10 seconds, then repeat puffs.

FIGURE 12-2   Diagram Illustrating Proper Technique for Inhaler Use

Evaluating Printed Materials

When evaluating printed materials, the following considerations should be kept in mind:

1. **Nature of the audience:**
   - What is the average age of the audience? For instance, children like short printed materials with many illustrations. Older adults tend to prefer printed materials that they can read at their leisure. Vision deficits are common in older adults, and short-term memory may be a problem for comprehension, so having simple materials that can be reread at their own pace can reinforce earlier learning and minimize confusion over treatment instructions.
   - What is the preferred learning style of the audience? Printed materials with many illustrations are best for patients who not only have difficulty reading, but also do not like to read. Graphs and charts can be included with the content of printed materials for those who are visual learners.

2. **Literacy level required:** Patient education materials are ineffective if the materials are written at a level beyond the comprehension of the learner. A survey in two urban, public hospitals by Williams et al. (1995) revealed a high proportion of

patients who were unable to read and understand the medical instructions given, including directions for taking medications, information about follow-up appointments, and informed consent forms for medical procedures. The Joint Commission on Accreditation of Healthcare Organizations mandates that health information must be presented in a manner that can be understood by patients and family members. A number of formulas (e.g., Fog, SMOG, Flesch, Fry) are available for determining readability (see Chapter 7 and Appendix A).

3. **Linguistic variety available:** Choices of printed materials in different foreign languages may be limited. The growth of the Hispanic population in the United States has led to increased attention to the need for Spanish-language teaching materials. Regional differences exist, so there may be more availability of Asian-language materials on the West Coast and more Spanish-language materials in the Southwest and Northeast than in other parts of the country.

4. **Brevity and clarity:** Simpler is better. Remind yourself of a revised form of the KISS rule: Keep it Simple and Smart. Address the critical facts only. What does the patient need to know? Choose words that tell the learner *what*, *when*, and *how*; the *why* can be explained during one-to-one or group discussion. Remember, instructional materials are only supplements to learning, not substitutes, so they shouldn't contain everything there is to know about a topic. Figure 12-3 is a good example of a clear, easy-to-follow instructional tool used to teach an asthma patient how to determine when a metered-dose inhaler is empty. Using simple graphics and minimal words, it leaves little room for misinterpretation and is suitable for a wide range of audiences.

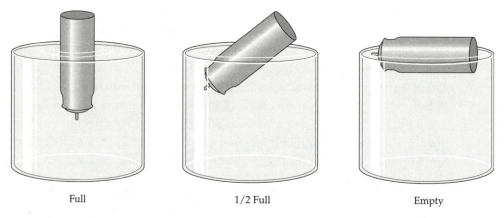

Full   1/2 Full   Empty

FIGURE 12-3   Example of a Clear, Easy-to-Follow Instructional Tool for an Asthma Patient

5. **Layout and appearance:** The appearance of written materials is crucial. If the tool is too wordy, with inadequate spacing, small margins, and numerous pages, the intended learner may ignore it, thinking that it is much too difficult and time-consuming to read. Again, Figure 12-1 illustrates the importance of the KISS principle.

Doak et al. (1996) point out that allowing plenty of white space is the most important step that should be taken to improve the appearance of written materials. This can be achieved by double-spacing, leaving generous margins, indenting important points, reducing the number of words to include only "need to know" information, using bold characters, and separating out key statements. In addition, a graphic in the middle of the text can break up the print and may be visually appealing. Redman (2001) states that pictorial learning is better than verbal learning for recognition and recall. An example used earlier in this chapter is teaching the psychomotor task of using a metered-dose inhaler (see Figure 12-2).

6. **Opportunity for repetition:** Written materials can be read later, again and again, to reinforce teaching. If information is presented in a question-and-answer format, particular topics can be easily found and reviewed as often as necessary.

7. **Concreteness and familiarity:** Using the active voice speaks to the reader in more immediate, straightforward, and concrete language. For example, "Shake the inhaler very well three times" is more effective than "The inhaler should be shaken thoroughly." Figure 12-4 illustrates use of the active voice. Using plain language instead of medical jargon cannot be over-emphasized. Byrne and Edeani (1984); Estey, Musseau, and Keehn (1994); and Lerner, Jehle, Janicke, and Moscati (2000)

STEPS FOR CORRECT INHALER TECHNIQUE

1. Shake the container well three times.
2. Remove cap and hold inhaler upright.
3. Hold the inhaler 1 to 2 inches from your mouth.
4. Tilt your head back slightly, and breathe out fully.
5. Press down on the inhaler and start to breathe in slowly.
6. Breathe in slowly (3 to 5 seconds) and deeply to pull medication down into the lungs.
7. Hold your breath for 10 seconds to keep the medicine in your lungs.
8. Take a few normal breaths.
9. Repeat puffs by following steps 1–8 again.

FIGURE 12-4 Example of Instructions Written in the Active Voice

surveyed knowledge of medical terminology among hospital patients and determined that poor patient understanding of common medical terms used by healthcare providers could be a significant factor in noncompliance with medical regimens. The studies indicate that patients understand medical terms far less than health professionals realize.

In summary, self-designed or commercially produced printed teaching materials are widely used for a broad range of audiences. They vary in literacy demand levels and may be written in several languages. Table 12-1 summarizes their major advantages and disadvantages.

Demonstration Materials

Demonstration materials include many types of nonprint media, such as models and real equipment, as well as displays such as posters, diagrams, illustrations, charts, bulletin boards, flannel boards, flip charts, chalkboards, photographs, and drawings. These aids primarily stimulate the visual senses but can combine the sense of sight with touch and sometimes even smell and taste. The nurse can choose one or more of these to complement teaching efforts. Just as with written tools, these aids must be accurate and appropriate for the intended audience. Ideally, these media forms bring learners closer to reality and actively engage them. The major forms of demonstration materials—displays and models—will be discussed in detail.

TABLE 12-1 Advantages and Disadvantages of Printed Materials	
Advantages	**Disadvantages**
Always available	Impersonal
Rate of reading is controlled by the reader	Limited feedback; absence of instructor lessens
Complex concepts can be explained both	opportunity to clear up misinterpretation
fully and adequately	Passive tool
Procedural steps can be outlined	Highly complex materials may be
Verbal instruction can be reinforced	overwhelming to the learner
Learner is always able to refer back to	Literacy skill of learner may limit
instructions given in print	effectiveness

Source: Adapted from Hinkle, Albanese, and McGinty, 1993.

Displays

Displays are found in almost any educational setting and are useful for a variety of teaching purposes. They can advertise events, convey simple or quick messages about healthcare issues, and clarify, reinforce, or summarize important topics and themes. Chalkboards, flip charts, and white markerboards are particularly helpful during brain-storming sessions in formal classes or group discussions. You can use them spontaneously to make drawings or diagrams (with contrasting colored chalk or markers if you wish) or to jot down ideas generated from participants while you are in the process of teaching. You can add, correct, or delete information quickly while the learners are actively following what you are doing or saying. These board devices are excellent in promoting participation. They are flexible tools for patient teaching that provide opportunities for the nurse to organize data, keep track of ideas, perform on-the-spot problem solving, and compare and contrast various points of view.

Babcock and Miller (1994) list guidelines for using chalkboards and white markerboards. The most important points include:

- Be sure your writing is legible.
- Step aside and face the audience after putting notations on the board to maintain contact with the audience and allow learners a chance to copy the message.
- Enlist a good note-taker to capture a creative design or record an idea before the board is erased.

Displays can be an effective way of achieving learning outcomes. Computer technology has made it easier to create attractive, up-to-date, and impressive displays as well as to revise ones already made (Bushy, 1991).

The following are some advantages of displays as teaching tools:

- A quick way to attract attention and get an idea across
- Flexible
- Portable (many posters can be folded for storage and unfolded for mounting)
- Reusable
- Stimulate learners' interest and participation
- Good for learning cognitive and affective behaviors

Some of the disadvantages of displays include the following:

- Can take up a lot of space
- Time-consuming to prepare, and for that reason tend to be reused again and again, increasing the risk of becoming outdated

- Unsuitable for large audiences if information is to be viewed simultaneously
- Limited amounts of information can be presented at one time
- Ineffective for teaching psychomotor skills
- Easily cluttered when too much information is placed on them
- May be ignored if posted too long or poorly arranged

Some displays, such as posters, are a combination of print and nonprint media because both the written word and graphic illustration are used. Posters have become an important teaching tool for patient education in clinical and home settings. Because the primary mode of the poster is visual stimulation, it must be designed to attract attention (Flournoy, Turner, & Combs, 2000). Effective posters leave a mental image long after they are seen. Much like a bumper sticker you see on a car in front of you while driving, effective poster displays can leave lasting impressions that are easily recalled at some future date.

The advantages of posters are that they can:

- help bring about a change of behavior by adding knowledge, reinforcing skill, or appealing to attitudes.
- convey a message quickly and simultaneously to an audience in a variety of settings.
- be used with individuals and small groups to transmit or reinforce information with or without the teacher present.
- be relatively inexpensive to produce.

The disadvantages of posters are that:

- the content is static and may become quickly dated.
- the message may begin to be ignored if the same poster is kept around too long.

The ability of a poster to influence behavior or increase awareness can be greatly enhanced by careful consideration of content, audience, and design elements. Because aesthetic appeal is critical in capturing learners' attention, the following tips, adapted from Bushy (1991); Moneyham, Ura, Ellwood, and Bruno (1996); Duchin and Sherwood (1990); and Haggard (1989) should be adhered to when making and critiquing a poster for use as a teaching tool:

- Use complementary (opposite-spectrum) color combinations.
- One color should make up as much as 70% of the display. No two colors should be used in equal proportions, and a third color should be used only to accent or highlight titles, subheadings, or credits. Too many colors make the design appear cluttered and complicated.

- Because a picture is worth a thousand words, graphics should be used to break up blocks of script or lettering.
- Use simple, high-quality drawings or graphics that can be easily interpreted.
- Balance script with white space (or another background color) and graphics to add variety and contrast.
- Convey the message in common, straightforward language, avoiding jargon and unfamiliar abbreviations or symbols.
- Adhere to the KISS principle (keep it simple and smart) when using words to decrease length, detail, and crowding. Simplicity and neatness attract attention.
- Include only essential information, but be sure the message is complete and not repetitious.
- Be sure content is current and free of spelling, grammar, and mathematical errors.
- Add textures by using a variety of paper and fabrics.
- Make titles catchy and crisp, using 10 words or less (no longer than two lines) and lettering large enough to read from a distance of at least 4 to 6 feet.
- Use a title that orients readers to the subject.
- Use letter-quality script or laser printing instead of dot matrix if using computer-generated type.
- Letters should be straight and at least one inch in height. Avoid using all-capital letters except for very short titles and labels.
- Use arrows, circles, or directional lines to merge the parts to achieve correct focus, flow, sequence, and unity.
- Achieve balance in visual weight on each side by positioning information around an imaginary central axis running vertically and horizontally.
- Handouts can be used to supplement, highlight, and reinforce the messages conveyed by the poster.
- If a poster is to be transported, use durable backboards and overlays (Styrofoam, heavy cardboard, lamination, or acrylic sprays).

The poster for AIDS awareness shown in Figure 12-5 is a stunning example of the ability of a poster to influence behavior through careful consideration of the content and design elements in attracting the attention of the intended audience. The key to this poster's success is its ability to connect the viewer with a message that lingers in memory.

Computers and printers have opened the door to very professional-looking productions of posters by almost any user. Software programs such as Print Shop Deluxe and Canvas are frequently used for these purposes.

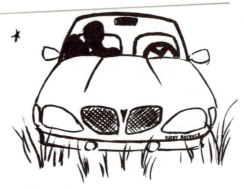

Last night Jennifer had a fatal accident.
She just doesn't know it yet

FIGURE 12-5   Example of an Effective Poster for AIDS Awareness.
Line drawing courtesy of Kathy Batruch-Meadows

Models

Models are three-dimensional instructional tools that allow the learner to immediately apply knowledge and psychomotor skills by observing, examining, manipulating, handling, assembling, and disassembling objects while the teacher provides feedback (Rankin & Stallings, 2001). In addition, these demonstration aids encourage learners to think abstractly and give them the opportunity to use many of their senses (Boyd, Gleit, Graham, & Whitman, 1998). Whenever possible, the use of real objects and actual equipment is preferred, but a model is the next best thing when the real object is not available, accessible, or feasible, or is too complex to use. The three specific types of models used for teaching and learning are replicas, analogues, and symbols. To differentiate the three types of models, Babcock and Miller (1994) suggest associating a replica with the word *resemble*, an analogue with the term *act like*, and a symbol with the words *stands for*.

Replica   A replica is a facsimile constructed to scale that resembles the features or substance of the original object. The dimensions of the reproduction may be decreased or enlarged to make demonstration easier and more understandable. A replica of the DNA helix is an example of a model used to teach the complex concept of genetics. Replicas are excellent for teaching psychomotor skills because they give the learner an opportunity for active participation through hands-on experience. Not only can the learner assemble and disassemble parts to see how they fit and operate, but the pace of learning can also be controlled by the learner (Babcock & Miller, 1994).

Replicas are used frequently by nurses when teaching anatomy and physiology. Models of the heart, kidney, ear, eye, joints, breast, and pelvic organs, for example, allow the learner to get a perspective on parts of the body not readily viewed without these teaching aids. Resuscitation dolls are a common type of replica used to teach the skills of cardiopulmonary resuscitation. Learners who regularly refresh their skills using demonstration models as instructional tools are more likely to maintain regular and effective use of the technique than learners who do not (Pinto, 1993).

For lessons aimed at psychomotor learning, skills checklists can be used to evaluate whether the learner has mastered the skill (Grier, Owens, Peavy, & Pelt, 1991). These checklists are easily used for observing return demonstrations.

Analogue   The second type of model is known as an *analogue* because it uses analogy to explain something by comparing it to something else. An analogue performs like the real object because it has the same properties. Mechanical devices such as extracorporeal and dialysis machines are good examples of analogues.

Symbol   The third type of model is a *symbol*, which is used more frequently in a teaching situation. Words, diagrams, musical notes, cartoons, and traffic signs are all examples of symbolic models that convey a message to the receiver. Symbols, such as international signs, are increasingly being used in multilingual or multicultural areas. However, abbreviations common to healthcare personnel, such as NPO, PRN, and PO, should be avoided when interacting with consumers because they may not be familiar with them.

The following are some advantages of models:

- Useful when the real object is too small, too large, too expensive, or too complex
- Allow learners to practice acquiring new skills without compromising themselves in the practice of self-care activities or risking damage to valuable equipment
- Learners become more actively involved, and the link between knowledge and skills is immediate
- Especially attractive and useful for the learner who prefers the hands-on approach
- Do not need to be expensive or elaborate to get concepts and ideas across (Rankin & Stallings, 2001)

Some disadvantages of models are:

- They are not suitable for the learner with poor abstraction abilities or for visually impaired audiences.
- Some can be fragile and very expensive, such as resuscitation models.

- Many are bulky to store and difficult to transport.
- Only a few learners can observe and manipulate them at any one time, although using teams or rotating learners between different "stations" for demonstration helps solve this problem (Babcock & Miller, 1994).

Table 12-2 summarizes the advantages and disadvantages of demonstration materials.

Audiovisual Materials

Technology has changed the traditional approach to teaching. Nowhere is this shift more evident than in the audiovisual arena. Audiovisual materials stimulate the learner's senses, add variety to the teaching-learning experience, and create visual memories, which are known to be more permanent than auditory memories (de Tornyay & Thompson, 1987). Some visual aids, such as pictures and diagrams, have been around for centuries. Recently, however, technology has provided access to sophisticated audiovisual tools. They are exceptional aids because many promote cognitive development, stimulate attitude change, and help to build psychomotor skills. Audiovisuals increase retention of information by combining what we hear with what we see.

Because we live in an increasingly technological age, nurses need to be aware of what audiovisual tools are available and how to effectively and efficiently use these tools. However, the nurse's comfort level and expertise in operating these technological devices must be considered. Not all nurses are oriented to the use of audiovisual aids, especially in light of the newness of some of the technology, such as computer-assisted instruction. Also, it should not be forgotten that some learners may have difficulty orienting to the newer modes of learning or have physical or cognitive limitations that may rule out the use of some types of audiovisual tools.

TABLE 12-2 Advantages and Disadvantages of Demonstration Materials	
Advantages	**Disadvantages**
Brings the learner closer to reality through active engagement	Content may be static, easily dated
Useful for cognitive reinforcement and psychomotor skill development	Can be time-consuming to make
	Potential for overuse
Effective use of imagery may impact affective domain	Not suitable for simultaneous use with large audiences
Many forms are relatively inexpensive	Not suitable for visually impaired learners or learners with poor abstraction abilities
Opportunity for repetition	

As with any teaching aids, audiovisuals must be carefully previewed for accuracy and appropriateness of content. Another major concern affecting media choice may be budgetary constraints for the purchase, rental, or repair of hardware equipment and software programs. Also, it is extremely costly and technologically demanding to self-produce audiovisual materials.

There are many nonprint media whose primary mode of presentation is visual or audio, or a blend of these two forms. Audiovisual materials can be categorized into five major types: projected, audio, video, telecommunications, and computer formats. Most of these learning resources are popular devices common to the general public. Others, like the computer, have only recently been applied to education; for this reason, many learners are not as accustomed to receiving information via this type of media.

The following is a summary of the various types of audiovisual tools available for teaching.

Projection Resources

The category of projection media, the best known of all audiovisual formats, includes overhead transparencies, computer outputs, and videos that can be projected on a screen. These media types are most frequently used with audiences of various sizes but can also be effective tools for teaching individuals.

PowerPoint   This computer-generated software program by Microsoft is rapidly replacing conventional slides for instruction. PowerPoint slides are easy to design, economical to produce, and an impressive medium by which to share information with a large or small audience. The program allows for flexibility to make changes whenever necessary as well as flexibility during a presentation to repeat slides or skip slides to move ahead to other content. Brown (2001) suggests the following important tips on how to use this innovative tool productively:

- Use this medium to generate interaction between the nurse and the learner rather than as a tool that provides an outline of content to be followed for presentation in a traditional lecture format.
- Open a blank slide and type in the main points as they emerge from interactive discussion.
- Use text sparingly on each slide to keep details to a minimum. Include no more than six points about any one idea per slide and limit the word count to approximately six words per point.
- Use contrasting but bold complementary colors so the text is clearly visible.
- Be sure the print size on each slide is large enough for the audience to read with ease at a distance. The Floor Test is one simple method to determine

appropriate print size. If you can read a printout of the slide placed on the floor in front of you when in a standing position, then the font size is adequate.
- Minimize or avoid animated text, sounds, and fancy transitions, which can distract the reader from the message.
- Use a master slide as a template for design unity of the entire set.
- Provide students with handouts of the slides (three slides per page) for note taking.
- The maximum number of slides to be projected for teaching should be no more than one to two slides per minute to avoid presenting too much content in a given period of time. This allows learners to internalize the concepts being presented and to have a chance to discuss content and ask questions.

PowerPoint slides must be used judiciously to avoid overuse and abuse of this medium as a tool for effective teaching and learning.

Overhead Transparencies   This medium is frequently used for teaching in a variety of settings. Their advantages are many:

- Large numbers of people can see the projected images at one time while information is being explained.
- They are a particularly useful tool to stimulate group discussion.
- They can be used to enlarge images.
- They can be shown in lighted rooms.
- They are inexpensive to produce or purchase.
- Multiple transparencies can be overlaid to illustrate changes in the content of teaching material.
- Colored felt pens can be used to provide contrast to images and lettering, which attracts attention and helps differentiate information for better retention and recall (Cooper, 1990).

Disadvantages of overhead transparencies are:

- You need both specialized equipment for projection and the support of verbal feedback. They are more useful in a classroom than for individual self-instruction.
- The projector itself is awkward to transport, and the noise given off by the fan of the machine can be distracting in a small room.
- Too much content on an overhead transparency will decrease its usefulness.

Babcock and Miller (1994) recommend the following helpful guidelines for the use of overhead projectors and transparencies:

- Do not block the audience's view of the screen by standing in front of the machine. Make a habit of sitting or standing to the side to avoid interference with the projected image.
- Turn the projector off when you have finished referring to the transparency to keep the learners' attention on you and away from what is being projected.
- Use letters at least 1/4 inch high so that words can be read at a distance of 10 feet.
- Keep the message on the transparency simple. Use handouts to cover complex information.
- Display only one point at a time by masking the rest with a piece of paper if you have listed several ideas on one transparency. This approach allows listeners to focus on what you are saying and gives them time for note taking.
- Use a screen large enough for the audience to read the information projected.
- Use a light-colored blank wall if a screen is unavailable or too small.
- Pull the projector closer or farther away from the screen to change the size of the projection.
- Use tinted film to reduce glare.
- Use colored pens to help organize information or make specific points.
- Use overlays to help illustrate complex or sequential ideas. Note, however, that too many overlays can make the picture fuzzy.

Table 12-3 summarizes the advantages and disadvantages of projected learning resources.

Audio Resources

Until recently, audio technology was primarily used as a tool for the blind or for those with serious visual or motor impairment. With significant advances in audio hardware and software and a turn away from the purely commercial use of this technology,

TABLE 12-3 Advantages and Disadvantages of Projection Resources	
Advantages	**Disadvantages**
Most effectively used with groups	Lack of flexibility due to static content for some forms
May be especially beneficial for hearing impaired or low-literate patients	Some forms may be expensive
Good for teaching skills in all domains	Requires darkened room for some forms
	Requires special equipment for use

however, audiotapes, compact discs (CDs), and radio have become more popular tools for teaching and learning. They are particularly helpful to learners who benefit from repetition, and are well suited for those who enjoy or prefer auditory learning. They are also useful in teaching persons who are illiterate or low literate.

Audiotapes   A popular format today is the cassette tape. Use of this medium by educators has been growing. The biggest advantage of cassettes is their practicality. They are small, portable, inexpensive, simple to operate, and easy to prepare or duplicate, and the required recorders are inexpensive.

Cassettes are now available on a variety of health topics, from stress reduction to programs to stop smoking, and can be prepared specifically to meet the needs of a learner by reinforcing facts, giving directions, or providing support. Information can be listened to at the leisure of the learner and reviewed as often as necessary. They can be used almost anywhere and can be listened to while simultaneously driving a car or fixing a meal. Developing a sizable library of tapes is well within the capability of most instructors, thanks to this medium's low cost and easy storage. Pictures, diagrams, and printed handouts can accompany these instructional tools.

The disadvantages of using audiotapes are few. The biggest drawback is that because audiotapes address only one sense—hearing—they cannot be used for hearing-impaired individuals. Also, some learners may not benefit without visuals to accompany the tapes. In addition, there is no opportunity for interactive feedback between the listener and the speaker.

Radio   The radio is the oldest form of audio technology. Due to its commercial nature and appeal to mass audiences, it has typically been used more for pleasure than for education. In recent years, however, the radio has been recognized as an effective vehicle for teaching and learning. Both public and private radio stations have begun airing community service and medical talk shows for public education on health issues.

The disadvantage of radio relates to the difficulty of consistently delivering information on major topics to general as well as specific populations. The nurse has little control over the variety and depth of topics or how regularly one listens to a program. Radio does not allow the opportunity for repetition of information.

Compact Discs   This modern form of media is rapidly replacing traditional audiotapes. The major advantage of CDs is their superior fidelity, which does not deteriorate over time. Other advantages and disadvantages of CDs are similar to those of audiotapes, except for the fact that not as many people or institutions have the recording hardware or the computer capability to accommodate the use of this tool. However, the versatility of CDs for application to education is currently growing at a rapid rate and will certainly affect patient education in the near future. The cost is becoming very reasonable, and the hardware availability for healthcare education will increase in the near future.

Table 12-4 summarizes the advantages and disadvantages of audio resources.

Video Resources

Videotapes, VCRs, and television sets have become commonplace in homes and healthcare settings. Camcorders and video cameras to make tapes are also owned by many people and institutions. People are becoming more accustomed to receiving information via this medium, and health educators are using it extensively for teaching in a variety of settings. Videotapes are one of the major nonprint media tools for enhancing patient/family education because tapes can be both entertaining and educational.

Videotapes are a good means to promote discussion because they can capture real-life situations. Their use as a critiquing instrument may provide direct feedback regarding learners' performances of interpersonal and psychomotor skills (Nielsen & Sheppard, 1988).

The combination of color, motion, different angles, and sound on videotapes enhances learning through visual as well as auditory senses. Videotaping has become very inexpensive, although whether the recorder is rented or owned by the user is a cost factor (Sternberger & Freiburger, 1996). The ready portability of recorders allows access to learning situations unavailable elsewhere.

The disadvantage of purchased tapes is that they may be beyond the viewers' level of understanding, inappropriate for learner needs, or too long. The ideal length of tapes in most instances is 15 to 20 minutes (Nielsen & Sheppard, 1988).

Another major disadvantage of this medium is that the quality of videotapes can deteriorate over time. For this reason alone, they are being replaced by the newer

Table 12-4 Advantages and Disadvantages of Audio Resources	
Advantages	**Disadvantages**
Widely available	Relies only on sense of hearing
May be especially beneficial for visually impaired or low-literacy patients	Some forms may be expensive
	Lack of opportunity for interaction between instructor and learner
May be listened to repeatedly	
Most forms are very practical, cheap, small, and portable.	

DVD technology. DVDs (digital video discs) incorporate the sound quality of CDs with video images by way of digital technology that allows for long-term storage and use. Unlike videotapes and audiotapes, DVDs will not deteriorate.

If you are planning to create your own videotapes or DVDs, strive for network-quality production by using the following guidelines (Williams, Wolgin, & Hodge, 1998):

- Write a script for the program. Rehearse thoroughly.
- Consider hiring a video technician on a per diem basis. This may be time- and cost-effective.
- For a small budget, a single camera with zoom capacity should be used. A larger budget may allow hiring a professional to edit the final product.
- Always be mindful of the program's objectives to avoid being seduced by the glamour of the process.
- Keep the program short. The longer the video, the more risk of losing viewer interest. Five to 15 minutes is ideal.

Table 12-5 summarizes the advantages and disadvantages of video learning resources.

Telecommunications Resources

Telecommunications includes television and telephone and their related modes of audio and video teleconferencing and closed-circuit, cable, and satellite broadcasting. Telecommunications devices have allowed messages to be sent to many people at the same time in a variety of places at great distances.

Television   The television has been used for many years as an entertainment tool. Today, there are more televisions than telephones in private residences. The TV is also well suited for educational purposes and has become a popular teaching-learning tool in homes, schools, businesses, and healthcare settings. The power to influence

TABLE 12-5 Advantages and Disadvantages of Video Resources	
Advantages	**Disadvantages**
Widely used educational tool	Viewing format limited, depending
Inexpensive, for the most part	on use of VHS or DVD
Uses visual and auditory senses	Some commercial products may
Flexible for use with different audiences	be expensive
Powerful tool for role modeling, demonstration,	Some purchased materials may be
and teaching psychomotor skills	too long or inappropriate for audience

cognitive, affective, and psychomotor behavior is well demonstrated by television commercials, whose messages are simple, direct, and repetitive to effectively influence the behavior of intended audiences.

Cable TV is legally obligated to provide public access programming by offering channels for community members to air their own programs. Health education, if placed on the cable system, can be seen in any home hooked up to cable. The advantage of this option is that distribution of programs is relatively inexpensive. The disadvantage is that one cannot control who is watching, and this medium cannot serve as an interactive question-and-answer experience unless call-in phone lines are provided.

Closed-circuit TV allows for education programs to be sent to specific locations, such as patient rooms. The learner can request a particular program at any given time, much like a guest in a hotel can choose from a variety of movies day and night. This telecommunications technology requires programs to be played intermittently or continuously, with program availability clearly advertised. Because the learner controls program viewing, the nurse must follow up to answer questions and determine whether learning has, in fact, occurred.

Satellite broadcasting, a newer form of telecommunications, can reach far more distant locations, and a number of programs can be carried at any one time. Because of its expense, not many institutions send health information via this mode, but many receive it.

Telephones   It is almost impossible to imagine being without the telephone as a daily tool. Americans have come to depend on it as a fundamental means of communication. It is not surprising, therefore, that the telephone can be used effectively for education. In recognition of this fact, many healthcare associations have begun to provide telephone services with messages about disease treatment and prevention. The American Cancer Society, for example, has established a toll-free number for the public to obtain short taped messages about various types of cancer.

The advantages are:

- These services are relatively inexpensive.
- They can be operated by someone with minimal medical knowledge because the taped message contains the substance of the content.
- This type of service is available around the clock in most cases.

The disadvantage is:

- There is no opportunity for questions to be answered directly.

Many hospitals and healthcare agencies have also established hotline consumer information centers, manned by knowledgeable healthcare personnel so that information can be personalized and appropriate feedback can be given on the spot. The Poison Control hotline is a good example of the use of this medium.

Table 12-6 summarizes the advantages and disadvantages of telecommunications learning resources.

Computer Resources

In our technological society, the computer has changed our lives dramatically and has found widespread use everywhere. The computer can store large amounts of information, and is designed to display pictures, graphics, and text. The presentation of information can easily be changed depending on user input.

Computer technology in education is becoming very common, especially with the rapid increase of computer literacy among professionals and the general public. There is a great deal of evidence that computer-assisted instruction (CAI) promotes learning in primarily the cognitive domain. More research needs to be done to establish its usefulness to change attitudes and behaviors or promote psychomotor skill development. Retention is improved by an interactive exchange between the learner and the computer, even though the instructor is not actually present. CAI simulates the feedback of a face-to-face exchange between individuals.

CAI has many advantages:

- You can individualize instruction to the learner on a moment-by-moment basis.
- Lessons can be varied readily.
- The learner controls the pace.
- The instructor can easily track the level of understanding of the learner.
- The computer can perform ongoing assessment of the learner and alter the content, pace, and examples presented.
- It can be programmed to provide feedback to the educator regarding the learner's grasp of concepts, the speed of learning, and what needs reinforcement.
- It can provide immediate feedback to the learner.

TABLE 12-6 Advantages and Disadvantages of Telecommunications Resources	
Advantages	**Disadvantages**
TV program distribution is relatively inexpensive to wide audiences	Complicated to set up interactive capability
Telephone is relatively inexpensive and widely available	Expensive to broadcast via satellite

- Many software packages are available, and even costly packages may be cost-effective if the potential audience is large (Gillespie & Ellis, 1993).
- The teacher has more time to devote to teaching other tasks not taught via computer, such as affective and psychomotor skills (Boyd et al., 1998).
- The content of CAI programs is consistent for all learners because they are exposed to the exact same information.
- It is a valuable tool for those with aphasia, hearing impairment, or learning disabilities (see Chapter 9 on special populations).

The major disadvantages of CAI are:

- Both hardware and software can be quite expensive.
- Most programs must be purchased because they are too time-consuming and too complex for the nurse to develop. Even if someone has programming skills, it can take up to 500 hours to produce 1 hour of instructional material (Boyd et al., 1998).
- Lack of computer literacy or a comfort level with computers may be a barrier to some learners and even some nurses.
- Many older adults are computer shy or computer illiterate.
- People with reading problems will likely have major difficulty making sense of the information on the screen (see Chapter 7 on literacy).
- Learners with physical limitations, such as arthritis, neuromuscular disorders, pain, fatigue, paralysis, or vision impairment, may find computer use difficult if not impossible (see Chapter 9 on special populations).
- Because the computer is a machine, the learner is deprived of the personal, compassionate, one-to-one interaction that only a teacher can provide to facilitate learning.
- Computer learning is not very suitable for nondirected or poorly motivated learners.
- Lack of access to computers may be a barrier, even for the computer-literate learner.
- Only a relatively small percentage of programs have dealt with patient education to date, and the quality of the products is uneven (Gillespie & Ellis, 1993).

More recently, the growth of the Internet has opened new doors for learners to gain access to libraries and to direct learning experiences, which can include online discussions with educators at great distances from the learner. Anyone with a computer and access to online technology can make use of this tremendous resource (see Chapter 13 on technology in education).

Table 12-7 summarizes the advantages and disadvantages of computer learning resources.

TABLE 12-7 Advantages and Disadvantages of Computer Resources	
Advantages	**Disadvantages**
Interactive potential promotes quick feedback and retention of learning	Primarily promotes learning in cognitive domain; less useful in changing attitudes and behaviors
Potential database is enormous	Both software and hardware are expensive, therefore less accessible to a wide audience
Instruction can be individualized to suit different types of learners or different paces for learning	Must be purchased—too complicated and time-consuming for most nurses to prepare
Time-efficient	Limited use for many elderly or low-literate learners and those with physical limitations

Evaluating Audiovisual Materials

Choosing the right audiovisual tools for patient education calls for judgment on the part of the nurse, who must take into consideration the *learner*, the *task*, and the *media* available to help patients learn. The method for selection of nonprint materials is the same, regardless of the domain of learning. Selection is based on the ability of materials to help with the instruction of a given behavioral objective. Materials should not be selected before the objectives are set. Always remember to consider the predetermined behavioral objectives. Ask yourself: Which materials will best support the teaching to meet these objectives with this audience? Also, remember that active is best, real is best, and instructional materials should be used only to support learning, not substitute for the teaching role of the nurse.

The evaluation of media involves evaluating the content, the instructional design, the technical production, and the packaging. Figure 12-6 depicts Discenza's (1993) checklist for selecting and evaluating audiovisual materials.

Table 12-8 provides a helpful, easy-to-use reference for evaluating the effectiveness of media in relationship to the various methods available for teaching.

SUMMARY

This chapter discussed the major categories of instructional materials and offered suggestions about how to select media from a range of possible options. Nurses are expected to be able to make appropriate choices of audiovisual tools every day to meet the needs of an individual learner or to satisfy a broader, more diverse group of

	Yes	No
A. Content		
Is the content valid?	___	___
Relevant?	___	___
Current?	___	___
Is the purpose of the program stated?	___	___
Are instructional objectives given?	___	___
B. Instructional Design		
Are the ideas and information presented logically?	___	___
Is the format of the program appropriate for the audience?	___	___
Does the instructor actively engage the learner?	___	___
Is there evidence of formative evaluation?	___	___
Is summative evaluation material provided?	___	___
C. Technical Production		
Is the visual material sharply focused and clear?	___	___
Is the image composition clear and uncluttered?	___	___
Is the text legible at the maximum viewing distance?	___	___
Is the audio clear and intelligible?	___	___
Is there any distracting background noise?	___	___
Is the pace of the narration appropriate for the audience?	___	___
D. Packaging		
Is the material available in a format for which equipment is available?	___	___
Is descriptive information provided?	___	___
Is a user's guide provided?	___	___
Has the instructional material won any awards?	___	___

FIGURE 12-6   A Checklist for Selecting and Evaluating Audiovisual Materials

Source: David J. Discenza. (1993). A systematic approach to selecting and evaluating instructional materials. *Journal of Nursing Staff Development, 9*(4), 198. Reprinted by permission of J.B. Lippincott Company.

learners. In this chapter, the importance of considering characteristics of the learner, the media, and the task when choosing instructional materials was emphasized. Several guidelines were put forth that would prove useful to nurses in selecting or developing print and nonprint materials appropriate to both the audience and the task. Also, the supplemental function of teaching materials was stressed.

The major categories of print and nonprint media were reviewed in full and comparisons were made of the advantages and disadvantages of each type. Examples of effective teaching tools were contrasted with examples of less effective instructional aids. Many audiovisual tools can influence all three domains of learning by promoting cognitive development, stimulating attitude change, and helping to build psychomotor skills. They vary in their ability to stimulate learners' visual and auditory senses, to actively engage learners, and to increase retention of information. Finally, comprehensive evaluation criteria were presented to assist the nurse in selecting effective tools for teaching and learning.

Table 12-8	Effectiveness of Teaching Tools and Methods		
Mode of Learning	**Retention**	**Media**	**Methods**
Reading	Learners retain 10% of what they read.	Leaflets, books, brochures, flip charts, chalkboards, instruction sheets	Self-instruction
Hearing	Learners retain 20% of what they hear.	Audiotapes, telephones	Lectures, discussion
Watching	Learners retain 30% of what they see.	Silent films, displays, photos, pictures, posters, cartoons, drawings	Demonstration, self-instruction
Watching and hearing	Learners retain 50% of what they see and hear.	Movies (films), TV, videotapes, DVDs, slides, overheads, models	Lecture or demonstration
Watching and speaking	Learners retain 70% of what they see and talk about.	Audiovisual media	Group discussion, 1:1 verbal interactions, demonstrations
Speaking and doing	Learners retain 90% of what they talk about and do.	Interactive media	Demonstration, return demonstration, gaming, role playing

Source: Adapted from Heinich, Malenda, and Russell (1992).

REVIEW QUESTIONS

1. How do instructional materials differ from teaching methods?
2. What are five general principles regarding the effectiveness of audiovisual tools?
3. What are the three major factors to consider when selecting, developing, and evaluating instructional materials?
4. What are the three primary components of media to be considered when evaluating appropriateness of audiovisual materials for instruction?
5. Which instructional tools are examples of realia and of illusionary representations?
6. What questions must be asked when reviewing commercially prepared print materials for possible use in instruction?

7. What are the major advantages and disadvantages of each type of print and non-print media as resources for patient education?
8. Why is the statement true that instructional materials should not be selected before behavioral objectives are determined?
9. What criteria must be considered when evaluating printed materials?

REFERENCES

Babcock, D. E. & Miller, M. A. (1994). *Client education: Theory and practice*. St. Louis: Mosby-Year Book.

Boyd, M. D., Gleit, C. J., Graham, B. A., & Whitman, N. J. (1998). *Health teaching in nursing practice: A professional model* (3rd ed.). Stamford, CT: Appleton & Lange.

Brown, D. G. (March 2001). *Judicious PowerPoint*. Retrieved from www.syllabus.com.

Brownson, K. (1998). Education handouts: Are we wasting our time? *Journal of Nurses in Staff Development, 14*(4), 176–182.

Bushy, A. (1991). A rating scale to evaluate research posters. *Nurse Educator, 16*(1), 11–15.

Byrne, T. J. & Edeani, D. (1984). Knowledge of medical terminology among hospital patients. *Nursing Research, 33*(3), 178–181.

Campbell, M. K., DeVellis, B., Strecher, V. J., Ammerman, A. S., DeVellis, R. S., & Sandler, R. S. (1994). Improving dietary behavior: The effectiveness of tailored messages in primary care settings. *American Journal of Public Health, 84*, 783–787.

Cooper, S. S. (1990). Teaching tips, one more time: The overhead projector. *Journal of Continuing Education in Nursing, 21*(3), 141–142.

de Tornyay, R. & Thompson, M. A. (1987). *Strategies for teaching nursing* (3rd ed.). Albany, NY: Delmar.

Discenza, D. J. (1993). A systematic approach to selecting and evaluating instructional materials. *Journal of Nursing Staff Development, 9*(4), 196–198.

Doak, C. C., Doak, L. G., Friedell, G. H., & Meade, C. D. (1998). Improving comprehension for cancer patients with low literacy skills: Strategies for clinicians. *CA-Cancer Journal for Clinicians, 48*(3), 151–162.

Doak, C. C., Doak, L. G., & Root, J. H. (1996). *Teaching patients with low literacy*. Philadelphia: J. P. Lippincott.

Duchin, S. & Sherwood, G. (1990). Posters as an educational strategy. *Journal of Continuing Education in Nursing, 21*(5), 205–208.

Estey, A., Musseau, A., & Keehn, L. (1994). Patient's understanding of health information: A multi-hospital comparison. *Patient Education and Counseling, 24*, 73–78.

Flournoy, E., Turner, G., & Combs, D. (2000). Innovative teaching: Read the writing on the wall. *Dimensions of Critical Care Nursing, 19*(4), 36–37.

Foster, S. D. (1987). Are commercial patient education materials right for you? *MCN: American Journal of Maternal Child Nursing, 12*(4), 287.

Frantz, R. A. (1980). *Selecting media for patient education. TCN/education for self-care*. Rockville, MD: Aspen.

Gillespie, M. O. & Ellis, L. B. (1993). Computer-based patient education revisited (review). *Journal of Medical Systems, 17*(3–4), 119–125.

Grier, E. C., Owens, C., Peavy, B. A., & Pelt, F. (1991). Use of a checklist to teach advanced technical skills. *Nurse Educator, 16*(5), 37–38.

Haggard, A. (1989). *Handbook of patient education.* Rockville, MD: Aspen.

Heinich, R., Malenda, M., & Russell, J. D. (1992). *Instructional media and the new technologies of instruction* (4th ed.). New York: Macmillan.

Hinkle, J. L., Albanese, M., & McGinty, L. (1993). Development of printed teaching materials for neuroscience patients. *American Association of Neuroscience Nurses, 25*(2), 125–129.

Lerner, E. B., Jehle, D. V. K., Janicke, D. M., & Moscati, R. M. (2000). Medical communication: Do our patients understand? *American Journal of Emergency Medicine, 18*(7), 764–766.

Moneyham, L., Ura, D., Ellwood, S., & Bruno, B. (1996). The poster presentation as an educational tool. *Nurse Educator, 21*(4), 45–47.

Nielsen, E. & Sheppard, M. A. (1988). Television as a patient education tool: A review of its effectiveness. *Patient Education and Counseling, 11*, 3–16.

Pinto, B. M. (1993). Training and maintenance of breast self-examination skills. *American Journal of Preventive Medicine, 9*(6), 353–358.

Rankin, S. H. & Stallings, K. D. (2001). *Patient education: Principles and practice* (4th ed.). Philadelphia: Lippincott.

Redman, B. K. (2001). *The practice of patient education* (9th ed.). St. Louis: Mosby.

Rice, V. H. & Johnson, J. E. (1984). Preadmission self-instruction booklets, postadmission exercise performance, and teaching time. *Nursing Research, 33*(3), 147–151.

Skinner, C. S., Strecher, V. J., & Hospers, H. (1994). Physician's recommendations for mammography: Do tailored messages make a difference? *American Journal of Public Health, 84*, 43–49.

Smith, C. E. (1987). *Patient education: Nurses in partnership with other health professionals.* Philadephia: Saunders.

Sternberger, C. S. & Freiburger, O. A. (1996). Faculty produced videos: An educational resource. *Journal of Nursing Staff Development, 12*(4), 173–178.

Weston, C. & Cranston, P. A. (1986). Selecting instructional strategies. *Journal of Higher Education, 57*(3), 259–288.

Williams, A. V., Parker, R. M., Baker, D. W., Parikh, N. S., Pitkin, K., Coates, W. C., & Nurss, J. R. (1995). Inadequate functional health literacy among patients at two public hospitals. *Journal of the American Medical Association, 274*(21), 1677–1682.

Williams, N. H., Wolgin, F., & Hodge, C. S. (1998). Creating an educational videotape. *Journal for Nurses in Staff Development, 14*(6), 261–265.

CHAPTER 13

Technology in Education

Deborah L. Sopczyk

CHAPTER HIGHLIGHTS

Health Education in the Information Age
The Impact of Technology on the Teacher
   and the Learner
Strategies for Using Technology in
   Healthcare Education
   The World Wide Web
   Healthcare Consumer Education and
     the World Wide Web

The Internet
   E-Mail
   Electronic Discussion Groups
   Other Forms of Online Discussion
Issues Related to the Use of Technology
   E-Learning

KEY TERMS

computer literacy
consumer informatics
Information Age

information literacy
Internet
World Wide Web

OBJECTIVES

After completing this chapter, the reader will be able to

1. Describe changes in education that have occurred as a result of Information Age technology.
2. Define the terms *Information Age, World Wide Web, Internet, information literacy*, and *computer literacy*.
3. Identify ways in which the resources of the Internet and World Wide Web could be incorporated into healthcare education.
4. Describe the role of the nurse as teacher in using technology in consumer education.
5. Recognize the issues related to the use of technology for teaching and learning.

Advances in technology have had a profound effect on the way we learn and the way we teach. Many adult learners can remember a time when finding information required traveling to the library to search a card catalog and spending countless hours looking through paper-based books and journals. Today, people have a world of information at their fingertips. Computers and the Internet have made it possible to get information from anyone, anywhere, anytime, within the blink of an eye. Not only is information readily available, but computer programs and simulations also allow today's learner to enter a virtual world where almost anything is possible. Like shiny new toys, educational technologies have captured the imagination and opened a world of opportunities for teachers and learners alike.

This chapter explores the tremendous potential of technology to transform teaching and learning experiences for nurses and healthcare consumers. However, technology is not a magic solution that can be implemented without careful planning, monitoring, and evaluation. Although computer programs have become easier to use and require less technical skill than they did in the past, the decision to use technology as a teaching strategy is likely to have many implications. Access, cost, support, and equipment must all be considered. It is important to remember that the application of technology in education is a means to an end, not an end in and of itself. "Without hard questions about learning, technology is like an unguided missile" (Ehrmann, 1995). Although it has incredible power, without careful planning, technology may take you to a place you did not want to go and give results you had not anticipated or desired. Therefore, the nurse who uses technology to enhance learning must not only have a basic understanding of the technology itself, but also be able to integrate the technology into a plan that is based on sound educational principles.

This chapter is designed as an introduction to technology-based resources and strategies appropriate for use with clients. Although it is not intended to provide detailed instruction on the mechanics of computers and other types of hardware and software, the chapter will provide a basic overview of the technology involved and implications for the teacher and the learner. Chapter 12 discusses the use of audiovisual materials for patient education. Hence, this chapter will focus primarily on the World Wide Web, the Internet, and computer-based hardware and software applications to enhance learning in traditional settings as well as with learners at a distance.

Before beginning this chapter, it is important to note that the World Wide Web, the Internet, and computer programs for teaching are developing at a rapid pace that is accelerating with each new generation of discoveries and applications (Cetron & Davies, 2001). Because of this phenomenon, consumers are often advised that the computers they buy today are not likely to reflect the "state-of-the-art" technology of tomorrow. Therefore, given the pace of technology, it is impossible to capture all that is new and cutting-edge in a textbook. This chapter is meant to serve as a starting point from which you can begin to investigate the resources currently available. Ideally, it will generate the interest and skill necessary for you to continue to search for new and exciting ways to integrate technology into your teaching and learning activities.

HEALTH EDUCATION IN THE INFORMATION AGE

We are in a period of history often referred as the *Information Age*, which Mitchel and McCullough (1995) describe as a place in time when sweeping advances in computer and information technology have transformed the economic, social, and cultural life of society. If you think about the many ways in which technology has changed the world we live in, it is clear that computers have become more than tools to make life easier—they have become part of our culture.

Computers have also become part of the culture of education and are as common in the educational environment today as chalk and blackboards were in years past. How has the Information Age changed health education? Consider the following. In the United States alone, more than 104 million adults report having Internet access (Rainie & Packel, 2001). By the year 2010, researchers predict that 95% of the people in the industrialized world and half of those in the developing world will be online and wired for high-speed access (Cetron & Davies, 2001). Much of the information available online is health-related, making it readily available to both consumers and healthcare professionals. For nurses who are providing health and healthcare education, it has never been easier to reach our clients, no matter where they live, and to provide interactive learning experiences that extend far beyond what was even imaginable in the recent past.

Despite the rapid growth of technology-based education programs and services, it is important to remember that electronic delivery of health information is in its infancy and many issues still need to be resolved. One major area of concern is the limited oversight and control over the content that is posted on the World Wide Web and Internet, two of the major vehicles for delivering information to a global audience. Many people believe that the lack of censorship on the World Wide Web is a freedom of speech issue. However, health professionals are concerned that consumers are making serious decisions about their health care based on information on the Web that has not been reviewed for accuracy, currency, or bias.

Recently, "codes" have been developed to guide practice and safeguard consumers who use the educational information and services that are delivered via the World Wide Web and the Internet. For example, the Internet Healthcare Coalition, a nonprofit group dedicated to quality health-related information on the Internet, established the *e-Health Code of Ethics* to ensure confident and informed use of the health-related information found on the Internet (Internet Healthcare Coalition, 2000). The e-Health Code of Ethics is based on the principles of candor, honesty, quality, informed consent, privacy, professionalism, responsible partnering, and accountability that are described in more detail in Table 13-1. Other codes have been established by the American Medical Association and by representatives of the United States–based Health.com organization (Foubister, 2000).

TABLE 13-1   Guiding Principles of the e-Health Code of Ethics

CANDOR
- Disclose information about the creators/purpose of the site that will help users make a judgment about the credibility and trustworthiness of the information or services provided.

HONESTY
- Be truthful in describing products/services, and present information in a way that is not likely to mislead the user.

QUALITY
- Take the necessary steps to ensure that the information provided is accurate and well supported and that the services provided are of the highest quality.
- Present information in a manner that is easy to understand and use.
- Provide background information about the sources of the information provided and the review process used to assist the user in making decisions about the quality of the information provided.

INFORMED CONSENT
- Inform users if personal information is collected and allow them to choose whether the information can be used or shared.

PRIVACY
- Take steps to ensure that the user's right to privacy is protected.

PROFESSIONALISM IN ONLINE HEALTH CARE
- Abide by the ethical code of your profession (e.g., nursing, medicine).
- Provide users with information about who you are, what your credentials are, what you can do online, and what limitations may be present in the online interaction.

RESPONSIBLE PARTNERING
- Take steps to ensure that sponsors, partners, and others who work with you are trustworthy.

ACCOUNTABILITY
- Implement a procedure for collecting, reviewing, and responding to user feedback.
- Develop and share procedures for self-monitoring compliance with the e-Health Code of Ethics.

Source: Adapted from the Internet Healthcare Coalition. (2000). *e-Health Code of Ethics.* e-Health Ethics Initiative, 2000, at http://www.ihealthcoalition.org/ethics/ehcode.html.

Technology will continue to make health and healthcare information more accessible and meaningful to consumers and healthcare professionals. It is important to note, however, that Information Age technology has done more than alter the way in which we teach and learn. As Mitchel and McCullough (1995) suggest in their definition of the Information Age, technology has and will continue to prompt dramatic, systemwide changes that will be evident in the roles played by nurses and clients, the relationships they establish, and the environments in which they interact.

THE IMPACT OF TECHNOLOGY ON THE TEACHER AND THE LEARNER ____

Information Age technology has influenced teaching and learning in two very important ways. First, the teacher is no longer the person who holds all of the answers or is solely responsible for imparting knowledge. Because information is so readily available, nurses are becoming facilitators of learning rather than providers of information, and are striving to create a collaborative atmosphere in their teaching and learning environments. Second, as information becomes more accessible, the need for memorization becomes less important than the ability to think critically. Therefore, it is essential that nurses help their clients to refine their problem, find the information they need, and evaluate the information they find.

As teachers, nurses also must know how and when to use technology, and how to modify their educational approaches to be consistent with the needs of Information Age clients. In addition, nurses must create learning environments in which clients are encouraged and supported in their attempts to seek the information they need to achieve optimum health. Technology and the increased accessibility to the information it offers have empowered consumers to form new partnerships with their healthcare providers (Kaplan & Brennan, 2001) and to assume more active roles in managing their care. As a result, today's consumers enter the healthcare arena with information in hand and are prepared to engage in a discussion about their diagnoses, treatments, and prognoses.

We can no longer assume that the clients we see in a hospital, home, or clinic setting have little information other than what we have given them. Whereas clients of the past were often isolated from others with similar diagnoses and dependent upon their providers for information, today they have the means to access networks of other patients and providers worldwide. Therefore, it is not surprising that the teaching needs of today's healthcare consumers and the expectations they hold for those who will be teaching them are changing. The role of the nurse has not been diminished, but it has been altered. Nurses must now be prepared not only to use technology in education, but also to help clients access, discuss, and evaluate the information that is available.

In addition, the Information Age has made a tremendous impact on professional education. Technology has given rise to a dramatic increase in educational opportunities for nurses. A 1999 survey of 281 colleges and universities, conducted by the American Association of Colleges of Nursing, revealed that nearly 2,000 courses are available using distance education technology, a number that is expected to continue to grow at a dramatic rate throughout the twenty-first century (Potema et al., 2001). Nurses seeking advanced degrees and credentials can now study at colleges and universities offering distance education programs in a wide range of subject areas. Computers have made it possible to provide "anytime, anywhere" access to job training and continuing education. Virtual reality and computer simulations can provide opportunities to learn hands-on skills and develop competencies in areas such as diagnostic reasoning and problem solving. Like consumers, healthcare professionals in the Information Age can use the World Wide Web and the Internet as vehicles for sharing resources and for gaining access to the most current information in their fields of practice.

STRATEGIES FOR USING TECHNOLOGY IN HEALTHCARE EDUCATION ____

The World Wide Web

One merely has to turn on a television to see the commercials for health-related Web sites or hear references to the Web on morning talk shows to appreciate the tremendous influence of the World Wide Web. A report produced by the Pew Foundation revealed that 52 million Americans, or more than half of all Americans with Internet access, have used the World Wide Web to obtain health-related information (Fox & Rainie, 2000). Consumers are bombarded with lures to the Web; once there, Web users can find anything from videos of surgical procedures to sites where they can ask questions as well as receive information. New sites are being introduced on a daily basis. It is estimated that more than 15,000 Web sites are devoted to healthcare issues and that these sites receive in excess of 22 million hits per month (Paris, 2001).

Having recognized the value of the World Wide Web, nurses and other healthcare providers are beginning to teach their clients how to use the Web to find the information they need. The nursing literature suggests that the Web is being incorporated into formal teaching plans with increasing frequency (Grandinetti, 2000; Leaffer & Gonda, 2000). Web pages are also being created by nurses as part of their outreach efforts to teach the community. Although health information on the Web is a relatively new phenomenon, so much interest has been generated that several professional publications, such as *Computers in*

Nursing, have a listing and review of Web sites devoted to a particular health- or nursing-related topic each month.

It is clear that the World Wide Web is an exceptionally rich educational resource for both professional and consumer use. However, despite people's familiarity with the Web, the terminology associated with it can be confusing. Therefore, some commonly used terms are clarified below:

- The World Wide Web is a virtual space for information. More than 1 billion Web pages covering a wide range of topics can be found on the Web, displaying a variety of formats including text, audio, graphics, and, in some cases, video (Why-not.com, 2001). Links on a Web page allow the user to easily move from one Web page to another with the click of a mouse.
- A Web browser is a special software program that locates and displays Web pages and enables a user to move around the World Wide Web. Netscape Navigator and Microsoft Internet Explorer are examples of Web browsers.
- Search engines and search directories are computer programs that allow the user to search the Web for particular subject areas. Google is an example of a search engine, and Yahoo! is an example of a search directory. The Web is so large that any one search engine or directory will cover only a small percentage of the Web pages available (Pandia.com, 1999).

The Internet is a huge global network of computers established to allow the transfer of information from one computer to another. Unlike the World Wide Web, which was created to display information, the Internet was created to exchange information. The World Wide Web resides on a small section of the Internet and would not exist without the Internet's computer network. Conversely, the Internet could exist without the World Wide Web and, in fact, flourished for many years before the World Wide Web was ever conceived.

Nurses or healthcare consumers need to go no farther than their computers if they wish to learn how to use the Internet or the World Wide Web. Getting into the Internet or the World Wide Web requires a computer with a modem or other telecommunication link and software to access an Internet service provider (ISP). Once connected, it is simple to find a wide range of Web sites devoted to teaching Internet or World Wide Web navigation skills. With a properly worded command (e.g., "World Wide Web" and "tutorial"), a search engine will uncover a number of self-paced tutorials designed to teach novice or intermediate users the desired skills. Most search engines even provide guidance in creating commands that will elicit the information needed.

Knowledge of the World Wide Web is critical for nurses who work with and educate consumers for several reasons:

- Nurses will be seeing an increase in the number of clients who have already searched the Web for information. Familiarity with the type of information found on the Web will help direct the assessment of clients prior to teaching to identify the needs of the learner and to determine whether follow-up is necessary.
- The World Wide Web is a tremendous resource for both consumer and professional education. The Web provides a mechanism for keeping up to date on professional and practice issues as well as a resource to be shared with clients. However, to use the Web effectively, nurses must possess information literacy skills and be prepared to teach these same skills to clients, including how to access the information on the Web and how to evaluate the information found.

Healthcare Consumer Education and the World Wide Web

Prior to teaching, a client must be assessed with questions about his or her computer use. It is important for nurses to determine whether a client has a computer, has access to the Internet, is knowledgeable about using a computer, and has interest in using a computer to obtain information. If a client does not have a computer but has interest in using one, libraries, senior centers, and community centers typically have computers with Internet access for public use, and often offer instruction and assistance for new users (Hendrix, 2000).

A Pew Foundation study found that approximately 21 million Web users in the United States located information on the Web that either:

1. Influenced their decisions about how to treat an illness
2. Led them to ask questions
3. Led them to seek a second medical opinion
4. Affected their decision about whether to seek the assistance of a healthcare provider (Fox & Rainie, 2000)

Therefore, it is important to determine if the information is not only accurate, complete, and unbiased, but also understandable. Since the World Wide Web contains information designed for both professional and public audiences, the lay consumer may not have the background necessary to comprehend information designed specifically for healthcare professionals. Consumers should not be discouraged from accessing these sites, but nurses must help clients find information written for them at their level of readability and comprehension (see Chapter 7 on literacy).

Unfortunately, much of the health information available on the Web is not written at a level that can easily be understood by the majority of the public (Graber, Roller, & Kaeble, 1999).

In addition to not fully understanding what they read, some clients may find that the Web has provided too much information, or information they are not ready to handle. For example, a patient newly diagnosed with a serious illness may be overwhelmed with the detailed information found on the Web regarding the course of the disease, prognosis, and treatment. Therefore, it is important to ask clients if they are using the Web to find health-related information and to explore the types of information they have found. Clients may or may not initially feel comfortable talking about what they have gathered. They may fear you will interpret their research as a lack of trust in your care. Some may be embarrassed to talk about information they do not fully understand. Others may be anxious about how to bring up information that conflicts with what they have been told or how they are being treated.

Also, readers must be warned that the Web contains information that may be biased, inaccurate, or misleading. Because the Web has the potential to change so quickly, it is difficult to regulate. Even Web pages sponsored by physicians, nurses, and university medical centers have been found to contain inaccurate information and treatment recommendations (Kiernan, 1998; Paris, 2001).

For these reasons, it is important to establish early in your relationships with clients that you are interested in talking with them about the information they have gathered from the Web or other resources they have available to them. Clients need to feel that you are open to discussing whatever they have found and that you are a partner in seeking the best information available. For clients who are being treated for a condition over an extended period of time, it is also important to continue the conversation about their Web searches throughout their treatment. Simply asking "Have you found any interesting information on the Web lately?" will keep the dialogue open and provide the nurse with the opportunity to respond to whatever questions or concerns they may have.

If possible, it is advantageous to conduct a teaching session in a place that has computer access. Having a computer available during a teaching session can accomplish several goals. You can:

- Introduce the client to Web sites that are relevant to his or her need.
- Review Web sites the client has been using to determine the type and amount of information to which the client has been exposed, assess the client's knowledge, and identify areas where the client may need further teaching. For example, a client may have visited a Web site that provides distressing information about

side effects of treatment, prognosis, or disease progression. Looking at the site together will give you the stimulus to talk with the client about what he or she has discovered and do additional teaching if needed.

- You can teach clients information literacy skills. *Information literacy* is defined as "the ability to access, evaluate, organize, and use information from a variety of sources" (Humes, 1999). If clients are going to make use of the vast array of information on the Web, they must be able to find what they are looking for, judge whether it is trustworthy, and decide how they will use it to meet their needs.

Information literacy is different from *computer literacy*, which is the ability to use the necessary computer hardware and software to take advantage of this technology (Association of Colleges and Research Libraries, 2000). A client who is information-literate knows how to find the information needed and can evaluate the information found for accuracy, currency, and bias. Although consumers may not have the background knowledge to evaluate health information to the same extent as a professional, they can be taught some simple steps to identify which Web sites are useful and which are problematic.

In years past, clients were not encouraged to search on their own for health information, but rather to rely on health providers for advice. Today, many consumers want to manage their own health care. More and more nurses are empowering their clients by teaching and encouraging them to take advantage of the available resources. For example, nurses are placing computers in patient waiting rooms with appropriate Web sites set up in a "point and click" format (Klemm, Hurst, Dearholt, & Trone, 1999). Others are preparing teaching materials on how to use the Web and what to look for once there.

There are many reasons why teaching clients where to go on the Web to find information is good practice. Web-based information can be obtained quickly, and the cost of Internet access in the home is minimal. Many consumers would benefit from having their questions answered quickly and inexpensively. For example, families with young children are likely to have frequent questions related to childhood illnesses, growth and development, and behavior problems and may not have the time or money to make a visit to the pediatrician. Senior citizens may have questions about problems encountered with aging but may have difficulty getting to a healthcare provider because of transportation and financial issues. People with chronic illness may gain some sense of control over their lives when they are able to access information about their conditions. Healthy people may have questions but few opportunities to talk with their provider. Even when they do, many of their questions go unanswered because they forget to ask, may be hesitant to ask, or may not be given sufficient time to ask the questions they may have.

The nurse can teach clients who access the Web to use it more effectively and encourage others to give it a try. A helpful approach is to compile lists of Web sites appropriate for the needs of different client populations. Table 13-2 provides examples of the various types of Web sites that are available for consumer use.

TABLE 13-2	Sample Web Sites for Healthcare Consumers		
Title	**URL**	**Sponsor/Author**	**Description**
Medline Plus	http://www.nlm.nih.gov/medlineplus/	National Library of Medicine	A government site that provides access to extensive information about specific diseases/conditions, links to consumer health information from the NIH, dictionaries, lists of hospitals and physicians, health information in Spanish and other languages, and clinical trials. There is no advertising on this site.
Virtual Hospital	http://www.vh.org	University of Iowa	A university site created to help meet the information needs of healthcare providers and patients. The digital information provided is all dated and reviewed for quality and accuracy.
Aplastic Anemia and MDS International Foundation	http://www.aplastic.org	Aplastic Anemia and MDS International Foundation, Inc.	A disease-specific site that provides a range of services, including free educational materials and access to a help line where consumer questions will be researched and answered.

(continued)

TABLE 13-2   Sample Web Sites for Healthcare Consumers (continued)

Title	URL	Sponsor/Author	Description
National Center for Infectious Diseases Travelers' Health	http://www.cdc.gov/travel	Centers for Disease Control and Prevention	A government site designed to provide a wide range of health-related information for travelers, including traveling with children, travelers with special needs, and specific disease information.
MayoClinic.com	http://www.mayoclinic.com	Mayo Clinic	A comprehensive hospital site that provides information as well as a variety of interactive tools to help healthcare consumers manage a healthy lifestyle, research disease conditions, and make healthcare decisions. Advertisement helps support this site.
Cancer Net	http://www.nci.nih.gov	National Cancer Institute	A government site devoted to all aspects of cancer. Provides both professional and consumer-oriented information and resources.
Bandaid®s and Blackboards	http://www.faculty.fairfield.edu/ fleitas/contents.html	Nursing faculty at Fairfield University	Site provides personal rather than factual information about growing up with health problems from the perspectives of kids, teens, and adults.
NetWellness	http://www.netwellness.org	University of Cincinnati, Ohio State University, and Case Western Reserve University	Nonprofit consumer health Web site that provides high-quality information created and evaluated by medical and health professional faculty at several universities.

In selecting Web sites to share with clients, it is important that the nurse first review them carefully. In recent years, multiple rating scales have been developed to assist in the evaluation of such sites. Table 13-3 summarizes the questions that should be asked in evaluating a health-related Web site (Kim, Eng, Deering, & Maxfield, 1999).

TABLE 13-3   Criteria for evaluating health-related Web sites

ACCURACY

- Are supportive data provided?
- Are the supportive data current and from reputable sources?
- Can you find the same information on other Web sites?
- Is the information provided comprehensive?
- Is more than one point of view presented?

DESIGN

- Is the Web site easy to navigate?
- Is the site "Bobby Approved"? (considered accessible to individuals with disabilities)
- Is there evidence that care was taken in creating the site? Do the links work? Are there typos?
- Is the information presented in a manner that is appropriate for the intended audience?
- Do the graphics serve a purpose other than decoration? Do they convey important messages?

AUTHORS/SPONSORS

- Are the sponsors/authors of the site clearly identified?
- Do the authors provide their credentials?
- Do the authors/sponsors provide a way to contact them or give feedback?
- Do the authors/sponsors clearly identify the purpose of the site?
- Is there reason for the sponsors/authors to be biased about the topic?

CURRENCY

- Is there a recent creation or modification date?
- Is there evidence of currency (e.g., updated bibliography reference to current events)?

AUTHORITY

- Are the sponsors/authors credible (e.g., is it a government, educational institution, or healthcare organization site versus a personal page)?
- Are the author's credentials appropriate to the purpose of the site?

THE INTERNET

The World Wide Web is merely a small component of a much larger computer network called the Internet. Although the Internet does not provide the eye-catching Web pages found on the World Wide Web, it does offer a wide range of services, many of which can be used to deliver health education to clients. The Internet can be used to enhance teaching by enabling individuals to interact with one another and with groups of people via the computer. Electronic mail (e-mail), real-time chat, and e-mail discussion or Usenet newsgroups are creative ways people can communicate with one another about issues related to health.

E-Mail

Despite the best efforts of health professionals to provide needed information to consumers, the factors of time, stress, fear, lack of experience, and simple human dynamics may result in clients walking away from a visit to a healthcare provider with incomplete or inaccurate information. Sometimes questions come up only after clients go home and try to follow the instructions they have been given. At other times, they may misunderstand what is being taught or be afraid or hesitant to admit that they do not understand. Unless there is a mechanism in place for clients to contact the nurse with questions, the client is at risk for making a mistake that may have serious consequences. Simply telling clients to call if they have questions is often inadequate. Calling a busy office or clinic usually results in having to wait a long time by the phone for an answer. Even calling hours can be problematic because they imply that the client is free to call at certain periods of the day or evening.

E-mail offers a quick, inexpensive way to communicate with clients. It has the advantage of being *asynchronous*, which means that the message can be sent at the convenience of the sender and the message will be read when the receiver is online and ready to read it. Messages can be sent and responded to anytime, day or night. However, despite the fact that electronic mail can provide a simple and efficient way to follow up with clients, nurses are just beginning to recognize its potential for teaching and learning. To date, little has been written in the literature about the purposes of and frequency with which nurses have used e-mail in communicating with clients. Some of the reasons nurses identify for not using e-mail include lack of instruction and support, limited access to computers, and preference for face-to-face communication (Hughes & Pakiesner, 2000).

E-mail for patient education is clearly a trend worth watching. In fact, in a discussion about healthcare delivery in the twenty-first century, the National Institute of

Medicine (2001) proclaimed that both patients and clinicians could benefit from increasing Internet-based communications. Studies suggest that patients are interested in interacting with their health providers via e-mail, and one survey found that one-third of online health seekers would consider switching health providers if they could communicate with them via this technology (Kassirer, 2000).

Given the opportunity e-mail provides for enhanced communication with clients, it is an approach worthy of further study by nurses. An e-mail message system gives clients who identify questions after they go home a chance to get answers from a reliable source familiar with their history. Clients who are not sure how to phrase a question or feel rushed when instructions are being given in a clinical setting have a chance to compose their thoughts at home and prepare an e-mail message. Also, from the nurse's perspective, an e-mail message system provides a simple way to check on clients to see whether they understood the instructions they were given and to respond to new questions that have arisen.

In some ways, an e-mail system is preferable to a voice messaging system. For clients who are anxious about asking questions, e-mail allows them all the time they need to gather their thoughts. In addition, clients do not have to remember the answers they are given by the nurse, as the e-mail message provides a written record of the nurse's response. In contrast, many voicemail systems are time-limited. Clients are sometimes cut off in the middle of a voice message if the message is long or if clients are struggling to make themselves understood. Other clients may hesitate to leave a voicemail in the evening or night hours when they know nobody is around to respond. However, by virtue of the way e-mail is designed, clients can feel comfortable sending messages of any length at any time.

An e-mail message system is simple to implement. Client e-mail addresses need to be identified as part of the routine information-gathering process for new clients. Because e-mail addresses are likely to change, they need to be updated, just like telephone numbers, whenever a client visits a physician's office, clinic, or other healthcare setting. It is a good idea to have more than one person be responsible for responding to e-mail messages, so that questions and concerns can be addressed even when a staff member is away due to vacation or time out of the office. One way to accomplish this goal is to have messages be sent to a mailbox rather than to an individual. Because more than one person can be given access to an electronic mailbox, continuous coverage can be established. If continuous coverage is not provided, it is important that clients know how long they can expect to wait to receive answers to their questions.

E-mail systems can be set up to serve a variety of purposes. If post-teaching follow-up is desired, e-mail offers one way for the nurse to initiate contact after the client has left the healthcare delivery system. The nurse can get in touch with the client via e-mail following a teaching session to convey interest in how he or she is doing with a medication regime, treatment, or other types of instructions given. The e-mail message could stress important points that were made during the teaching session—for example, "Remember to take your pill around the same time every day." An e-mail message could also be used to assess the client's understanding of what was taught; for example, a client might be asked: "What time of day will you be giving your child his medication?" In all cases, the nurse should encourage the client to get in touch if questions remain. Any follow-up system will take time, resolve, and commitment on the part of the organization for the system to work effectively. An e-mail system also can be established as a mechanism to answer questions and exchange health-related information with every client who receives services at a particular healthcare organization. An "e-mail question box" can provide simple access to all nurses available to provide a reliable source of information. For this type of system to work, the e-mail address for the mailbox needs to be widely distributed and easy to remember. For example, a mailbox address such as Questions@RDClinic.org would be easy to remember because it includes the purpose of the mailbox and the name of the organization. This address should then be placed on the bottom of written instructions, teaching materials, appointment cards, and other sources of communication with the client. A description of the service and instructions for use should also be distributed. For example, it may be helpful for clients to know who will be answering their questions, the types of questions that can be submitted, and the typical response time. Also, it is very important that clients understand that an e-mail message system is not intended to replace a visit or phone call when they need to see or talk with a healthcare provider about an immediate problem.

When sending e-mail messages, it is important to remember that electronic communication differs in several ways from face-to-face communication:

- Electronic communication lacks context. Without cues like facial expressions, tone of voice, and body posture, e-mail messages can appear cold and unfeeling. Although emoticons (symbols like "smiley faces" used to express emotion) are commonly used by people who send e-mail messages, they may not be appropriate for all professional correspondence. However, a carefully constructed e-mail message can convey the intent of the sender.
- Although electronic communication is convenient, it may take hours or days before the message is received and answered. For this reason, it is very important that an e-mail response to a client question be clear and of sufficient detail so that it does not generate more questions that cannot be answered immediately.

- E-mail messages provide a written record. A printed copy can serve as a handy reference for a client, but it can also serve as documentation of having provided either sufficient teaching or inaccurate or inappropriate information. When responding to a client question, it is vital that the client's record be reviewed and that the response to the question be accurate and carefully thought out. Copies of the e-mail messages sent to clients should be placed in the client's record.
- Electronic communication can never be assumed to be private. Therefore, it is important that both nurses and clients understand that violations of privacy can occur in many ways. For example, clients who send e-mail messages from work may not be aware of the fact that their messages may be stored on servers and hard drives even after they have been deleted from their personal computer. In some cases, the employer may have legal access to this information (Kassirer, 2000). E-mail messages can also be easily forwarded. Therefore, the nurse should assume that the client may choose to share a response with others.

E-mail communication between nurse and client has tremendous potential to enhance teaching. However, despite the increased use of e-mail among the general population, it is important to remember that not every client has a computer, computer skills, or access to e-mail. A backup system such as voicemail should therefore be made available so that the needs of all clients will be met.

Electronic Discussion Groups

The Internet provides many opportunities for clients and health professionals to participate in electronic discussion groups with other people who share a common interest, such as cancer. Although different types of electronic discussion groups are available, they all share the ability to connect people asynchronously from various locations via computer. Many people like electronic discussion groups because they are easy to use, are available 24 hours a day, and involve "faceless" communication with strangers from all over the world, so there is a sense of anonymity even when real names are used. Electronic discussion groups fall into two main categories: those that distribute mail to individual subscribers and those that post messages in a way that make them accessible to group participants. In the first case, messages are sent to the individual; in the second case, the subscriber seeks out the messages that have been posted. Electronic discussion groups can be structured in many different ways. Some are moderated, whereas others have little or no oversight. Some electronic discussion groups have thousands of subscribers, whereas others are very small closed groups created for specific purposes.

For the nurse, electronic discussion groups can serve as an effective vehicle for teaching. Whether the group is large or small, the asynchronous nature of electronic discussion groups makes it possible for people to communicate with one another despite different time zones and work schedules. Whether the nurse chooses to create an electronic discussion group or uses one already in existence, this form of online communication provides a creative way to teach and to learn. The two major formats used to create electronic discussion groups, those that distribute mail (mailing lists) and those that post it (newsgroups), are discussed next.

Mailing Lists

Automated mailing lists are one of the most common means of setting up an electronic discussion group. With an automated mailing list, people communicate with one another by sharing e-mail messages. The principle by which these groups work is simple. Individuals who have subscribed to the mailing list send their e-mail messages to a designated address, where a software program then copies the message and distributes it to all subscribers. Therefore, when a message is sent to the group, everyone gets to see it.

The most popular of these automated software programs is called "Listserv." In fact, the Listserv program is so commonly used that automated mailing lists are often referred to as "listservs." Other automated programs include Majordomo, Mailbase, and Listproc.

Listservs are wonderful for the nurse as a teaching tool or learning resource. Mailing lists are easy to use once a user understands how the system works. With more than 100,000 listservs and mailing lists available, it is possible to find an online group to cover almost any issue. The quality of the messages is usually very high in both health-related and professional mailing lists.

Because mailing lists facilitate group rather than individual communication, they work especially well with groups that are interested in collaborative learning or learning from the experiences of others. Most lists are quite active and, at any given time, several discussion topics can be addressed by the group. Members post questions, ask advice, and comment on current issues. Relationships between active members are established over time, and group members come to count on others in the group for their counsel. For these reasons, listservs and other types of automated mailing lists have become popular as mechanisms for online support for health consumers (Bliss, Allibone, Bontempo, Flynn, & Valvano, 1998; Han & Belcher, 2001; Klemm, Reppert, & Visich, 1998). The Association of Cancer Online Resources, Inc. (ACOR) has been a major player in the move to bring online support to healthcare consumers (Han & Belcher, 2001). This nonprofit organization devoted to assisting people with cancer has established more than 70 different online support groups since 1996, each devoted to a particular type of cancer or cancer-related problem. Its Web page states that ACOR delivers almost 2 million messages per week to the almost 70,000 people who subscribe to one of its online groups (Association of Cancer Online Resources, 2000). Memberships in the various groups range from about 25 people in the smaller groups to almost 2,000 individuals in the larger groups. Other individuals and organizations have established similar online groups covering a wide range of healthcare issues. Sometimes groups are started by individuals who have been unable to find the information and support they need in their home communities (Bliss et al., 1998). Others are started by advocacy groups interested in providing service to a particular group of people. A review of the purposes and goals of several online support groups revealed education and information sharing as the reasons for starting and maintaining a group.

Many people join online support groups after they or their loved ones have been diagnosed with a serious illness. They come to the support group not only to receive reassurance and encouragement, but also to gather as much information as possible so that they can begin to make necessary decisions about treatment. By joining an online support group, they are turning to people who know what they are going through and who can give practical advice based on real-life experience. The desire to share the most current information is commonly what brings group members together (Han & Belcher, 2001). Nurses may wish to teach their clients about the benefits of online support groups, or, if an appropriate group is not available, nurses can start an online support group of their own. These groups may be especially helpful to people who find it difficult to leave home because of illness or care responsibilities.

Clients who are unfamiliar with online communication should be reassured that there is no pressure for them to contribute to the discussion and that many people benefit just by reading the comments of others (Klemm et al., 1998). Clients who are insecure about their ability to express themselves in written format can take the time to think about what they want to say and use the spelling and grammar check functions to edit their remarks. Clients who are unsure if an online support group will meet their needs should be encouraged to give one a try. There are no costs involved other than the cost of being online, and there is no obligation to continue. Subscribers can withdraw from a group at any time.

Nevertheless, online support groups have some disadvantages that should be shared with clients who are thinking about joining a group. The most common disadvantages include the following:

- The volume of messages received each day can be problematic (Han & Belcher, 2001; Klemm et al., 1998). Some lists report an average of 50 or more messages per day. Experienced users learn to sort messages and delete the unnecessary or irrelevant ones quickly. Others find requesting that messages be sent in digest form (all messages received in a day are combined and sent in one mailing) helps control the volume of e-mails received. In any case, the daily volume of messages initially can be overwhelming, and may present a problem for people with low literacy levels or for people for whom English is a second language.

- Most online groups do not have a professional facilitator. Online groups are often run by someone who is interested in the health problem being discussed because he or she either has the condition or has a family member with the healthcare problem. As a consequence, inaccurate information may be shared and problems with group dynamics may not be addressed.

- If clients are connected to the Internet via the sole phone line into their homes, time spent on the computer may be a problem. Family members cannot call into the home when the client is online reading or responding to messages. An open phone line is often critical in the home when someone is seriously ill. If busy phone lines become a problem, it may help to go online at the same time every day and let significant others know that the phone will be unavailable during that time.

Although this chapter classifies online support groups as part of the category of automated mailing groups, it should be noted that online support groups take many forms, such as scheduled and unscheduled chats, bulletin boards, mailing lists, and electronic newsletters. Regardless of the format, online support groups provide a mechanism for meeting the teaching and learning needs of many different client populations.

Usenet

Usenet is a global online discussion system that distributes and archives messages posted to topic-specific electronic discussion groups called newsgroups. Although referring to Usenet newsgroups as electronic bulletin boards is technically incorrect, the analogy works well because newsgroups work in a manner similar to a bulletin board. People "post" messages to the newsgroup, and anyone who has access to a newsreader can then subscribe to the newsgroup and read the messages that have been posted. There are thousands of Usenet newsgroups in existence, many of which are devoted to health topics. Similar to e-mail addresses and Web addresses (URLs), the names assigned to newsgroups follow a set of rules that define the group. A newsgroup name consists of several words or labels, each followed by a period—for example, sci.med.diseases.lyme. In this, the category "sci" indicates that this newsgroup falls under the broad category of science. Seven major categories are commonly used in Usenet newsgroup names: comp (computers), misc (miscellaneous), sci (science), soc (social or cultural), talk (debate-oriented), news (news network), and rec (recreation). In the example sci.med.diseases.lyme, each word that follows the major category "sci" narrows the focus. Therefore, this newsgroup falls under the category of science and is devoted to discussion of medical diseases—specifically, Lyme disease.

Like Web sites and listservs, Usenet newgroups are a source of healthcare information for both consumers and health professionals. However, unlike health-related Web sites that are informational or educational in nature, newsgroups are designed to provide a way for people to talk about health-related issues and to answer questions posted by members of the group. Although the volume of messages is problematic (some subscribers are frequent contributors, whereas others are "lurkers" who log on and read messages but never post one of their own), many people subscribe because they enjoy the interaction and like to read the various messages that have been posted. Unlike listservs that send newly posted messages to subscribers every day, newsgroups require subscribers to come to them whenever they want to read messages. Newsgroups may or may not be moderated, and the subscribers who post messages range from the very knowledgeable to the uninformed.

Although clients may find newsgroups to be a source of support and practical information, they may also be a source of misinformation. Therefore, it is important for clients to understand the need to verify the information they receive from a newsgroup, either by bringing questions to the nurse or by doing further research on the Web or in a library. Nurses who work with clients in a particular area of care may find it helpful to subscribe to relevant newsgroups to discover the types of messages that are being posted. Not only will this exercise provide the nurse with data about the types of information clients are receiving, but it will also provide insight into the kinds of issues, concerns, and unanswered questions clients may have.

Other Forms of Online Discussion

Online forums, message boards, and bulletin boards are systems that provide a way for people to post messages for others to read and respond to. They differ from newsgroups in two important ways. First, whereas newsgroups are found on the Internet and use e-mail as the means by which messages are sent to the group, online forums, message boards, and bulletin boards are found on a Web site. Because users of this type of discussion board are posting directly to the discussion board rather than indirectly via e-mail, many people may find this system easier to use. Second, although most discussion board-type forums require some system of registration, users can often select a user name of their choosing and e-mail addresses are not displayed. This added privacy is a boon to many people who are reluctant to share their names and e-mail addresses with strangers. Online forums, message boards, and bulletin boards for healthcare consumers and healthcare professionals can be found on many health-related sites on the World Wide Web.

Chat differs from e-mail and the other forms of electronic communication previously discussed in that it provides an opportunity for online conversation to take place in real time. Although chat conversations take the form of text rather than audio, a chat session shares many features with a telephone conference call. Several people from different locations participate in a conversation at the same time and can join or leave the session as needed. For example, the award-winning Web site called MentalHealth.Net (http://www.mentalhealth.net) sponsors a wide range of scheduled chats for professionals, the general public, and persons dealing with mental illness. In addition to public chat rooms, many organizations sponsor chats for their own clients or staff as a way to offer ongoing educational programs or information exchange among groups.

When leading or facilitating a chat group, it is important for the nurse to plan ahead. Without adequate control systems in place, a number of communication problems can occur such as multiple ongoing conversations, lack of focus, and periods of silence. The discussion in a chat room can move quickly, and it is very easy to get so involved in the process of chatting that the content to be covered gets lost or forgotten. The following suggestions may help to organize a successful chat session:

- E-mail or post the purpose and/or the agenda of the chat session several days in advance.
- Make a list of the discussion points to be covered during the session that is well organized, easy to follow, and placed so that it can be easily seen during the chat.
- Depending on the topic and the experience of the facilitator, it may be appropriate to limit the number of participants. The larger the group, the more difficult the challenge of running a smooth and productive online chat.
- Sign on to the chat session early. You want to be able to handle unexpected problems before the session begins.
- Watch the clock. Time in a busy chat session goes by quickly. If the chat was designed as a question and answer period, it may be helpful to ask people to e-mail important questions ahead of time so they are not forgotten.

- Help the group to follow the conversation taking place. For example, it is easy for chat discussions to become disjointed or off-topic. When responding to a question, refer to the query and the person asking it. If the group is losing focus, bring the participants back to the agenda and the points being discussed.
- Limit the amount of time spent discussing the detailed questions or concerns of one participant. If someone in the group needs individualized attention, suggest that they e-mail or call you after the chat has ended.
- If appropriate, ask participants who have not offered comments if they have any questions. A statement such as "Our conversation moved very quickly tonight so I want to give those who haven't had a chance some time to ask their questions" may slow down the conversation long enough for everyone to have an opportunity to contribute.
- Begin to wrap up the session about 10 minutes before the scheduled end time.

It may also help to prepare participants for the chat experience. Chat sessions can be overwhelming for new users. The following guidelines for chat participation should be shared with clients or colleagues who will be joining a chat session for the first time:

- Be prepared to choose a user name. Participants in public chats with strangers are often advised not to use their real names so as to protect their privacy.
- Keep comments short and to the point.
- Be prepared for "chat lingo" in public chat rooms. Abbreviations like BTW (by the way) and emoticons (symbols that represent emotions, such as ;) = winking) are commonly used.
- Do not worry about typos and grammar. Chat programs do not have spell checks and not everyone is an experienced typist. People who are frequent chat users learn to overlook spelling errors.

Some limitations of chat must be considered. Because chat requires that people be online at the same time, scheduling conflicts and time-zone issues result in less accessibility than asynchronous forms of electronic discussion. Due to the fast pace of most chat discussions, it may be difficult for some clients to keep up with the dialogue. Clients with certain disabilities, clients who are ill, and clients with low literacy levels may have trouble participating if the group moves along too quickly.

The future for electronic communication is exciting. The technology to add audio and video components to online conferencing is available and is becoming more refined and less expensive every day. It is likely that both audio and video online options will be commonplace in the near future.

ISSUES RELATED TO THE USE OF TECHNOLOGY

Despite the power of computer and Internet technology to enhance teaching and learning, it does present some unique challenges. Think for a moment about the many ways in which patient education differs via the computer from more traditional classroom education. The characteristics of the learners, the setting, and the access to hardware, software, and technological support are all likely to be different. Teaching and learning take place in a wide range of settings, many of which are unstructured. Access to resources and support varies considerably among healthcare consumers and in healthcare organizations, and clients participating in education programs may cover a wide range of ages, abilities, and limitations. Therefore, it is important for the nurse to consider these factors when using technology in healthcare education.

Although the latest available national statistics indicate that the percentage of households with Internet access was 42% in 2000 (compared with 26% in 1998), only about 18% of adults over the age of 65 had access to the Internet. That percentage increased significantly in the 45- to 64-year-old age group, 47% of whom have Internet access, largely because many people between these ages are still in the work-force (U.S. Census Bureau, 2001; Lenhart, 2000). Despite the statistics, it would be a mistake to discount computer-delivered education as a possibility for the senior population. Studies have found wide diversity among older adults. Although some seniors report believing that there is little reason for them to go online, others are taking the initiative to learn computer and Internet skills and are joining online communities (Alder, 1996; Lenhart, 2000). Although large numbers of older adults have only limited incomes, numerous government and private initiatives are available to provide free or low-cost computer and Internet access for the senior population. Some older adults have physiologic and neurologic problems that make computer use difficult, but many other seniors enjoy good health and functionality.

Computer- and Internet-based technology holds much promise as a means of educating this segment of the population. Therefore, it is important that the nurse be prepared to support computer-based learning among older clients. The following interventions may be helpful in encouraging senior citizens to engage in learning activities via the computer:

- Reinforce principles of ergonomics by making suggestions about equipment and posture that will minimize physical problems related to computer use. Proper posture, correct positioning of the keyboard and monitor, adjusted screen colors and font size, a supportive chair, and a reminder to get up and walk around three to four times per hour will help older adults to avoid discouraging physical symptoms that may interfere with computer use.

- Identify resources that will provide computer access and support in the senior citizen's home community. Supply seniors with a comprehensive resource list containing places where free computer and Internet access is available, places where computer training is provided for seniors, and contact people who will assist if problems are encountered. For example, SeniorNet (http://www.seniornet.org) is an organization created for the purpose of supporting computer use among senior citizens.

- Motivate older adults to use a computer by helping them to identify how the computer can meet their needs. "Older people perform best when the task is relevant to their lives" (Hendrix, 2000, p. 66). It is important to talk to seniors about their needs and abilities. Matching a computer program or Web site to the individual's unique circumstances will encourage computer use. For example, a senior who is caring for a spouse with cancer might enjoy an online support group if he or she enjoys interacting with and learning from the experiences of others.

- Create a supportive and nonthreatening environment to teach older adults about using a computer for health education. Seniors did not grow up with computers and may not have confidence in their ability to learn this new skill at this point in their lives. Avoid computer jargon, define new terms, pace your teaching according to their responses, provide opportunities for practice and reinforcement of skills, and write the instructions down.

Computers can open up a whole new avenue of support and information to older adults who are struggling with their own health problems and those of their partners. Seniors who enjoy good health can find resources to help them maintain their health and to become educated consumers. It is important that older adults be given the same opportunities to take advantage of the Information Age resources that are available to younger clients. The nurse can play a key role in promoting digital inclusion among this segment of the population.

People with disabilities make up another special population that may require additional planning before using technologies for health education. Not only are people with disabilities less likely to have computer and Internet access than are members of the general population, but they also may have difficulty using hardware and software.

An individual with a hearing problem may not be able to hear the sounds that are often used as prompts when a wrong key is struck or when an e-mail message is delivered. Accessibility for individuals with hearing impairments will become a bigger issue in the future when it becomes easier to send audio signals across the Web and audio messages become more commonplace. Many of the learning platforms used to deliver online courses are inaccessible to people with visual impairments.

Despite the protections offered by the Americans with Disabilities Act and other federal legislation, accessibility issues on the Web and constraints with hardware and software persist. Federal legislation requires government agencies and institutions receiving government funding to make their Web sites accessible to people with disabilities. To date, only a small percentage of these required Web sites accommodate the disabled or have been approved by disability organizations (West, 2000).

E-Learning

Technology has had such an impact on workforce training that it has given birth to a new industry and a new set of buzzwords that define an Information Age approach to staff education. Professional development and training organizations have capitalized on the power of computer technology to provide businesses with learning solutions referred to as *e-learning*, an abbreviation for electronic learning. Although no consensus of opinion has been reached on a precise definition for the term *e-learning*, there is some agreement that it involves the use of technology-based tools and processes to provide for customized learning anytime or anywhere. The emphasis in e-learning is on outcomes, with the goal of providing an individual with the information or practice opportunities required to perform a task or solve a problem at the point of need. E-learning has been well received in health care because it is cost-effective, promotes positive patient outcomes, and leads to greater staff satisfaction. The nature of the work of health care makes workforce training a critical issue, and e-learning appears to have provided a solution to the problem of keeping staff current in a world where new treatments and new techniques are always on the horizon.

SUMMARY

This chapter focused on Information Age technology for education. Specifically, the chapter discussed ways in which the World Wide Web and the Internet can be used by nurse educators to enhance teaching for consumers. The impact of technology on teachers and learners was addressed, and special considerations for older adults and other client groups were identified.

Information Age technology has the potential to transform the delivery of health education. This powerful tool must be used thoughtfully and carefully, however. Education is about learning, not about technology. Technology is merely a vehicle to deliver educational programs and to promote learning. The benefits of technology-based education are numerous, as are the challenges for teachers and learners. As nurses, we have a responsibility to learn how to use this new tool to promote health in our clients. The future for health education via the computer looks very bright, and we can help to shape it by continuing to think creatively about how to use technology in education and by participating in research about its effectiveness.

REVIEW QUESTIONS

1. What is the "Information Age," and how has it influenced the delivery of health education?
2. What Information Age skills are required by nurses and consumers to participate in computer-based teaching and learning?
3. What standards that have been established to ensure the quality of and access to technology for health education?
4. What resources on the World Wide Web and the Internet facilitate electronic communication between and among nurses and consumers? What are the advantages and disadvantages of each of these resources?
5. What steps are being taken to address the issues of limited access and special population needs to obtain health education via the computer?

REFERENCES

Alder, J. (1996). Older adults and computers: Report of a national survey. Retrieved April 2001, from http://www.seniornet.org/research/survey2.html

Association of Cancer Online Resources. (2000). About ACOR.org. Retrieved May 2001, from http://www.acor.org/about/index.html

Association of Colleges and Research Libraries. (2000). Information literacy competency standards for higher education. Retrieved April 2001, from www.ala.org/acrl/ilintro.html

Bliss, J., Allibone, C., Bontempo, B., Flynn, T., & Valvano, N. (1998). Creating a Web site for online social support: Melanocyte. *Computers in Nursing, 16*(4), 203–207.

Cetron, M. J. & Davies, O. (2001). Trends now changing the world. *The Futurist, 35*(2), 27–40.

Ehrmann, S. C. (1995). Asking the right question: What does research tell us about technology and higher learning? *Change, 27,* 20–27. Retrieved April 2001, from http://www.learner.org/edtech/rscheval/rightquestion.html

Foubister, V. (2000). Developing rules for the Web. Amednews.com. Retrieved October 2000, from http://www.ama-assn.org/sci-pubs/amnews/pick_00/prsa0731.htm

Fox, S. & Rainie, L. (2000). The online healthcare revolution: How the Web helps Americans take better care of themselves. Pew Internet and American Life Project: Online Life Report. Retrieved April 2001, from http://www.pewinternet.org/reports/toc.asp?Reports=26

Graber, M. A., Roller, C. M., & Kaeble, B. (1999). Readability levels of patient education materials on the World Wide Web. *Journal of Family Practice, 48*(1), 58–61.

Grandinetti, D. A. (2000). Help patients surf the Net safely. *RN Online, 63*(8), 51–63.

Han, H. R. & Belcher, A. (2001). Computer-mediated support group use among parents of children with cancer. An exploratory study. *Computers in Nursing, 19*(1), 27–33.

Hendrix, C. (2000). Computer use among the elderly. *Computers in Nursing, 18*(2), 62–67.

Hughes, J. A. & Pakiesner, R. A. (2000). Factors that impact nurses' use of electronic mail (e-mail). *Computers in Nursing, 17*(6), 251–259.

Humes, B. (1999). *Understanding Information Literacy.* Office of Educational Research, National Institute on Postsecondary Education, Libraries, and Lifelong Learning. Retrieved October 2001, from http://www.ed.gov/pubs/UnderLit/

Internet Healthcare Coalition. (2000). e-Health Code of Ethics. Retrieved October 2001, from http://www.ihealthcoalition.org/ethics/ehcode.html

Kaplan, B. & Brennan, P. F. (2001). Consumer informatics: Supporting patients as co-producers of quality. *Journal of the American Medical Informatics Association, 8*(4), 309–315.

Kassirer, J. P. (2000). Patients, physicians and the Internet. *Health Affairs, 19*(6), 115–123.

Kiernan, V. (1998). Study finds errors in medical information available on the Web. *Chronicle of Higher Education, XLIV*(40), A25.

Kim, P., Eng, T., Deering, M. J., & Maxfield, A. (1999). Published criteria for evaluating health-related Web sites: Review. Retrieved April 2000, from http://bmj.org/cgi/contents/short/318/7184/647

Klemm, P., Hurst, M., Dearholt, S. L., & Trone, S. R. (1999). Cyber solace: Gender differences on Internet cancer support groups. *Computers in Nursing, 17*(2), 65–72.

Klemm, P., Reppert, K., & Visich, L. (1998). A nontraditional cancer support group: The Internet. *Computers in Nursing, 16*(1), 31–36.

Leaffer, T. & Gonda, B. (2000). The Internet: An underutilized tool in patient education. *Computers in Nursing, 18*(1), 47–52.

Lenhart, A. (2000). Who's not online: 57% of those without Internet access say they do not plan to log on. Pew Internet and American Life Project: Online Life Report. Retrieved April 2001, from http://www.pewinternet.org/reports/pdfs/Pew_Those_Not_Online_Report.pdf

Mitchel, W. J. & McCullough, M. (1995). Digital Design Media: Online. Retrieved September 2001, from http://www.gds.harvard.edu/~malcolmDDM/DDMain.html

National Institute of Medicine, Committee on Quality of Health Care in America. (2001). *Crossing the Quality Chasm: A New Health System for the 21st Century.* Washington, DC: National Academy Press.

Pandia.com. (1999). A short and easy Web search tutorial. Retrieved April 2001, from http://www.pandia.com/goalgetter/index.html

Paris, J. J. (2001). Ethical issues in cybermedicine. *America, 184*(4), 15–22.

Potema, K., Stanley, J., Davis, B., Miller, K. L., Hassett, M. R., & Pepicello, S. (2001). Survey of technology use in AACN member schools. *Journal of Professional Nursing, 17*(1), 7–13.

Rainie, L. & Packel, D. (2001). More online doing more. Pew Internet and American Life Project: Online Life Report. Retrieved April 2001, from http://www.pewinternet.org/reports/pdfs/PIP_Changing_Population.pdf

West, D. M. (2000). Assessing e-Government: The Internet, democracy, and service delivery by state and federal governments. Retrieved April 2001, from http://www.brown.edu/Departments/Taubman_Center/polreports/egovreport00.html#Executive Summary

Why-not.com. (2001). World Wide Web user statistics. Retrieved May 17, 2001, from http://www.why-not.com/company/stats.htm

U.S. Census Bureau. (2001). Home computer and Internet use in the United States: August 2000. Retrieved March 2005, from http://www.census.gov/prod/2001pubs

CHAPTER 14

Evaluation in Healthcare Education

Priscilla Sandford Worral

KEY TERMS

assessment
content evaluation
evaluation
impact evaluation

outcome (summative) evaluation
process (formative) evaluation
program evaluation

OBJECTIVES

After completing this chapter, the reader will be able to

1. Define the term *evaluation*.
2. Compare and contrast evaluation and assessment.
3. Identify purposes of evaluation.
4. Distinguish between five basic types of evaluation: process, content, outcome, impact, and program.
5. Discuss characteristics of various models of evaluation.
6. Assess barriers to evaluation.
7. Examine methods for conducting an evaluation.
8. Select appropriate instruments for various types of evaluation data.
9. Identify guidelines for reporting results of evaluation.

Evaluation is the process that can justify that what we do as nurses makes a value-added difference in the care we provide. Planning for evaluation has never been more critical than in today's healthcare environment. Crucial decisions regarding learners rest on the outcomes of learning. Does the patient's family know how to care for the patient after discharge? Can the patient safely give himself medication? If education is to be shown as a value-added activity, education of the patient must be able to be linked to positive patient outcomes. The outcomes of education, for the learner and for the organization, must be measurably effective.

Evaluation is defined as a systematic process by which the worth or value of something—in this case, teaching and learning—is judged. Evaluation is a process within a process—an important part of the nursing process, the decision-making process, and the education process. Evaluation is the final component of each of these processes. Because these processes are cyclical, evaluation serves as the critical bridge at the end of one cycle that guides direction of the next cycle.

The sections of this chapter follow the steps in conducting an evaluation. These steps include (1) determining the focus of the evaluation; (2) designing the evaluation; (3) conducting the evaluation; (4) analyzing data collected; (5) reporting results of the evaluation; and (6) using evaluation results. Each aspect of the evaluation process is important, but all of them are meaningless if the results of evaluation are not used to guide future action in planning and carrying out patient education activities.

EVALUATION VERSUS ASSESSMENT

While assessment and evaluation are highly related to one another, they are not one and the same. The process of *assessment* is to gather, summarize, interpret, and use data to decide a direction for action. The process of *evaluation* is to gather, summarize, interpret, and use data to determine the extent to which an action was successful. The primary differences between the two terms are those of timing and purpose. For example, an education program begins with an assessment of learners' needs. While the program is being conducted, periodic evaluation lets the nurse educator know whether the program and learners are proceeding as planned. After program completion, evaluation identifies whether and to what extent identified needs were met.

An important note of caution: You may conduct an evaluation at the end of your program, but always plan an evaluation at the same time as you are assessing the learner's needs. Evaluation as an afterthought is, at best, a poor idea. Data used for evaluation may be impossible to collect, may be incomplete, or may even be misleading. When possible, use the same data collection methods and instruments for both assessment and evaluation. This approach is especially appropriate for outcome and impact evaluations, as will be discussed later in this chapter. "If only . . ." is an all-too-frequent lament, which can be minimized by planning ahead.

DETERMINING THE FOCUS OF EVALUATION

In planning any evaluation, the first and most crucial step is to determine the focus of the evaluation. The focus then will guide evaluation design, conduct, data analysis, and reporting of results. The importance of a clear, specific, and realistic evaluation focus cannot be emphasized enough. How useful and accurate the results of an evaluation will be depend on how well the evaluation is initially focused.

Evaluation focus includes five basic components: audience, purpose, questions, scope, and resources (Ruzicki, 1987). To determine these components, ask the following questions:

1. For whom is the evaluation being conducted?
2. Why is the evaluation being conducted?
3. What questions will be asked in the evaluation?
4. What is the scope of the evaluation?
5. What resources are available to conduct the evaluation?

The person or group for whom the evaluation is being conducted is known as the *audience* (Ruzicki, 1987). This individual or group includes, first, who requested the evaluation and, second, all those who will use evaluation results or who might benefit from the evaluation. The audience might include your patients, your peers, your supervisor, or the nursing director. When you report results of the evaluation, you will provide feedback to all members of the audience.

The *purpose* of the evaluation answers the question "Why is the evaluation being conducted?" The purpose might be to decide whether to continue a particular education program or to determine the effectiveness of teaching. If a particular individual or group has a primary interest in results of the evaluation, use input from them to clarify the purpose.

An important note of caution: Why you are conducting an evaluation is not the same as with whom or what you are evaluating. For example, nursing literature on patient education commonly distinguishes among three types of evaluation: learner, teacher, and program. This distinction answers the question of who or what will be evaluated and is extremely useful in designing and conducting an evaluation. Why learner evaluation might be undertaken is answered by the reason or purpose for evaluating learner performance. For example, can the patient correctly return a demonstration of a dressing change that she will be doing herself after discharge from the hospital? Determining teaching or program effectiveness is another reason or purpose for undertaking evaluation. An example in this case would be to determine whether teaching a group of patients is as effective as teaching patients one-on-one to help them learn the proper use of crutches.

An excellent rule of thumb in stating the purpose of an evaluation is: Keep it singular. In other words, state, "The purpose is . . . ," not "The purposes are . . . ." Keeping the purpose audience focused and singular will help avoid the all-too-frequent tendency to attempt too much in one evaluation.

The *questions* to be asked in the evaluation are specific, measurable, and directly related to the purpose for conducting the evaluation. Examples of questions are "To what extent are patients satisfied with the cardiac discharge teaching program?" and "How many signs and symptoms of insulin shock is the patient with diabetes able to correctly list?" Asking the right questions is essential if the evaluation is to serve the purpose intended. As will be discussed later in the chapter, stating specific evaluation questions is both the first step in selecting an evaluation design and the basis for eventual data analysis.

The *scope* of an evaluation answers the question "How much will be evaluated?" "How much" includes "How many aspects of education will be evaluated?", "How many individuals or groups will be evaluated?", and "What time period is to be evaluated?" For example, will the evaluation focus on one class or on an entire program; on the learning experience for one patient or for all patients being taught a particular skill? Evaluation could be limited to the teaching process during a particular patient education class or could be expanded to encompass both the teaching process and related patient outcomes of learning. The scope of an evaluation is determined in part by the purpose for conducting the evaluation and in part by available resources. For example, an evaluation addressing patient satisfaction with instructors for all childbirth classes conducted in a given year is an evaluation that is broad and long-term in scope and will require expertise in data collection and analysis. An example of an evaluation that is narrow in scope and at a point in time, and will require expertise by the teacher in clinical practice and observation, is whether a patient understands each step in a learning session on how to self-administer insulin injections.

The *resources* needed to conduct an evaluation include time, expertise, personnel, materials, equipment, and facilities. A realistic appraisal of what resources are accessible and available compared to what resources are required is very important in focusing any evaluation. Remember to include the time and expertise required to collect, organize, analyze, and interpret data and to prepare the report of evaluation results.

Evaluation can be classified into different types based on one or more of the five components described above. The most common types of evaluation identified include process, content, outcome, impact, and program evaluation. A number of evaluation models have been developed that help to clarify differences among these evaluation types as well as how they relate to one another (Abruzzese, 1978; Haggard, 1989; Koch, 2000; Puetz, 1992; Rankin & Stallings, 2001; Walker & Dewar, 2000).

EVALUATION MODELS

Abruzzese (1978) developed the Roberta Straessle Abruzzese (RSA) Evaluation Model for classifying educational evaluation into different categories or levels. Although developed more than 20 years ago and from the perspective of staff development education, the RSA Model remains useful for classifying types of evaluation from a patient education perspective. The RSA Model levels five basic types of evaluation in relation to one another based on purpose and related questions, scope, and resource components of evaluation focus (Figure 14-1). The five types of evaluation are process, content, outcome, impact, and program. Abruzzese describes the first four types as levels of evaluation leading from the simple (process evaluation) to the complex (impact evaluation). Total program evaluation includes and summarizes all four levels.

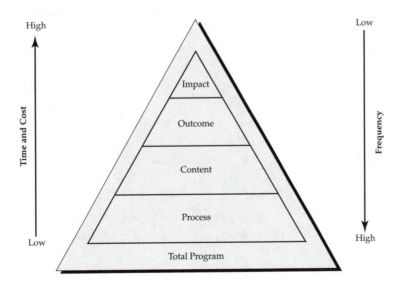

FIGURE 14-1 RSA Evaluation Model.
Reprinted by permission of Roberta S. Abruzzese.

Process (Formative) Evaluation

The purpose of *process evaluation* is to make adjustments in a patient education activity as soon as they are needed, whether those adjustments be in personnel, materials, facilities, learning objectives, or even one's own attitude. Adjustments may need to be made after one class or session before the next is taught or even in the middle of a single learning experience. Consider, for example, evaluation of the process of teaching a newly diagnosed juvenile insulin-dependent diabetic and her parents how to administer insulin. Would you facilitate learning better by first injecting yourself with normal saline so they can see you maintain a calm expression? If you had planned to have the parent give the first injection, but the child seems less fearful, might you consider revising your teaching plan to let the child first perform self-injection?

Process evaluation, also called *formative evaluation,* "forms" an educational activity because evaluation is an ongoing component of assessment, planning, and implementation. As part of the education process, this ongoing evaluation helps the nurse anticipate and prevent problems before they occur or identify problems as they arise.

Consistent with the purpose of process evaluation, the guiding question is, "How can teaching be improved to help patients learn more successfully?" The nurse's teaching effectiveness, the teaching process, and the learner's responses are monitored on an ongoing basis. While teaching and learning are occurring, learners are asked their opinions about the instructor, learning objectives, content, teaching and learning methods, and physical facilities. Specific questions could include: Am I giving the patient time to ask questions? Is the information I am giving in class consistent with information included in the handouts? Does the patient look bored? Is the room too warm? Should I include more opportunities for return demonstration?

The scope of process evaluation generally is limited in breadth and time period to a specific learning experience, such as a group or a single one-to-one interaction. Learner behavior, teacher behavior, learner–teacher interaction, learner response to teaching materials and methods, and characteristics of the environment are all aspects of the learning experience within the scope of process evaluation. If resources are limited and a number of different groups are included as participants, a representative number of individuals from each group rather than everyone from each group may be included in the evaluation.

Resources usually are less costly and more readily available for process evaluation than for other levels of evaluation, such as impact or total program evaluation. Although process evaluation occurs more frequently during and throughout every learning experience than does any other level, it occurs at the same time as teaching. As a result, the need for additional time, facilities, and dollars to conduct process evaluation is decreased.

Content Evaluation

The purpose of *content evaluation* is to determine if learners have acquired the knowledge or skills taught during the learning experience. Abruzzese (1978) describes content evaluation as taking place immediately after the learning experience to answer the guiding question, "To what degree did the learners learn what was taught?" or "To what degree did learners achieve the specified objectives?" Asking a patient to give a return demonstration or asking a parent to describe the steps in cleaning and dressing their child's wound are common examples of content evaluation.

Content evaluation is depicted in the RSA Model as the level "in between" process and outcome evaluation levels. In other words, content evaluation focuses on how the teaching-learning process affected immediate, short-term outcomes. To answer the question "Were specified objectives met as a result of teaching?" requires that the evaluation be designed differently from an evaluation to answer the question "Did learners achieve specified objectives?" Evaluation designs will be discussed in some detail later in this chapter. An important point to be made here, however, is that evaluation questions must be carefully considered and clearly stated because they dictate the basic framework for evaluation design and conduct.

The scope of content evaluation is limited to a specific learning experience and to specifically stated objectives for that experience. Content evaluation occurs immediately after completion of teaching and includes all teaching-learning activities included in the patient education experience. Data are obtained from all learners in a specific class or group. For example, if both parents and their child with asthma are taught how to use a spacer with an inhaler, all three are asked to complete a return demonstration.

Resources used to teach content can also be used to carry out evaluation of how well that content was learned. For example, equipment included in teaching a patient how to change a dressing can be used again by the patient to perform a return demonstration.

Outcome (Summative) Evaluation

The purpose of *outcome evaluation* is to determine effects or outcomes of teaching efforts. Outcome evaluation is also referred to as summative evaluation because its intent is to "sum" what happened as a result of education. Guiding questions in outcome evaluation include, "Was teaching appropriate?", "Did the individual(s) learn?",

"Were behavioral objectives met?", and "Did the patient who learned a skill before discharge use that skill correctly once home?" Just as process evaluation occurs at the same time as the teaching-learning experience, outcome evaluation occurs after teaching has been completed.

Outcome evaluation measures changes occurring as a result of teaching and learning. Abruzzese (1978) differentiates outcome evaluation from content evaluation by focusing outcome evaluation on measuring more long-term change that "persists after the learning experience" (p. 243). Changes can include instituting a new process, habitual use of a new technique or behavior, or integration of a new value or attitude. Which changes you will measure usually will be decided based on the objectives established as a result of initial needs assessment.

The scope of outcome evaluation depends in part on the changes being measured, which, in turn, are dependent on objectives established for the educational activity. As has already been discussed, outcome evaluation focuses on a longer time period than does content evaluation. Whereas evaluating accuracy of a patient's return demonstration of a skill prior to discharge may be appropriate for content evaluation, outcome evaluation should include measuring a patient's competency with a skill in the home setting after discharge. Abruzzese (1978) suggests that outcome data be collected six months after baseline data to determine whether a change has really taken place.

Resources required for outcome evaluation are more costly and sophisticated than for process or content evaluation. Compared to resources required for the first two types of evaluation in the RSA Model, outcome evaluation requires greater expertise to develop measurement and data collection strategies, more time to conduct the evaluation, knowledge of baseline data establishment, and ability to conduct reliable and valid comparative data after the learning experience. Postage to mail surveys and time and personnel to carry out observation of patients during a home visit or to complete patient/family telephone interviews are specific examples of resources that may be necessary to conduct an outcome evaluation.

Impact Evaluation

The purpose of *impact evaluation* is to determine the relative effects of education on the institution or the community. Put another way, the purpose of impact evaluation is to obtain information to decide whether continuing an educational activity is worth its cost. Examples of questions appropriate for impact evaluation include "What is the effect of a bicycle safety program on subsequent emergency room or urgent clinic visits by children who attended the program or whose family member(s) attended the program?" and "What is the effect of the cardiac discharge teaching program on long-term frequency of rehospitalization among patients who have completed the program?"

The scope of impact evaluation is broader, more complex, and usually more long-term than that of process, content, or outcome evaluation. For example, outcome evaluation would focus on whether specific teaching resulted in achievement of specified outcomes, whereas impact evaluation would go beyond that to measure the effect or worth of those outcomes. Consider, for example, a program on healthy diet and regular exercise for young adults at high risk for cardiac disease. The outcome objectives are that the participants will change eating and exercise habits to be consistent with what they learned. The goal is to prevent or delay onset of symptoms of cardiac disease among those who attended the program. This distinction between outcome and impact evaluation may seem subtle, but it is important to the appropriate design and conduct of an impact evaluation.

Resource requirements for conducting an impact evaluation are extensive and most likely beyond the scope of an individual nurse. Literature on evaluation describes impact evaluation as most like evaluation research (Abruzzese, 1978; Hamilton, 1993; Waddell, 1992). A discussion of evaluation research is beyond the scope of this chapter. The point here is that "good" science is rarely inexpensive and is never quick; good impact evaluation has the same characteristics. Resources needed to design and conduct an impact evaluation generally include reliable and valid instruments, trained data collectors, personnel with research and statistical expertise, equipment and materials necessary for data collection and analysis, and access to populations who may be culturally or geographically diverse. Because impact evaluation is so expensive and time-intensive, this type of evaluation should be targeted toward courses/programs where learning is critical to patient well-being or to safe, high-quality, cost-effective healthcare delivery (Puetz, 1992).

Conducting an impact evaluation may seem a monumental task, but do not let that stop you from participating in the effort. The current managed-care environment requires justification for every health dollar spent. The value of patient education may be intuitively evident, but the positive impact of education must be demonstrated if it is to be funded.

Program Evaluation

Using the framework of the RSA Model (Abruzzese, 1978), the purpose of total *program evaluation* is to determine the extent to which all activities for an entire department or program over a specified period of time meet or exceed goals originally established. A guiding question appropriate for a total program evaluation from this perspective might be "How well did patient education activities implemented throughout the year meet annual goals established for a clinic's patient education program?"

The scope of program evaluation is broad, generally focusing on overall goals rather than on specific objectives. Abruzzese (1978) describes the scope of program evaluation as including all aspects of educational activity (e.g., process, content, outcome, impact) with input from all the participants (e.g., learners, teachers, institutional representatives, community representatives). The time period over which data are collected may extend from several months to one or more years, depending on the timeframe established for meeting the goals to be evaluated.

Resources required for program evaluation may include the sum of resources necessary to conduct process, content, outcome, and impact evaluations. A program evaluation may require significant expenditures for personnel if the evaluation is conducted by an individual or team external to the organization. Additional resources required include time, materials, equipment, and personnel necessary for data entry, analysis, and reporting.

As stated earlier, the RSA Model remains useful as a general framework for categorizing basic types of evaluation: process, content, outcome, impact, and program. As shown in the model, differences between these types are, in large part, a matter of degree. For example, process evaluation occurs most frequently; impact evaluation occurs least frequently. Content evaluation focuses on immediate effects of teaching; outcome on more long-term effects of teaching. Carrying out process evaluation requires fewer resources compared with impact evaluation, which requires extensive resources for implementation. The RSA Model further describes one way that process, content, outcome, and impact evaluations can be considered together as components of total program evaluation.

Clinical examples of how different types of evaluation relate to one another can be found in Haggard's (1989) description of three dimensions in evaluating teaching effectiveness for the patient and in Rankin and Stallings's (2001) four levels of evaluation of patient learning. The three dimensions described by Haggard and four levels identified by Rankin and Stallings are consistent with the basic types of evaluation included in the RSA Model, as shown in Table 14-1. As can be seen from Table 14-1, models developed from an education theory base, such as the RSA Model, have much in common with models developed from a patient care theory base, such as Haggard's and Rankin and Stallings's evaluation models for patient education.

TABLE 14-1	Comparison of Levels/Types of Evaluation Across Staff/Patient Education Evaluation Models	
Abruzzese (1978)	**Haggard (1989)**	**Rankin & Stallings (2001)**
Process	Patient assimilation of information during teaching	Patient-education intervention
Content	Patient information retention after teaching	Patient/family performance following learning
Outcome	Patient use of information in day-to-day life	Patient/family performance at home
Impact	N/A	Overall self-care and health maintenance
Program	N/A	N/A

At least one important difference between the RSA and other models needs to be mentioned, however. That difference can be seen in the learner evaluation model shown in Figure 14-2. This learner-focused model emphasizes the continuum of patient health performance, from needs assessment to patient health performance, once an adequate level of health status/performance has been regained or achieved. These models have value in focusing and planning any type of evaluation, but are especially important for impact and program evaluations.

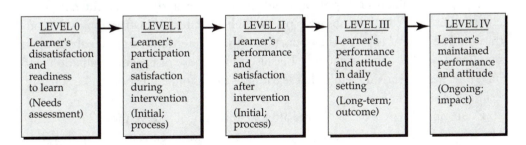

FIGURE 14-2   Five Levels of Learner Evaluation
Source: Based on S. H. Rankin & K. D. Stallings (2001). *Patient education: Principles and practices,* 4th ed. Philadelphia: Lippincott.

DESIGNING THE EVALUATION

The design of an evaluation is created within the framework, or boundaries, already established by focusing the evaluation. In other words, the design must be consistent with the purpose, questions, and scope and must be realistic given available resources. Evaluation design includes at least three interrelated components: structure, methods, and instruments.

Designing Structure

An important question to be answered in designing an evaluation is "How rigorous should the evaluation be?" The obvious answer is that all evaluations should have some level of rigor. In other words, all evaluations should be systematic and thoroughly planned or structured before they are conducted. How rigor is translated into design structure depends on the questions to be answered by the evaluation, the complexity of the scope of the evaluation, and the expected use of evaluation results. The more the questions address cause and effect, the more complex the scope. And, the more critical and broad-reaching the expected use of results, the more the evaluation design should be rigorous.

How are decisions about level of rigor of an evaluation actually translated into an evaluation structure? The structure of an evaluation design depicts the number of groups to be included in the evaluation, the number of evaluations or periods of evaluation, and the time sequence between an educational intervention and evaluation of that intervention. A "group" can comprise one individual, as in the case of one-to-one nurse–patient teaching, or several individuals, as in the case of a nurse teaching a group of patients or a patient plus family members.

A process evaluation might be conducted during a single patient education activity where the educator observes patient behavior during instruction or demonstration. The patient is given the opportunity to ask questions or get feedback upon completion of each new instruction. Because the purpose of process evaluation is to encourage better learning while that learning is going on, education and evaluation occur at the same time.

Evaluation also may be conducted after an educational intervention. This is probably the most common structure used in conducting educational evaluations, although it is not necessarily the most appropriate. On completion of an educational activity, participants may be asked to complete a satisfaction survey to provide data for a process evaluation. Participants also may be given a cognitive test to provide data for a content evaluation.

If the purpose for conducting a content evaluation is to determine whether learners know the content just taught, a cognitive posttest or immediate return demonstration is adequate. A structure that begins with collection of baseline data is more appropriate, however, if the purpose for conducting the evaluation is to determine whether learners know specific content following a class that they did not know before attending that class. Collection of baseline data, which can be compared with data collected at one or more points in time after learners have completed the educational activity, provides an opportunity to measure whether change has occurred. The ability to measure change in a particular skill or level of knowledge, for example, also requires that the same instruments be used for data collection at both points in time. Data collection will be discussed in more detail later in this chapter.

If the purpose for conducting an evaluation is to determine whether learners know content or can perform a skill as a result of an educational intervention, the most appropriate structure is one that includes at least two groups, one receiving education and one not receiving education. Both groups are evaluated at the same time even though only one group receives education. For example, patients on Nursing Unit A may receive an educational pamphlet to read prior to attending a class, while patients on Nursing Unit B attend the class without first reading the pamphlet. Because patients on the two units probably are different in many ways—age and diagnosis, for example—besides which educational intervention they received, the evaluation must take these differences into account.

Another design for conducting an evaluation might include only one group of learners from which evaluative data are collected at several points in time both before and after receiving an educational intervention. For example, if data collected before the education consistently demonstrate lack of learner ability to comply with a treatment regimen, and data collected after the education consistently demonstrate a significant improvement in patient compliance with that regimen, the evaluator could argue that the education was the reason for the improvement.

A detailed description of evaluation designs is not the intent of this chapter. What is intended is to increase awareness that evaluations can be designed in a number of different ways. When the results of an evaluation are to be used to make major financial or personnel decisions, the design selected is likely to require more resources and expertise. The literature on evaluation of patient education has become an increasingly rich source of examples of how to conduct rigorous evaluation. A literature search that includes many or all of the following journals is a must for planning evaluation of healthcare education in a cost-conscious and outcome-focused healthcare environment: *Evaluation and the Health Professions, Journal of Continuing Education in Nursing, Adult Education Quarterly, Health Education Quarterly,* and *Nurse Educator.*

Evaluation Methods

Evaluation focus provides the basis for determining the evaluation design structure. The design structure, in turn, provides the basis for determining evaluation methods. Evaluation methods include those actions that are undertaken to carry out the evaluation according to the design structure. All evaluation methods deal in some way with data and data collection. Answers to the following questions will assist in selecting the most appropriate, feasible methods for conducting a particular evaluation in a particular setting and for a specified purpose:

1. What types of data will be collected?
2. From whom or what will data be collected?
3. How, when, and where will data be collected?
4. By whom will data be collected?

Types of Data to Collect

Evaluation of healthcare education includes collection of data about people, about the educational program or activity, and about the environment in which the educational activity takes place. Process, outcome, impact, and program evaluations require data about all three: the people, the program, and the environment. Content evaluations may be limited to data about the people and the program, although this limitation is not necessary. Types of data that are collected about people can be classified as physical, cognitive, affective, or psychomotor. Data that are collected about educational activities or programs generally include such program characteristics as cost, length, number of instructors required, amount and type of materials required, teaching-learning methods used, and so on. Data that are collected about the environment in which a program or activity is conducted generally include such environmental characteristics as temperature, lighting, location, layout, space, and noise level.

Given the possibility that an unlimited and overwhelming amount of data could be collected, how do you decide what data should be collected? The most straightforward answer to this question is that data should be collected that will answer evaluation questions posed in focusing the evaluation. The likelihood that you will collect the right amount of the right type of data to answer evaluation questions can be significantly improved, first, by remembering that you are obligated to use any data you collect, and second, by using definitions that are written in measurement terms.

Patient compliance, for example, can be theoretically defined as the patient's regular and consistent adherence to a prescribed treatment regimen. For use in an outcome evaluation of a particular educational activity, patient compliance might be measurably defined as the patient's demonstration of unassisted and error-free completion of all steps in the sterile dressing change as observed in the patient's home on three separate occasions at two-week time intervals. As you can see from this example, a definition in measurement terms states exactly what data will be collected. The measurable definition of patient compliance includes where and how many times the patient's performance of the dressing change is to be observed, as well as stating that criteria for compliance include both unassisted and error-free performance on each occasion.

From Whom or What to Collect Data

Data can be collected directly from the individuals whose behavior or knowledge is being evaluated, from representatives of these individuals, or from documentation or databases already created. Whenever possible, plan to collect at least some data directly from the individuals being evaluated. In the case of process evaluation, data should be collected from all learners and all educators participating in the educational activity. Content and outcome evaluations should include data from all learners. Because impact and program evaluations have a broader scope than do the first three types of evaluation, collecting data from all individuals who participated in an educational program over an extended period of time may be impossible due to the inability to locate participants or lack of sufficient resources to gather data from such a large number of people. When all participants cannot be counted or located, data may be collected from a subset, or sample, of participants who are considered to represent the entire group. If an evaluation is planned to collect data from a sample of participants, be careful to include participants who are representative of the entire group.

Preexisting databases should never be used as the only source of evaluative data unless they were created for the purpose of that evaluation. Even though these data were collected for a different purpose, they may be helpful for providing additional information for the evaluation. Data already in existence generally are less expensive to obtain than are original data. The decision whether to use preexisting data depends on whether they were collected from people of interest in the current evaluation and whether they are consistent with measurement definitions used in the current evaluation.

How, When, and Where to Collect Data

Methods for how data can be collected include the following:

- Observation
- Interview
- Questionnaire or written test
- Patient record review

Evaluations also may use data that already have been collected for another purpose, if appropriate. Which method is selected depends, first, on the type of data being collected, and second, on available resources. Whenever possible, data should be collected using more than one method. Using multiple methods will provide the evaluator, and consequently others who are interested, with more complete information about the program or performance being evaluated than could be accomplished using a single method.

Observations can be conducted by the evaluator in person or can be videotaped for viewing at some later time. In the combined role of teacher-evaluator, the nurse who is conducting a process evaluation can directly observe a learner's physical, verbal, psychomotor, and affective behaviors so that they can be responded to in a timely manner. Use of videotape or a second observer also can be beneficial for picking up the nurse's own behaviors. The nurse who is doing the teaching might not be aware of how her or his behaviors are influencing the learner.

The timing of data collection, or when data collection takes place, already has been addressed both in discussion of different types of evaluation and in descriptions of evaluation design structures. Process evaluation, for example, generally occurs during and immediately after an educational activity. Content evaluation takes place immediately after completion of education. Outcome evaluation occurs sometime after completion of education, when learners have returned to the setting where they are expected to use new knowledge or perform a new skill. Impact evaluation generally is conducted from weeks to years after the educational program has been offered. This is because the purpose of impact evaluation is to determine what change has occurred within the community or institution as a whole as a result of an educational program.

Timing of data collection for total program evaluation is less obvious than for other types of evaluation. As discussed earlier, Abruzzese (1978) describes data collection for total program evaluation as occurring over a prolonged period because program evaluation includes process, content, outcome, and impact evaluations already conducted.

Where an evaluation is conducted can have a major effect on evaluation results. Be careful not to make the decision about where to collect data on the basis of convenience for the data collector. An appropriate setting for conducting a content evaluation may be in the patient's room or a classroom where patients have just finished learning new information or a new skill. An outcome evaluation to determine whether discharge teaching in the hospital enabled the patient to provide self-care at home requires that data collection, or observation of the patient's performance, be conducted in the home. What if available resources are insufficient to allow for home visits by the evaluator? To answer this question, keep in mind that the focus of the evaluation is on performance by the patient, not performance by the evaluator. Training a family member or the patient to observe and record patient performance at home is preferable to bringing the patient to a place of convenience for the evaluator.

Who Collects the Data

Evaluative data are most commonly collected by the teacher who is conducting the class or activity being evaluated because that nurse is already present and interacting with learners. Combining the role of evaluator with that of teacher is one correct method for conducting a process evaluation because evaluative data are actually a part of the teaching-learning process. Inviting another nurse or a patient representative to observe a class can provide additional data from the perspective of someone who does not have to divide attention between teaching and evaluating. Input from this second person can strengthen the usefulness of evaluation results because the input is likely to be more objective.

Data also can be collected by the patients themselves, by other nurses within the department or institution, or by someone from outside the institution. For example, patients who have learned a new dietary regimen might be asked to keep diaries of their intake over a two- or four-week period. The diary can be shared with the nurse at the patient's next clinic visit.

When deciding who will collect data, keep in mind that the individuals chosen to collect data become an extension of the evaluation instrument. If the data that are collected are to be reliable, unbiased, and accurate, the data collector must be unbiased and sufficiently expert at the task. Use of unbiased expert data collectors is especially important for collecting observation and interview data. This is because these types of data are in part dependent on how the data collector interprets what she or he sees during observation or hears during the interview. Other data also can be affected by who collects those data. Consider, for example, an outcome evaluation to determine whether a series of biofeedback classes given to young executives can reduce stress as measured by pulse and blood pressure. How might some executives' pulse and blood pressure results be affected by a data collector who is extremely physically attractive or who seems rushed or impatient?

The potential for a data collector to bias data can be minimized. First, limit as much as possible the number of data collectors, as this automatically will decrease person-based variation. Ask individuals helping you with data collection to wear similar neutral colors and to speak in a moderate tone. Because "moderate tone," for example, may not be interpreted the same way by everyone, hold at least one practice session or "dry run" with all data collectors prior to actually conducting the evaluation.

Whenever possible, ask for help with data collection from someone who has no particular interest in the results and who will be seen as unbiased and nonthreatening by the individuals providing the data. Interview scripts to be read word-for-word by the interviewer can ensure that all patients being interviewed will be asked the same questions.

With the emphasis on continuous quality improvement as an expectation of daily activity in healthcare organizations, nurses are obligated to become more knowledgeable about principles of measurement and how to implement measurement techniques in their work setting (Joint Commission on Accreditation of Healthcare Organizations, 1995). One benefit this change in practice has for the nurse in the role of teacher is that more people within the organization have some expertise in data collection and are motivated to help with data collection activities. Another potential benefit is that data collection activities are likely to be already a part of nursing practice. Other colleagues may be able to help with data collection. Also, the educator might already have available instruments and data that can be used to measure outcomes of patient education interventions.

Evaluation Instruments

This chapter is intended to present key points to consider in selection, revision, or construction of evaluation instruments. Whenever possible, an evaluation should be conducted using existing instruments. Instrument development requires considerable expertise, time, and expenditure of resources. Construction of an original evaluation instrument, whether it is in the form of a questionnaire or a type of equipment, requires rigorous testing to establish reliability and validity. Conducting an evaluation in a timely manner rarely allows the luxury of the several months to several years needed to develop a reliable, valid instrument.

The first step in choosing an instrument is to conduct a literature search for evaluations similar to the evaluation being planned. A helpful place to begin is with the same journals listed earlier in this chapter. Instruments that have been used in more than one study should be given preference over an instrument developed for a single use. Instruments used many times generally have been more thoroughly tested for reliability and validity. Once a number of potential instruments have been identified, each instrument must be carefully examined to determine whether it is, in fact, appropriate for the evaluation you are planning.

First, the instrument must measure the performance being evaluated exactly as that performance has been defined for the evaluation. For example, if satisfaction with a patient education program is defined to include a score of 80% or higher on five specific program components, such as nurse responsiveness to questions, relevance of content, and so on, then the instrument selected to measure patients' satisfaction with the program must include exactly those five components and must be able to be scored in percentages.

Second, an appropriate instrument should have documented evidence of reliability and validity with individuals who are as identical as possible to those from whom you will be collecting data. If you will be evaluating the ability of elderly patients to complete activities of daily living, for example, you would not want to use an instrument developed for evaluating the ability of young orthopedic patients to complete routine activities. Similarities in reading level and visual acuity also should exist if the instrument being evaluated is a questionnaire or scale that participants will complete themselves.

Existing instruments being considered for selection also must be affordable, must be feasible for use in the location planned for conducting data collection, and should require minimal training on the part of data collectors.

Barriers to Evaluation

If evaluation is so crucial to healthcare education, why is evaluation often an after-thought or even overlooked entirely? The reasons given for not conducting evaluations are many and varied but can be overcome. To overcome barriers to evaluation, they first must be identified and understood. Then the evaluation must be designed and conducted in a way that will lessen or remove as many identified barriers as possible.

Barriers to conducting an evaluation can be classified into three broad categories:

1. Lack of clarity
2. Lack of ability
3. Fear of punishment or loss of self-esteem

Lack of Clarity

Lack of clarity most often is the result of an unclear, unstated, or poorly defined evaluation focus. Undertaking any action is difficult if the nurse does not know the purpose for taking that action. Undertaking an evaluation certainly is no different. Often evaluations are attempted to determine the quality of an educational program or activity, yet quality is not defined beyond some vague sense of "goodness." What is goodness, and from whose perspective will goodness be determined? Who or what has to demonstrate evidence of goodness? What will happen if goodness is or is not evident? Inability to answer these or similar questions creates a significant barrier to conducting an evaluation. Not knowing the purpose of an evaluation or what will be done with evaluation results, for example, can become a barrier for even the most seasoned evaluator.

Barriers in this category are perhaps the easiest to overcome because the best solution for lack of clarity is to provide clarity. You will recall that evaluation focus includes five components: audience, purpose, questions, scope, and resources. To overcome a potential lack of clarity, all five components must be identified and made available to those conducting the evaluation. A clearly stated purpose must include why the evaluation is being conducted. Part of the answer to why conduct an evaluation is a statement of what decisions will be made on the basis of evaluation results. Clear identification of who asked that the evaluation be done is as important as a clear statement of purpose. It is from the perspective of the most interested person or group that terms such as quality should be defined and measured. Although results of the evaluation will provide the information on which decisions will be made, the person or group who asked for the evaluation will actually make those decisions.

Lack of Ability

Lack of ability to conduct an evaluation most often is the result of not knowing how to conduct the evaluation or not having the resources necessary to conduct the evaluation. Clarification of evaluation purpose, questions, and scope is often the responsibility of the person or group who initially requested the evaluation be done. This person or group also is accountable for providing the necessary resources—personnel, equipment, time, facilities, and so on—to conduct the evaluation they are requesting. Unless these individuals have some expertise in evaluation, they may not know what resources are necessary. The nurse conducting the evaluation, therefore, must accept responsibility for knowing what resources are necessary and for giving that information to the person or group requesting the evaluation.

Lack of knowledge of what resources are necessary or lack of actual resources to conduct an evaluation are barriers that can be difficult, although not impossible, to overcome. Lack of knowledge can be resolved by asking for and receiving help from those who are expert in evaluation. Lack of other resources—time, money, equipment, facilities, and so on—should be documented, justified, and presented to those requesting the evaluation.

Fear of Punishment or Loss of Self-Esteem

Evaluation may be seen as a judgment of personal worth. Those being evaluated (patients, family members of patients, or nurses in practice) may fear that anything less than a perfect performance will result in punishment or that their mistakes will be seen as evidence of failing to accomplish what is expected of them. These fears form one of the greatest barriers to conducting an evaluation. Unfortunately, the fear of punishment or of being seen as unworthy may not easily be overcome, especially if the individual being evaluated has had past negative experiences. Consider, for example, traditional quality assurance monitoring where results of evaluation were used to correct deficiencies in nursing practice through punitive measures. To give another example, how many times has a nurse interpreted patient dissatisfaction with a teaching style as patient dislike for the nurse as a person? Or, how many times have parents of pediatric patients said, "If you don't do it right, the doctors and nurses won't let you go home . . . and we will be very disappointed in you"?

The first step in overcoming this barrier is to realize that the potential for its existence may be close to 100%. Individuals whose skill or knowledge is being evaluated are not likely to admit that evaluation represents a threat to them. They are far more likely to demonstrate self-protective behaviors or attitudes. These can range from claiming that they are too ill to learn, to providing socially desirable answers on a questionnaire, to responding with hostility to evaluation questions. An individual may intentionally choose to "fail" an evaluation as a method for controlling the uncertainty of success.

The second step in overcoming the barrier of fear or threat is to remember that "the person is more important than the performance or the product" (Narrow, 1979, p. 185). If the purpose of an evaluation is to facilitate better learning, as in process evaluation, focus on the process. Consider the example of teaching a patient newly diagnosed with diabetes how to administer insulin. The nurse has carefully and thoroughly explained each step of insulin administration, observing the patient's level of attention and frequent head nods during the explanation. When the patient tries to demonstrate the steps, however, he is unable to begin. Why? One answer may be that the use of an auditory teaching style does not match the patient's visual learning style. Another possibility might be that too many distractions are present in the immediate environment, making concentration on learning all but impossible.

A third step in overcoming the fear of punishment or threatened loss of self-esteem is to point out achievements, if they exist, or continue to encourage effort if learning has not been achieved. Give praise honestly, focusing on the task at hand.

Finally, and perhaps most importantly, use communication of information to prevent or minimize fear. Lack of clarity exists as a barrier for those who are the subjects of an evaluation as much as for those who will conduct the evaluation. If learners or teachers know and understand the focus of an evaluation, they may be less fearful of being evaluated than if such information is left to their imaginations. Remember, however, that providing certain information may be unethical or even illegal. For example, any evaluation data about an individual that can be identified with that individual should only be collected with the person's informed consent and should remain confidential. The ethical and legal importance of confidentiality as a protection of human rights is a central concern of healthcare institutions and is the primary focus of the Health Information Portability and Accountability Act (HIPAA) enacted in 2003.

CONDUCTING THE EVALUATION

To conduct an evaluation means to implement the evaluation design by using the instruments chosen according to the methods selected. How smoothly an evaluation is carried out depends primarily on how carefully and thoroughly the evaluation was planned. Planning is not a complete guarantee of success, however. Three methods to lessen the effects of unexpected events that occur when carrying out an evaluation are:

1. Conduct a pilot test or "dry run" first.
2. Include "extra" time to do an evaluation.
3. Keep a sense of humor during the entire process.

Conducting a pilot test of the evaluation means to try out the data collection methods, instruments, and plan for data analysis with a few individuals who are the same as or very similar to those who will be included in the full evaluation. A pilot test should be conducted prior to implementing a full evaluation that will be expensive or time-consuming to conduct or on which major decisions will be made. Process evaluation is the one type of evaluation for which pilot testing generally is not conducted. Pilot testing should be considered prior to conducting outcome, impact, or program evaluations, however.

Including "extra" time to do an evaluation means to leave room for the unexpected delays that almost always occur during evaluation planning, data collection, and reporting of evaluation results that will be meaningful and usable by decision makers.

Because delays not only will occur, but also are likely to occur at inconvenient times during the evaluation, keeping a sense of humor is vitally important. An evaluator with a sense of humor, for example, is more likely to maintain a realistic perspective in reporting results that are lower than expected.

ANALYZING AND INTERPRETING DATA COLLECTED

The purposes for conducting data analysis are, first, to organize data so that they can provide meaningful information and, second, to provide answers to evaluation questions. The terms *data* and *information* are not synonymous. In other words, a mass of numbers or a mass of comments does not become information until that mass has been organized and summarized into meaningful tables, graphs, or categories that clearly show the results of an evaluation. Table 14-2 presents an example of how such information might be displayed.

Basic decisions about how data will be analyzed depend on the type of data collected and the questions used to focus the evaluation. Data collected during an evaluation may be numeric, such as scores on a test, or may be verbal, such as comments obtained during interviews. Numeric data are summarized using statistics such as frequencies and percentages. For example, Table 14-2 shows that learners who were included in a survey had an average age of 27.5 years. Verbal comments obtained during interviews and written comments obtained from open-ended questionnaires are summarized into categories of similar comments. A useful suggestion for deciding how data will be analyzed is to enlist the assistance of someone with experience in data analysis.

REPORTING EVALUATION RESULTS

Results of an evaluation must be reported if the evaluation is to be of any use. Such a statement seems obvious, but how many times have you heard that an evaluation was being conducted and then never heard anything more about it? How many times have you participated in an evaluation but never saw the final report? How many times have you conducted an evaluation yourself but have not provided anyone with a report on findings? Almost all of us, if we are honest, would likely answer "yes" to even the last question.

TABLE 14-2	**Demographic Comparison of Survey Respondents to Total Course Participants Using Group Averages**	
Learner demographics	**Survey Respondents (n = 50)**	**All Course Participants (n = 55)**
Age	25.5 years	27.5 years
Length of hospital stay	3.5 days	4.0 days
Number of previous hospitalizations	2	2

Reasons for not reporting evaluation results are diverse and numerous. The four basic reasons for why evaluative data may never be reported are:

- Not knowing who should receive the results
- Belief that the results are not important or will not be used
- Inability to translate results into language useful for producing the report
- Fear that results will be misused

A few guidelines established in planning an evaluation will significantly increase the likelihood that results of the evaluation will be reported to the appropriate individuals or groups, in a timely manner, and in usable form.

1. Focus on those who asked for the evaluation.
2. Stick to the evaluation purpose.
3. Stick to the data.

Focus on Those Who Asked for the Evaluation

The purpose for conducting an evaluation is to provide information for decision making by those who requested the evaluation. The report of evaluation results must be consistent with that purpose. One rule of thumb to use: Always begin an evaluation report with a summary that is no longer than one page. No matter who the decision makers are, their time is important to them. A second important guideline is to present evaluation results in a format that decision makers can easily understand and use. This does not mean that technical information should be excluded from a report to a lay audience; it means that such information should be written using nontechnical terms. Graphs and charts generally are easier to understand than are tables of numbers, for example. Third, make every effort to present results in person as well as in writing. A direct presentation provides an opportunity for the evaluator to answer questions and to assess whether the report meets the needs of the decision makers. Finally, include specific recommendations or suggestions for how evaluation results might be used.

Stick to the Evaluation Purpose

Keep the main body of an evaluation report focused on information that fulfills the purpose for conducting the evaluation. Provide answers to the questions asked. Include the main aspects of how the evaluation was conducted, but avoid a diary-like chronology of the activities of the evaluators.

Stick to the Data

Do not go beyond the actual data when reporting and interpreting findings. Keep in mind that a question not asked cannot be answered, and data not collected cannot be interpreted. If you did not measure or observe a patient's family member's performance, for example, do not draw conclusions about adequacy of that performance. Similarly, if the only measures of patient performance were those conducted in the hospital, do not interpret successful inpatient performance as successful performance by the patient at home or at work. These examples may seem obvious; however, "conceptual leaps" from the data collected to the conclusions drawn from those data are a common occurrence.

A discussion of any limitations of the evaluation is an important part of the evaluation report. For example, if several patients were unable to complete a questionnaire because they could not understand it or because they were too fatigued, say so. Knowing that evaluation results do not include data from patients below a certain educational level or physical status will help the decision makers realize that they cannot make decisions about those patients based on the evaluation. Discussion of limitations also will provide useful information for what not to do the next time a similar evaluation is conducted.

SUMMARY

The process of evaluation in healthcare education is to gather, summarize, interpret, and use data to determine the extent to which an educational activity is efficient, effective, and useful for those who participate in that activity as learners, teachers, or sponsors. Five types of evaluation discussed in this chapter include process, content, outcome, impact, and program evaluations. Each of these types focuses on a specific purpose, scope, and questions to be asked of an educational activity or program to meet the needs of those who ask for the evaluation or who can benefit from its results. Each type of evaluation also requires some level of available resources for the evaluation to be conducted.

The number and variety of evaluation models, designs, methods, and instruments are experiencing a tremendous growth as the importance of evaluation becomes more evident in today's healthcare environment. A number of guidelines, rules of thumb, and suggestions have been included in the discussion of how a nurse might go about selecting the most appropriate model, design, methods, and instruments for a particular type of evaluation. Perhaps the most important point to remember, however, is one made at the beginning of this chapter: Each aspect of the evaluation process is important, but all of them are meaningless if the results of evaluation are not used to guide future action in planning and carrying out educational interventions.

REVIEW QUESTIONS

1. How is the term *evaluation* defined?
2. How does the process of evaluation differ from the process of assessment?
3. What is the first and most crucial step in planning any evaluation?
4. What are the five basic components included in deciding the focus of an evaluation?
5. What is the purpose of each type (level) of evaluation as described by Abruzzese in her RSA Evaluation Model?
6. What are the three major barriers to conducting an evaluation?
7. What are the three guidelines to follow in reporting the results of an evaluation?

REFERENCES

Abruzzese, R. S. (1978). *Nursing Staff Development: Strategies for Success*. St. Louis: Mosby-Year Book.

Haggard, A. (1989). *Handbook of Patient Education*. Rockville, MD: Aspen.

Hamilton, G. A. (1993). An overview of evaluation research methods with implications for nursing staff development. *Journal of Nursing Staff Development, 9*(3), 148–154.

Joint Commission on Accreditation of Healthcare Organizations. (1995). *Accreditation manual for hospitals*. Oakbrook Terrace, IL: Author.

Koch, T. (2000). "Having a say": Negotiation in fourth-generation evaluation. *Journal of Advanced Nursing, 31*(1), 117–125.

Narrow, B. (1979). *Patient teaching in nursing practice: A patient and family-centered approach*. New York: Wiley.

Puetz, B. E. (1992). Evaluation: Essential skill for the staff development specialist. In K. J. Kelly (ed.), *Nursing Staff Development: Current Competence, Future Focus* (pp. 183–201). Philadelphia: Lippincott.

Rankin, S. H., & Stallings, K. D. (2001). *Patient education: Principles and practices*, 4th ed. Philadelphia: Lippincott.

Ruzicki, D. A. (1987). Evaluating patient education—a vital part of the process. In C. E. Smith (ed.), *Patient Education: Nurses in Partnership with Other Health Professionals* (pp. 223–248). Philadelphia: Saunders.

Waddell, D. (1992). The effects of continuing education on nursing practice: A meta-analysis. *Journal of Continuing Education in Nursing, 23*(4), 164–168.

Walker, E. & Dewar, B. J. (2000). Moving on from interpretivism: An argument for constructivist evaluation. *Journal of Advanced Nursing, 32*(3), 713–720.

Readability and Comprehension Tests

HOW TO USE THE FLESCH FORMULA

1. To test a whole piece of writing, take three to five 100-word samples of an article or twenty-five to thirty 100-word samples of a book. For short pieces, test the entire selection. Do not pick "good" or "typical" samples, but choose every third paragraph or every other page. In a 100-word sample, find the sentence that ends nearest to the 100-word mark; that may be, for example, at the 94th or the 109th word. Start each sample at the beginning of a paragraph, but do not use an introductory paragraph as part of the sample. Count contractions and hyphenated words as one word; count numbers and letters separated by space as words.

2. Figure the average sentence length (SL) of each sample by counting the number of words and dividing by the number of sentences. In counting sentences, follow units of thought marked off by periods, colons, semicolons, question marks, or exclamation points.

3. Determine word length (WL) of each sample by counting the number of syllables in each word as it is normally read aloud (i.e., two syllables for $ ["dollars"] and four syllables for 1918 ["nineteen-eighteen"]). It helps to read silently aloud while counting. Divide the syllables by the number of words in the sample and multiply by 100.

4. Determine the average SL and WL of the samples and then apply the formula:

$$RE = 206.835 - 0.846 \ (WL) - 1.015 \ (SL)$$

where RE is the reading ease score, WL is the average word length measured as syllables per 100 words, and SL is the average sentence length in words (Flesch, 1948; Spadero, 1983; and Spadero et al., 1980).

The reading ease score ranges from zero (practically unreadable) to 100 (very easy for any literate person) with interpretations in between (Table A-1).

TABLE A-1	Reading Ease Scores			
READING EASE SCORE	SYLLABLES PER 100 WORDS	AVERAGE SENTENCE LENGTH	DIFFICULTY LEVEL	GRADE LEVEL
0–30	192 or more	29 or more	Very difficult	College grad
30–50	167	25	Difficult	College
50–60	155	21	Fairly difficult	10–12
60–70	147	17	Standard	8–9
70–80	139	14	Fairly easy	7
80–90	131	11	Easy	6
90–100	123 or less	8 or less	Very easy	5

Source: Adapted from Flesch, R. (1948). A new readability yardstick. *Journal of Applied Psychology, 32*(3), 230; and Spadero, D. C. (1983). Assessing readability of patient information materials. *Pediatric Nursing, 9*(4), 275.

HOW TO USE THE FOG FORMULA

1. Count 100 words in succession (W). If the selection is long, choose several samples of 100 words from the text, and average the results.
2. Count the number of complete sentences (S). If the 100th word falls past the midpoint of a sentence, include this sentence in the count.
3. Divide the words (W) by the number of sentences (S).
4. Count the number of words having three or more syllables (A), but do not count verbs ending in -*ed* or -*es* that make a word have a third syllable, do not count capitalized words, and do not count combinations of simple words, such as *butterfly*.
5. Apply the formula:

$$GL = (W/S + A) \times 0.4$$

In other words, to find the GL (grade level), divide the number of words (W) by the number of complete sentences (S) in the sample 100-word passage, add the number of words having three or more syllables (A), and multiply the result by a constant of 0.4 (Gunning, 1968; Spadero, 1983; Spadero et al., 1980).

HOW TO USE THE FRY READABILITY GRAPH _____

1. Select three 100-word sample passages from near the beginning, middle, and end of a book, article, pamphlet, or brochure. Skip all proper nouns as part of the 100-word count. Fewer than three samples and passages of less than 30 sentences can be used, but the user should be aware that there is necessarily a sacrifice in both reliability and validity.
2. Count the total number of sentences in each 100-word sample (estimating to the nearest tenth of a sentence for partial sentences).
3. Average the sentence counts of the three sample passages.
4. Count the total number of syllables in each 100-word sample. Count one syllable per vowel sound; for example, *cat* has one syllable, *blackbird* has two, and *continental* has four. Caution: Do not be fooled by word size (e.g., *polio* [three syllables], *through* [one syllable]). Endings such as *-y*, *-ed*, *-el*, or *-le* usually make a syllable (e.g., *ready* [two syllables], *bottle* [two syllables]). Graph users sometimes have trouble determining syllables. The clue is to believe what you hear (speech sounds), not what you see (e.g., *wanted* is a two-syllable word, but *stopped* is a one-syllable word). Count proper nouns, numerals, and initials or acronyms as words. A word is a symbol or group of symbols bounded by a blank space on either side. Thus, *1945*, *&*, and *IRS* are all words. Each symbol should receive a syllable count of one (i.e., the date *1945* is one word with four syllables, and the initials *IRS* is one word with three syllables).
5. Average the total number of syllables for the three samples.
6. Plot on the graph the average sentence count and the average word count to determine the appropriate grade level of the material. For example,

	NUMBER OF SYLLABLES	NUMBER OF SENTENCES
1st hundred words	153	6.3
2nd hundred words	161	5.9
3rd hundred words	139	5.2
Average count =	453 ÷ 3 = 151	17.4 ÷ 3 = 5.8

In the example, the average number of syllables is 151, and the average number of sentences is 5.8. When plotted on the graph (Figure A-1), the point falls within the

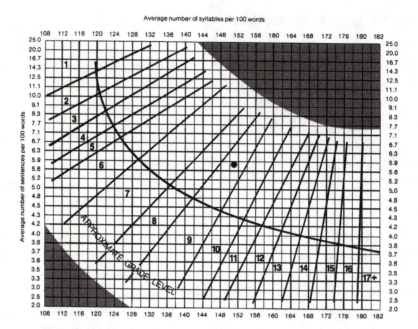

FIGURE A-1   Fry Readability Graph—Extended
Source: Edward Fry, Rutgers University Reading Center, New Brunswick, NJ.

approximate grade level of 9, which shows the materials to be at the ninth-grade readability level. If the point when plotted falls in the gray area, grade-level scores are invalid (Fry, 1968; Fry, 1977; Spadero et al., 1980).

HOW TO USE THE SMOG FORMULA

Printed Materials Longer Than 30 Sentences

1. Count 10 consecutive sentences near the beginning, 10 consecutive sentences from the middle, and 10 consecutive sentences from the end of the selection to be assessed. A sentence is any independent unit of thought punctuated by a period, question mark, or exclamation point. If a sentence has a colon or semi colon, consider each part as a separate sentence.

2. From the 30 randomly selected sentences, count the words containing three or more syllables (polysyllabic), including repetitions. Abbreviated words should be read aloud to determine their syllable count (e.g., *Sept.* = *September* = three syllables). Letters or numerals in a string beginning or ending with a space or

punctuation mark should be counted if, when read aloud in context, at least three syllables can be distinguished. Do not count words ending in *-ed* or *-es* if the ending makes the word have a third syllable. Hyphenated words are counted as one word. Proper nouns should be counted.

3. Approximate the reading grade level from the SMOG Conversion Table (Table A-2), or calculate the reading grade level by estimating the nearest perfect square root of the number of words with three or more syllables and then adding a constant of 3 to the square root. For example, if the total number of polysyllabic words was 53, the nearest perfect square would be 49. The square root of 49 would be 7. By adding a constant of 3, the reading level would be tenth grade.

Table A-2   SMOG Conversion Table

WORD COUNT	GRADE LEVEL
0–2	4
3–6	5
7–12	6
13–20	7
21–30	8
31–42	9
43–56	10
57–72	11
73–90	12
91–110	13
111–132	14
133–156	15
157–182	16
183–210	17
211–240	18

Source: Developed by: Harold C. McGraw, Office of Educational Research, Baltimore County Public Schools, Towson, MD.

Figure A-2 is an example of how to count all the words containing three or more syllables in a set of 10 sentences taken from one of the many pamphlets designed and distributed by the National Cancer Institute of the National Institutes of Health, Public Health Service, U.S. Department of Health and Human Services, entitled *Mastectomy: A Treatment for Breast Cancer* (1987, p. 1).

In Figure A-2, there are 20 words with three or more syllables. Note, the word *United* is not counted as a three-syllable word because only the *-ed* ending makes it polysyllabic (see rule 2).

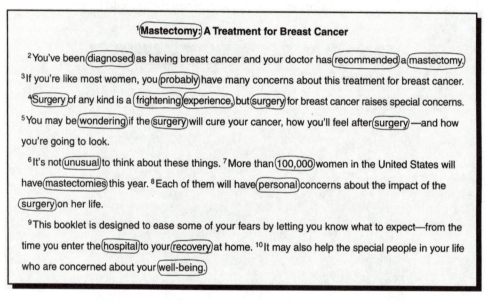

FIGURE A-2   Example of Counting Words with Three or More Syllables

Printed Materials Shorter Than 30 Sentences

1. Count the number of sentences in the material and the number of words containing three or more syllables.
2. In the left-hand column of Table A-3, locate the number of sentences. Then in the column opposite, locate the conversion number.
3. Multiply the word count found in Step 1 by the conversion number. Locate this number in Table A-2 to obtain the corresponding grade level.
   Example: If the material is 25 sentences long and 15 words of three or more syllables were counted in this material, the conversion number in Table A-3 for

25 sentences is 1.2. Multiply the word count of 15 by 1.2 to get 18. For the word count of 18, the grade level in Table A-2 is 7. Therefore, the material is at a seventh-grade reading level.

Table A-3 SMOG Conversion for Samples with Fewer Than 30 Sentences	
NUMBER OF SENTENCES IN THE SAMPLE MATERIAL	**CONVERSION NUMBER**
29	1.03
28	1.07
27	1.1
26	1.15
25	1.2
24	1.25
23	1.3
22	1.36
21	1.43
20	1.5
19	1.58
18	1.67
17	1.76
16	1.87
15	2.0
14	2.14
13	2.3
12	2.5
11	2.7
10	3

HOW TO USE THE CLOZE TEST

How to Construct a Cloze Test

1. Select a prose passage (one without reference to figures, tables, charts, or pictures) from printed educational materials currently in use such as pamphlets, brochures, manuals, or instruction sheets. Be sure the material is typical of what is normally given to patients but has not been previously read by them. The chosen passage should include whole paragraphs so that readers benefit from complete units of thought.

2. Leave the first and last sentences intact, and delete every fifth word from the other sentences for a total of about 50 word deletions. Do not delete proper nouns, but delete the word following the proper noun. Replace all deleted words with a line or blank space, all of equal length.

High Blood Pressure

High blood pressure, also called hypertension, affects 37 million Americans—many of them older than 55. A dangerous, silent killer, __1__ can lead to stroke, __2__ attack and heart or __3__ failure. Yet, in most __4__, no one knows what __5__ high blood pressure. Body __6__, emotions, heredity, overweight, and __7__ high-sodium (salt) diet may __8__ something to do with __9__ blood pressure, but scientists __10__ uncertain. It has long __11__ recognized as a major __12__ factor in stroke and __13__ attack—cardiovascular diseases which __14__ nearly 1 million deaths __15__ year.

To understand high __16__ pressure, it is necessary __17__ know something about how __18__ heart and blood vessels __19__. Your heart is a __20__ that acts like a __21__. The left side of __22__ heart receives oxygen-rich blood __23__ the lungs and pumps __24__ through the arteries to __25__ parts of your body, __26__ it with nutrients and __27__. Blood that has distributed __28__ nutrients and oxygen returns __29__ the right side of __30__ heart which pumps it __31__ the pulmonary artery to __32__ lungs where it absorbs __33__, and then the process __34__ again.

The force exerted __35__ your blood flowing against __36__ walls of the blood __37__ is blood pressure. The __38__ action of your heart __39__ the force. Your blood __40__ varies from moment to __41__ depending upon the situations __42__ activities in which you __43__ involved. For example, when __44__ become excited, the small __45__ that nourish your tissues __46__. The heart must pump __47__ harder to force the __48__ through the arteries, causing __49__ blood pressure to rise. __50__ the blood pressure will __51__ to normal when you __52__. Because of these changes in blood pressure, the doctor will usually take several blood pressure readings over a period of time before making a diagnosis of high blood pressure.

FIGURE A-3 Sample Cloze Test

Source: Adapted from American Heart Association (1983) *An older person's guide to cardiovascular health*, National Center, 7320 Greenville Avenue, Dallas, TX 75231. The information from this booklet is not current and is used for illustrative purposes only.

How to Score a Cloze Test

1. Count as correct only those words that *exactly* replace the deleted words (synonyms are not to be counted as a correct answer).
2. Inappropriate word endings such as *-s*, *-ed*, *-er*, and *-ing* should be counted as incorrect. Hyphenated words are counted as one word; words in parentheses are counted as a word.
3. The raw score is the number of exact word replacements.
4. Divide the raw score by the total number of blank spaces to determine the percentage of correct responses. For example, if the passage has 50 blanks and the patient correctly filled in 25 blanks (of the other 25 blanks, 10 were incorrect responses and 15 spaces were left blank), divide 25 by 50, and the percentage score would be 50%.
5. A score of 60% or above indicates the patient is fully capable of understanding the material. A score of 40% to 60% indicates the patient needs supplemental instruction. A score below 40% indicates that the material as written is too difficult for the patient to understand.

The following are the missing words that were deleted from the sample Cloze test in Figure A-3.

1. it	14. cause	27. oxygen	40. pressure
2. heart	15. a	28. its	41. moment
3. kidney	16. blood	29. to	42. or
4. cases	17. to	30. your	43. are
5. causes	18. the	31. through	44. you
6. chemistry	19. work	32. the	45. arteries
7. a	20. muscle	33. oxygen	46. constrict
8. have	21. pump	34. begins	47. even
9. high	22. your	35. by	48. blood
10. remain	23. from	36. the	49. your
11. been	24. it	37. vessels	50. usually
12. risk	25. all	38. pumping	51. return
13. heart	26. supplying	39. creates	52. relax

Resources and Organizations for Special Populations

Blindness

National Diabetes Information Clearinghouse
Box NDIC
9000 Rockville Pike
Bethesda, MD 20892
(301) 468-2162

Resource Persons for Diabetes and Vision Impairment
VIP Special Interest Group
AADE
444 North Michigan Avenue
Suite 1240
Chicago, IL 60611-3901

Lists members of American Association of Diabetes Educators (AADE) who possess specialized skills for working with visually impaired persons. List is compiled by the Visually Impaired Persons (VIP) Special Interest Group for the AADE and is available from that special interest group.

Resources for Visually Impaired Diabetics
Vision Foundation Inc.
818 Mt. Auburn Street
Watertown, MA 02172

The Vision Foundation publication is revised annually and is available for $4 prepaid for either large-print or cassette edition.

Deafness

The National Academy of Gallaudet College
Florida Avenue at 7th Street N.E.
Washington, DC 20002

Training programs; assistance in developing training programs; publications on working with deaf patients.

The National Center for Law and the Deaf
Gallaudet College
Florida Avenue at 7th Street N.E.
Washington, DC 20002

Guidelines for services for deaf patients; assistance in developing such guidelines.

The Registry of Interpreters for the Deaf
814 Thayer Avenue
Silver Spring, MD 20910

Information on interpreting and interpreters; referral to local agencies and state chapters of the Registry of Interpreters for the Deaf for assistance in locating interpreters.

Disability Services

Clearinghouse on Disability Information
U.S. Department of Education
Switzer Building Room 3132
Washington, DC 20202
(202) 731-1241

Information Center for Individuals with Disabilities
Fort Point Place First Floor
27-43 Wormwood Street
Boston, MA 02210-1606
(617) 727-5540

Library of Congress National Library Service for the Blind and Physically Handicapped
1291 Taylor Street NW
Washington, DC 20542

(202) 707-5100
(800) 424-9100
(TDD 202) 707-0744

Brain Injury

National Head Injury Foundation
1776 Massachusetts Avenue NW
Suite 100
Washington, DC 20036
(202) 296-6443

Healthcare-Related Federal Agencies

National Institute on Disability and Rehabilitation Research
U.S. Department of Education
400 Maryland Avenue SW
Room 3060
Washington, DC 20202
(202) 732-1134

Rehabilitation Services Administration
Department of Human Services
605 G Street NW
Room 101M
Washington, DC 20001
(202) 727-3211

Learning Disabilities

A.D.D. Warehouse
300 Northwest 70th Avenue
Suite 102
Plantation, FL 33317
(305) 792-8944

Association for Children and Adults with Learning Disabilities
4156 Library Road
Pittsburgh, PA 15234
(412) 341-8077

Attention Disorders Association of Parents and Professionals Together (ADAPPT)
P.O. Box 293
Oak Forest, IL 60452
(312) 361-4330

Neuromuscular Disorders

Amyotrophic Lateral Sclerosis Association
21021 Ventura Boulevard
Suite 321
Woodland Hills, CA 91364
(818) 990-2151

Epilepsy Foundation of America
4351 Garden City Drive
Landover, MD 20785
(301) 459-3700

Guillain-Barré Syndrome Foundation International
P.O. Box 262
Wynnewood, PA 19096
(215) 667-0131

Muscular Dystrophy Association
810 7th Avenue
New York, NY 10019
(212) 586-0808

Myasthenia Gravis Foundation, Inc.
53 W. Jackson Boulevard
Suite 660
Chicago, IL 60604
(312) 427-6252

National Ataxia Foundation
15500 Wayzata Boulevard
Suite 750
Wayzata, MN 55391
(612) 473-7666

National Multiple Sclerosis Society
205 E. 42nd Street
New York, NY 10017
(800) 624-8236

Parkinson's Disease Foundation
William Black Medical Research Building
Columbia Presbyterian Medical Center
650 W. 168th Street
New York, NY 10032
(212) 923-4700
(800) 457-6676

United Cerebral Palsy Foundation Associations
7 Penn Plaza, Suite 804
New York, NY 10001
(212) 268-6655

Stroke

National Institute of Neurological and Communicative Disorders and Stroke
Building 31
Room 8A52
9000 Rockville Pike
Bethesda, MD 20892

National Stroke Association
300 E. Hampden Avenue
Suite 240
Englewood, CO 80110-2654
(303) 762-9922

Stroke Clubs International
805 12th Street
Galveston, TX 77550
(409) 762-1022

ADAPTIVE COMPUTERS

The following is a partial list of computer software and other adaptive equipment available to people with disabilities.

The Alliance for Technology Access (ATA), formerly called the National Special Education Alliance, is a growing network of nonprofit resource centers located around the country that specializes in using computers to help individuals with disabilities. For more information on the ATA contact:

Foundation for Technology Access
1307 Solano Avenue
Albany, CA 94706
(415) 528-0747

TSI/VTEK
455 N. Bernardo Avenue
Mountain View, CA 94039-7455
(800) 227-8418

Large Print Display Processor, Braille Display Processor, Optacon II

Blindness

Some Braille printers are able to print both Braille and standard text on the same page. This feature enables individuals who are blind to share their printed work with people who are sighted.

American Thermoform Corp.
2311 Travers Avenue
City of Commerce, CA 90040
(213) 723-9021

Ohtsuki Printer (Braille)

Enabling Technologies
3102 S.E. Jay Street
Stuart, FL 33497
(407) 283-4817

Romeo Brailler

Duxbury Systems, Inc.
435 King Street
P.O. Box 1504
Littleton, MA 01460
(508) 486-9766

Duxbury Braille Translator (software)

Head-Controlled Mouse
Prentke Romich Company
1022 Heyl Road
Wooster, OH 44691
(800) 642-8255

Headmaster Workstation

Pointer Systems, Inc.
One Mill Street
Burlington, VT 05401
(800) 537-1562

Freewheel

Outliners (Thought Processors)

In many instances, outlining software can be used in place of a word processor, and for people with learning disabilities, outlining software may be the best place to start almost any kind of writing.

Symmetry Corporation
761 E. University Drive, #C
Mesa, AZ 85203
(800) 624-2485

Acta Advantage

MECC
3490 Lexington Avenue North
St. Paul, MN 55126
(612) 481-3500

MECC Outliner

Computerized Speech Tools

American Speech-Language and Hearing Association
10801 Rockville Pike
Rockville, MD 20852
(301) 897-5700

United States Society for Augmentative and Alternative Communication
c/o Barkley Memorial Center
University of Nebraska
Lincoln, NE 68588
(402) 472-5463

Voice Recognition Systems

Voice recognition systems hold enormous potential for individuals with movement limitations; they effectively control the computer without any physical interaction taking place between the person and computer.

Articulate Systems, Inc.
2380 Ellsworth Street
Berkeley, CA 94720
(415) 549-1013

Voice Navigator

Voice Connection
17835 Skypark Circle
Suite C
Irvine, CA 92714
(714) 261-2366

IntroVoice

Newsletters and Magazines

Assistive Device News
Central Pennsylvania Special Education
Regional Resource Center
150 South Progress Avenue
Harrisburg, PA 17109
(717) 367-1161

The Assistive Device News is published by the Pennsylvania Assistive Device Center located at the Elizabethtown Hospital and Rehabilitation Center. The newsletter contains information about technology solutions for individuals with physical impairments.

Augmentative Communication News
One Surf Way
Suite 215
Monterey, CA 93940
(408) 649-3050

The Augmentative Communication News is a professional journal that focuses on augmentative communication, integration theory, technology, assessment, treatment, and the education of users who rely on augmentative communication systems.

abstract conceptualization   A term used by Kolb to describe a dimension of perceiving information; known as the "thinking" mode.

accommodator   One of the four learning style types according to Kolb's theory, combining the learning modes of concrete experience and active experimentation.

acculturation   The willingness of an individual to adapt to the customs, values, beliefs, and behaviors of another culture.

active experimentation   A term used by Kolb to describe a dimension of processing information; known as the "doing" mode.

adaptive computing   The professional services and the technology (both hardware and software) that make computing technology accessible for persons with disabilities.

adherence   Commitment or attachment to a prescribed, predetermined regimen.

affective domain   One of three domains in the taxonomy of behavioral objectives; deals with attitudes, values, and beliefs.

ageism   Prejudice against the older adult that perpetuates the negative stereotyping of aging as a period of decline.

aids   See *instructional materials/tools*.

analogue   A type of model that uses analogy to explain something by comparing it to something else. The model performs like the real object, although its actual appearance may differ. A dialysis machine and the use of a description of a pump to explain how the kidneys and heart work respectively are examples of analogues.

andragogy   The art and science of helping adults learn; a term coined by Malcolm Knowles to describe his theory of adult learning.

animistic thinking   The tendency of preschoolers to think nonliving objects are alive and conscious; the belief that objects possess human characteristics.

assess   To gather, summarize, and interpret pertinent data about the learner to make a decision or plan.

assessment   The process of systematically collecting data to determine the relative magnitude, importance, or value of needs, problems, and strengths of the learner to decide a direction for action.

assessment phase   The first phase of the educational cycle, which provides the foundation for the rest of the educational process.

assimilation   The willingness of a person emigrating to a new culture to gradually adopt and incorporate the characteristics of the prevailing culture.

assimilator   One of the four learning style types, according to Kolb's theory, combining the learning modes of abstract conceptualization and reflective observation.

attention deficit disorder (ADD)   A disorder of children with prominent attentional difficulties as demonstrated by inattention and impulsivity that are signs of developmentally inappropriate behavior.

audio resources   Instructional tools whose chief characteristic is exploitation of the learners' sense of hearing as a mechanism for teaching. Audiotapes and recorders are examples.

audiovisual materials (tools)   Nonprint instructional media that can influence all three domains of learning and stimulate the senses of hearing and/or sight to help convey the message to the learner. This category includes five major types: projected, audio, video, telecommunications, and computer formats.

augmented feedback   An opinion or conveyance of a message through oral or body language by the teacher to the learner about how well he or she performed a psychomotor skill; often referred to as extrinsic feedback.

autonomy   The right to self-determination.

barriers to teaching   Those factors that impede the nurse's ability to deliver educational services.

behavioral (learning) objectives   Intended outcomes of the education process that are action oriented rather than content oriented and learner centered rather than teacher centered.

behaviorist learning   One of the five major learning theories. According to behaviorists, the focus for learning is mainly on what is directly observable, and learning is viewed as the product of the stimulus conditions (S) and the responses (R) that follow. It is sometimes termed the S-R model of learning.

beneficence   The principle of doing good.

bodily-kinesthetic intelligence   A term used by Gardner to describe children who learn by processing knowledge through bodily sensations.

causal thinking   The ability of school-aged children to understand cause and effect through logic, concrete thinking, and inductive and deductive reasoning.

chronic illness   A disease or disability that is permanent and can never be completely cured. It constitutes the number one medical malady of people in this country and affects the physical, psychosocial, economic, and spiritual aspects of an individual's life.

Cloze procedure   A standardized test to measure comprehension of written materials (particularly recommended for health education literature) based on systematically deleting every fifth word from a portion of a text and having the reader fill in the blanks.

cognitive ability   The extent to which information can be processed, indicative of the level at which the learner is capable of learning; of major importance when designing instruction.

cognitive development   The process of acquiring more complex and adaptive ways of thinking as an individual grows from infancy to adulthood according to Piaget's four stages of cognitive maturation: sensorimotor, preoperational, concrete operations, and formal operations.

cognitive development perspective Focuses on the qualitative changes in perceiving, thinking, and reasoning as individuals grow and mature based on how external events are conceptualized, organized, and represented within each person's mental framework or schema.

cognitive domain   One of three domains in the taxonomy of behavioral objectives; deals with aspects of behavior focusing on the way in which someone thinks in acquiring facts, concepts, principles, etc.

cognitive learning   One of the five major learning theories. According to a cognitive theorist's perspective, in order to learn, individuals change as a result of the way they perceive, process, interpret, and organize information based on what is already known; the reorganization of information leads to new insights and understanding.

commercially prepared materials Predesigned, cost-effective printed educational materials that are widely available on a wide range of topics for purchase by educators as supplements to teaching-learning, such as brochures, pamphlets, books, and posters.

compliance   Submission or yielding to predetermined goals through regimens prescribed or established by others.

comprehension   The degree to which individuals understand what they have read or heard; the ability to grasp the meaning of a verbal or nonverbal message.

computer literacy   The ability to use the necessary computer hardware and software to meet the needs for information.

concrete experience   A term used by Kolb to describe a dimension of perceiving; known as the "feeling" mode.

concrete operations period   As defined by Piaget, this is the third stage in the cognitive development of children when the school-aged child (ages 6 to 12 years) is capable of logical thought processes and the ability to reason but is still incapable of abstract thinking.

confidentiality   A binding social contract or covenant; a professional obligation to respect privileged information between the health professional and the client.

content   The actual information that is communicated to the learner through various teaching methods and tools.

content evaluation   A systematic assessment taking place immediately after the learning experience to determine the degree to which learners have acquired the knowledge or skills taught during a teaching/learning session.

converger   One of the four learning style types according to Kolb's theory, combining the learning modes of abstract conceptualization and active experimentation.

corpus callosum   The connector between the two hemispheres of the brain.

cosmopolitan orientation   Persons with a worldly perspective on life who are receptive to new ideas and opportunities to learn new ways of doing things; a component of experiential readiness.

cost benefit   "Money well spent." Cost of services (e.g., education) ensures return of satisfied clients and stability of the economic base of a healthcare facility.

cost-benefit analysis   The relationship between cost and outcomes that can be expressed in monetary terms; also called a *cost-benefit ratio*.

cost-benefit ratio   Relationship (expressed as a ratio) of program costs to economic benefits gained by the healthcare institution.

cost-effectiveness analysis   The efficiency of an educational offering when an actual monetary value cannot be assigned to a program.

cost recovery   Occurs when revenues generated are equal to or greater than expenditures.

cost savings   Monies realized through decreased use of expensive services, shortened length of stay, or fewer complications resulting from preventive services or patient education.

crystallized intelligence The intellectual ability developed over a lifetime, which includes such elements as vocabulary, general information, understanding of social interactions, arithmetic reasoning, and capacity to evaluate experiences, which tends to increase over time as a person ages.

cuing Using prompts and reminders to get a learner to perform routine tasks by focusing on an appropriate combination of time and situation.

cultural assessment An organized, systematic appraisal of beliefs, values, and practices of an individual or group to determine client needs as a basis for planning nursing care interventions.

cultural awareness The process of becoming sensitive to the interactions with other cultural groups by examining one's biases and prejudices toward others of another culture or ethnic background.

cultural competence The ability to demonstrate knowledge and understanding of another person's culture and accept and respect cultural differences by adapting interventions to be congruent with that specific culture when delivering care.

cultural encounter The process of exposing oneself in nursing practice to cross-cultural interactions with clients of diverse cultural backgrounds.

cultural knowledge The process of acquiring an educational foundation about various cultural world views.

cultural literacy The ability of knowing how to communicate with someone from another culture without having to explain undertones, voice intonations, and message contexts during a conversation.

cultural phenomena Six factors (communication patterns, personal space, social organization, time perspective, environmental control, and biological variations) that need to be taken into account when assessing a client's cultural response to health care.

cultural skill The process of learning how to conduct an accurate cultural assessment.

Culturally Competent Model of Care A model for conducting a thorough and sensitive cultural assessment that includes the four components of cultural awareness, cultural knowledge, cultural skill, and cultural encounter.

culture A complex concept that is an integral part of each person's life and includes knowledge, beliefs, values, morals, customs, traditions, and habits acquired by the members of a society.

delivery system The physical form of instructional materials, including durable equipment used to present these materials, such as film and projectors, audiotapes and tape players, and computer programs and computers.

demonstration   A traditional instructional method by which the learner is shown by the teacher how to perform a particular psychomotor skill.

demonstration materials   Tools that stimulate the senses by combining sight with touch, smell, and sometimes even taste with the advantage of helping to teach cognitive and psychomotor skill development. Major forms of media in this category include many types of nonprint media, such as models, real equipment, diagrams, charts, posters, displays, photographs, and drawings.

desirable needs   Learning needs of the client that are not life dependent but related to well-being and can be met by the overall ability of nursing staff to provide quality care.

determinants of learning   Consist of learning needs, readiness to learn, and learning styles.

developmental stages   Milestones marking changes in the physical, cognitive, and psychosocial growth of an individual over time from infancy to old age.

direct costs   Tangible, predictable costs associated with expenditures for personnel, equipment, etc.

disability   Inability to perform some key life functions; often used interchangeably with the term functional limitation.

discharge planning   An interdisciplinary process, highly dependent on patient educational interventions for effectiveness, by which members of the healthcare team (often led by nurses) plan and coordinate services for the purpose of providing continuity of care to patients and their families between various care settings.

displays   Type of demonstration materials, frequently regarded as static, which may be permanently installed or portable. Included in this category are chalkboards, flip charts, and posters.

distance learning   A flexible telecommunications method of instruction using video or computer technology to transmit live, online, or taped messages directly between the instructor and the learner who are separated from one another by time and/or location.

diverger   One of the four learning style types according to Kolb's theory, combining the learning modes of concrete experience and reflective observation.

domains of learning   Cognitive, psychomotor, and affective are the three domains in which learning occurs.

Dunn and Dunn Learning Style   Identification of how individuals prefer to function, learn, concentrate, and perform in learning activities based on five basic stimuli.

duty　Responsibility; professional expectation.

dysarthria　Difficulty with voluntary muscle control of speech due to damage to the central or peripheral nervous system that controls muscles essential to speaking and swallowing. Types of dysarthria include flaccid, spastic, ataxic, hypokinetic, or mixed. Persons with degenerative neurologic diseases often suffer with this disorder.

education　An umbrella term used to describe the process, including the components of teaching and instruction, of producing observable or measurable behavioral changes (in knowledge, attitudes, and/or skills) in the learner through planned educational activities.

education process　A systematic, sequential, planned course of action that parallels the nursing process and consists of two interdependent operations, teaching and learning, which form a continuous cycle to include assessment of the learner, establishment of a teaching plan, implementation of teaching methods and tools, and evaluation of the learner, teacher, and education program.

e-mail　An Internet-based activity that is a quick, inexpensive, and increasingly popular way to communicate asynchronously via the computer.

emoticons　Symbols commonly used to represent emotions, such as a :) (smiley face) or ;) (winking), by people who are sending e-mail messages.

emotional readiness　A state of psychological willingness to learn, which is dependent on such factors as anxiety level, support system, motivation, risk-taking behavior, frame of mind, and psychosocial developmental stage.

ethical rights and duties　A term that refers to the norms or standards of behavior of healthcare professionals.

ethics　Guiding principles of human behavior.

ethnocentrism　A concept in which the belief is held that one's own culture is superior and all other cultures are less sophisticated.

evaluation　A systematic and continuous process by which the significance of something is judged; the process of collecting and using information to determine what has been accomplished and how well it has been accomplished to guide decision making.

experiential readiness　A state of willingness to learn based on such factors as an individual's past experiences with learning, cultural background, previous coping mechanisms, and locus of control.

expressive aphasia　An absence or impairment of the ability to communicate through speech or writing due to a dysfunction in the Broca's area of the brain, which is the center of the cortex that controls motor abilities.

external locus of control   An individual's motivation to learn comes from outside oneself, attributing success or failure of an action to luck, the nature of the task, or to the efforts of someone else.

extraversion-introversion (EI)   Terms used to describe behavior that reflects an orientation to either the outside world of people or to the inner world of concepts and ideas; one of four dichotomous preference dimensions in the Myers-Briggs Typology.

fixed costs   Predictable and controllable expenses that remain stable over time.

Flesch formula   An objective, statistical measurement tool for readability of written materials between fifth grade and college level, based on a count of the two basic language elements of average sentence length and of average word length (measured as syllables per 100 words) of selected samples.

fluid intelligence   The intellectual capacity to perceive relationships, to reason, and to perform abstract thinking, which declines over time as degenerative changes occur with aging.

Fog formula   An index appropriate for use in determining readability of materials from fourth grade to college level based on average sentence length and the percentage of multisyllabic words in a 100-word passage.

formal operations period   As defined by Piaget, this is the fourth and final stage of cognitive development in which the adolescent (ages 12 to 18 years) is capable of abstract thought, internalization of ideas, complex logical reasoning, and understanding causality.

formative evaluation   Also referred to as *process evaluation*. It is a systematic and continuous assessment of success of the teaching process made during the implementation of materials, methods, and activities to control, ensure, or improve the quality of performance in delivery of an educational program.

Fry formula   A measurement tool for testing the readability of materials (especially books, pamphlets, and brochures) at the level of first grade through college by using a graph to plot the number of syllables of words and the number of sentences in three 100-word samples.

functional illiteracy   The lack of fundamental education skills needed by adults to read, write, or comprehend information below the fifth-grade level of difficulty to function effectively in today's society; the inability to read well enough to understand and interpret written information for use as intended.

functional magnetic resonance imaging (FMRI) A type of advanced technology that has revolutionized the field of neuroscience by making colorful images on computer monitors of the brain to determine the possible areas of nerve activity involved in the processes of thinking, emotions, and recall.

gaming A nontraditional instructional method requiring the learner to participate in a competitive activity (which may or may not reflect reality) with preset rules.

Gardner's seven types of intelligence A theory that describes the styles of learning in children.

gender-related cognitive abilities A comparison between the sexes as to how males and females act, react, and perform in situations affecting every sphere of life as a result of genetic and environmental influences on behavior.

gerogogy The art and science of teaching the elderly.

goal A desirable outcome to be achieved by the learner at the end of the teaching-learning process; goals are global and more future oriented and long-term in nature than the specific, short-term objectives that lead step by step to the final achievement of a goal.

group discussion A commonly employed, traditional method of instruction whereby a group of learners (ideally 3 to 20 people) gather together to exchange information, feelings, and opinions with each other and the teacher; the activity is learner centered and subject centered.

habilitation Includes all the activities and interactions that enable individuals with a disability to develop new abilities to achieve their maximum potential.

hardware Part of the delivery system for many types of media (e.g., computers, projectors, tape players).

Health Belief Model A framework or paradigm used to explain or predict health behavior composed of the interaction among individual perceptions, modifying factors, and likelihood of action.

health education A participatory educational approach, often used interchangeably with the term *patient education* or client education, aimed at preventing disease, promoting positive health, and incorporating the physical, mental, and social aspects of learning needs.

health literacy   Refers to how well an individual can read, interpret, and comprehend health information for maintaining an optimal level of wellness.

Health Promotion Model   A framework that describes the interaction of health-promoting factors including cognitive perceptual factors, modifying factors, and likelihood of participation in health promoting behaviors.

healthcare setting   One of three classifications of instructional settings, in which the delivery of health care is the primary or sole function of an institution, organization, or agency. Examples: hospitals, visiting nurse associations, public health departments, outpatient clinics, physician offices, health maintenance organizations, extended-care facilities, and nurse-managed centers.

healthcare-related setting   One of three classifications of instructional settings, in which healthcare-related services are offered as a complementary function of a quasihealth agency. Examples: American Heart Association, American Cancer Society, Muscular Dystrophy Association, and Leukemia Society of America.

healthcare team   An interdisciplinary group of healthcare professionals and nonprofessionals who provide services to the patient and family members in an attempt to maximize optimal health and well-being of the client to whom their activities are directed.

hearing impairment   A general term used to categorize an auditory sensory deficit that includes either complete loss or a reduction in sensitivity to sounds by persons who are deaf or hard of hearing.

hidden costs   Costs that cannot be predicted or accounted for until after the fact.

hierarchy of needs   Theory of human motivation based on integrated wholeness of the individual and levels of satisfaction of basic human needs organized by potency.

humanistic learning   One of the five major learning theories, which views learning as being facilitated by curiosity, needs, a positive self-concept, and open situations where freedom of choice and individuality are promoted and respected.

illiteracy   The total inability of adults to read, write, or comprehend information.

illusionary representations   A category of instructional materials that lack realism, such as dimensionality. Examples are photographs, drawings, and audiotapes, which depend on imagination to fill in the gaps and offer the learner experiences that simulate reality.

imaginary audience A belief or obsession by adolescents that everyone is focusing on them and their activities, which has considerable influence over teenagers' behavior.

impact evaluation The process of assessing outcomes or effects of an educational activity that extend beyond the activity itself to address organizational and/or societal effects.

indirect costs Costs that may be fixed but are not necessarily directly related to an educational activity (e.g., heating, electricity, housekeeping).

informal teaching Unplanned or spontaneous sessions in which teaching-learning takes place.

Information Age The present period of time, in which sweeping advances in computer and information technology have transformed the economic, social, and cultural life of society.

information literacy The ability to access, evaluate, organize, and use information from a variety of sources.

information processing perspective Emphasizes the process of memory functioning in the way information is encountered, organized, stored, and retrieved.

input disability A general category of learning disability that refers to problems of receiving and recording information in the brain, which includes visual, auditory, perceptual and integrative processing, such as dyslexia and short-and long-term memory disorders.

instructional materials/tools The resources or vehicles used to help communicate information, which include both print and non-print media, to aid teaching-learning by stimulating the various senses such as vision and hearing. These are intended to supplement, not replace, actual teaching. Synonymous terms are educational aids or *audiovisual materials*.

instructional setting A situation or area in which health teaching takes place as classified on the basis of what relationship health education has to the primary function of an organization, agency, or institution in which the teaching occurs.

instructional strategy See *teaching strategy*.

internal locus of control Individuals are motivated from within to learn, attributing success or failure to their own ability or effort.

Internet A huge global computer network, of which the World Wide Web is a component, established to allow transfer (exchange) of information from one computer to another; it provides a diverse range of services used to deliver information to large numbers of people and to enable people to communicate with one another, such as via e-mail, real-time chat, electronic discussion groups, or Usenet newsgroups.

interpersonal intelligence   A term used by Gardner to describe children who learn best in groups.

intrapersonal intelligence   A term used by Gardner to describe children who learn well with independent self-paced instruction.

intrinsic feedback   A response that is generated within the self, giving learners a sense of or a feel for how they have performed; often used in relation to a psychomotor skill performance.

judgment-perception (JP)   Terms used to describe behavior that reflects the way a person comes to a conclusion about something or becomes aware of something; one of four dichotomous preference dimensions in the Myers-Briggs Typology.

justice   The equal distribution of benefits and burdens.

knowledge deficit   A gap in what a learner needs or wants to know; this category of nursing diagnosis can include learning needs in the cognitive, affective, and psychomotor domains.

knowledge readiness   A state of willingness to learn dependent on such factors as the learner's present knowledge base, the level of

learning capability, and the preferred style of learning.

Kolb's Cycle of Learning   An experiential learning model that includes four modes of learning reflecting the dimensions of perception and processing.

law   A clearly stated pronouncement of a binding custom, enforceable by a controlling body.

layout   The arrangement of printed and/or graphic information on a flat surface. Effective use of white space, graphics, and wording will depend heavily on this arrangement.

learner characteristics   One of the three major variables that refers to the learner's perceptual abilities, reading ability, self-direction, and learning style, which must be considered when making appropriate choices of instructional materials.

learning   A conscious or unconscious permanent change in behavior as a result of a lifelong, dynamic process by which individuals acquire new knowledge, skills, and/or attitudes that can be measured and can occur at any time or in any place due to exposure to environmental stimuli.

learning curve   Also sometimes referred to as the experience curve, it is a record of an individual's improvement in psychomotor skill development made by measuring his or her ability at different stages during a specified time period, which includes six stages: negligible progress, increasing gains, decreasing gains, plateau, renewed gains, and approach to limit.

learning disability (LD)   A generic term that refers to a heterogeneous group of disorders manifested by significant difficulties with learning. Inattention and impulsivity are signs indicating developmentally inappropriate behavior.

learning needs   Gaps in knowledge that exist between a desired level of performance and the actual level of performance; what the learner needs to know.

learning styles   The manner by which (how) individuals perceive and then process information. Certain characteristics of style are biological in origin, whereas others are sociologically developed as a result of environmental influences.

learning theory   A coherent framework and set of integrated constructs and principles that describe, explain, or predict how people learn.

lecture   The oldest, most commonly used, and most traditional instructional method by which the teacher verbally transmits information in a highly structured format directly to a group of learners.

legal rights and duties   A term that refers to rules governing behavior or conduct of health care professionals that are enforceable under threat of punishment or penalty, such as a fine, imprisonment, or both.

legally blind   A person's vision is 20/200 or less in the better eye with correction, or if visual field limits in both eyes are within 20 degrees diameter.

linguistic intelligence   A term used by Gardner to describe children who have highly developed auditory skills and think in words.

listening test   A standardized test to measure comprehension using a selected passage from an instructional material written at approximately the fifth-grade level that is read aloud at a normal rate to determine what a person understands and remembers when listening.

listserv   An automated mailing list software program that copies messages and distributes them to all subscribers.

literacy   The ability of adults to read, understand, and interpret information written at the eighth-grade level or above. An umbrella term used to describe socially required and expected reading and writing abilities; the relative ability of persons to use printed and written material commonly encountered in daily life.

locus of control (LOC)   The location of control of behaviors as either self-directed or directed by others.

Persons with internal or external locus of control differ particularly in the degree of responsibility taken for their own actions (see also *internal locus of control* and *external locus of control*).

logical-mathematical intelligence   A term used by Gardner to describe children who are strong in exploring patterns, categories, and relationships of objects.

low literacy   The ability of adults to read, write, and comprehend information between the fifth- and the eighth-grade level of difficulty (also referred to as marginally literate or marginally illiterate).

magnetic resonance imaging (MRI)   See *functional magnetic resonance imaging (FMRI)*.

malpractice   Failure to exercise an accepted degree of professional skill or learning by one rendering professional services that results in injury, loss, or damage to the recipient of those services.

mandatory needs   Requisites to be learned for survival or situations where the learner's life or safety is threatened.

marginally literate   A term to describe a person with low literacy skills; also known as marginally illiterate.

media characteristics   One of the three major variables that refers to the form through which information will be communicated, which must be considered when making appropriate choices of instructional materials.

media/medium   The form in which information or ideas are conveyed to learners.

models   Three-dimensional instructional tools that allow the learner to immediately apply knowledge and psychomotor skills by observing, examining, manipulating, handling, assembling, and disassembling objects while the teacher provides feedback. Replicas, analogues, and symbols are all types of models that enhance instruction by means that range from concrete to abstract.

moral rights and duties   A term that refers to an internal value system, a certain "moral fabric," that is expressed externally in ethical behaviors of healthcare professionals; often used interchangeably with the terms morality and *morals*.

morals   Synonymous with *ethics*; a value system.

motivation   A psychological force that moves a person to take action in the direction of meeting a need or goal, evidenced by willingness or readiness to act.

motivational axioms   Premises on which an understanding of motivation is based, such as a state of optimum anxiety, learner readiness, realistic goal setting, learner satisfaction/-

success, and uncertainty-reducing or uncertainty-maintaining dialogue.

motivational incentives   Factors that influence motivation in the direction of the desired goal.

MRI   See *functional magnetic resonance imaging (FMRI).*

musical intelligence   A term used by Gardner to describe children who are talented in playing musical instruments, singing, dancing, and keeping rhythm and who often learn best with music playing in the background.

Myers-Briggs Typology   A self-report inventory that uses forced-choice questions and word pairs to measure four dichotomous dimensions of behavior.

needs assessment   The process of determining through data collection what a person, group, organization, or community must learn or wants to learn to provide appropriate education programs to meet the required or desired needs of the learners.

negligence   Conduct that falls below professional legal standards and puts a person at risk for harm. Doing or nondoing of an act, pursuant to a duty, that a reasonable person in the same circumstances would or would not do; the acting or the nonacting is the proximate cause of injury to another person or property.

noncompliance   Nonsubmission or resistance of the individual to follow a prescribed, predetermined regimen.

non-healthcare setting   One of three classifications of instructional settings in which health care is an incidental or supportive function of an organization, such as a business, industry, or school system.

nonmalfeasance   The notion of doing no harm.

nonprint instructional materials   Include the full range of audio and visual instructional materials, including demonstrations and displays.

numeracy   The ability to read and interpret numbers.

Nurse-Client Negotiations Model   A model developed for the purpose of cultural assessment and planning for care of culturally diverse people that recognizes the popular, professional, and folk arenas (sectors) as concepts to bridge the gap between the scientific perspectives of the nurse and the cultural perspectives of the client.

nurse practice acts   Legal provisions of each state defining nursing and the standards of nursing practice, usually including patient teaching as a professional responsibility to protect the public from incompetent practitioners.

nursing process   A model for nursing practice using the problem-solving approach, which includes the phases of assessment, nursing diagnosis, planning, implementation, and evaluation of patient care that parallels the *education process*.

objectives (behavioral)   Statements defining specific health activities, quantitatively measurable and descriptive of the intended results (rather than the process) of instruction, to be competently achieved by the learner in a finite period of time. Well-stated objectives reflect the characteristic components of performance, condition, and criteria.

obstacles to learning   Those factors that negatively affect the ability of the learner to attend to and process information.

one-to-one instruction   A common, traditional instructional method for exchange of information whereby the teacher delivers individual verbal instruction of learning activities in a format designed specifically to meet the needs of a particular learner.

operant conditioning   Focuses on the behavior of an organism as a result of a positive or negative reinforcer (stimulus or event) applied after a response that strengthens the probability that the response will be performed again; nonreinforcement and punishment decrease the likelihood that a response will continue to be performed.

outcome   The result of actions that may be intended or unintended; synonymous with stated goals.

outcome evaluation   See *summative evaluation*.

output disability   A general category of learning disability that refers to orally responding and performing physical tasks, which include language and motor disorders.

pacing   The speed at which information is presented to a learner.

parochial orientation   Persons who tend to be more conservative in thinking, are less willing to accept change, and place trust in traditional authority figures; a component of experiential readiness.

patient education   A process of assisting consumers of health care to learn how to incorporate health-related behaviors (knowledge, skills, and/or attitudes) into everyday life with the purpose of achieving the goal of optimal health.

pedagogy   The art and science of helping children to learn.

PEMs   See *printed education materials*.

personal fable   A belief by adolescents that they are invincible and invulnerable to outside forces.

physical maturation   Change in an individual's physical characteristics as a result of normal body growth and development during the aging process.

physical readiness   A state of willingness to learn that is dependent on such factors as measures of physical ability, complexity of task, health status, and gender.

pooled ignorance   Lack of knowledge or information about issues or problems prior to a group discussion session, whereby clients cannot adequately learn from one another if they do not possess a basic, accurate understanding of a subject to draw on for purposes of discourse.

positron emission tomography (PET)   A type of technology that has revolutionized the field of neuroscience by making images of the brain to detect which possible areas of the brain are used for cognating, feeling, and remembering.

possible needs   "Nice to know" information that is not essential at a given point in time or in situations in which learning is not directly related to daily activities.

posters   A type of display that combines print and nonprint media to help convey a message.

poverty circle (cycle of poverty)   A process whereby parents who are of low income and educational level produce children of low income and educational attainment, who grow up and repeat the process with their own children; a situation in which generation after generation are born into poverty by many factors, such as poor health care, limited resources, family stress, and low-paying jobs.

precausal thinking   Unawareness by preschoolers of causation by invisible and mechanical forces.

preoperational period   As defined by Piaget, this is the second key milestone in the cognitive development of children when the child of the preschool age group (3 to 6 years) is acquiring language skills and gaining experience but thinking is precausal, animistic, egocentric, and intuitive, with only a vague understanding of relationships and multiple classifications of objects.

presentation   The form in which the message (content) is put forth, occurring along a continuum from real objects to symbols.

printed education materials (PEMs)   As the most common type of teaching tools, these include handouts, leaflets, books, pamphlets, brochures, and instruction sheets, which may be purchased or instructor developed.

process evaluation   See *formative evaluation*.

Prochaska's Change Model   See *Stages of Change Model*.

program evaluation   A systematic assessment to determine the extent to which all activities for an entire department or program over a specified time period have accomplished the goals originally established.

projection resources   Audiovisual instructional formats that depend primarily on the learners' sense of sight as the means through which messages are received. These resources require equipment to project images, usually in a darkened room, and include movies, slides, overhead transparencies, and others.

psychodynamic learning   One of the five major learning theories. Largely a theory of motivation stressing emotions rather than cognition and responses; this perspective emphasizes the importance of conscious and unconscious forces derived from earlier childhood experiences and conflicts that guide and change behavior.

psychomotor domain   One of three domains in the taxonomy of behavioral objectives, which is concerned with the physical activities of the body, such as coordination, reaction time, and muscular control, related to the acquisition of a skill or task.

psychosocial development   The process of psychological and social adjustment as an individual grows from infancy to adulthood according to Erickson's eight stages of the psychological and social maturation of humans: trust versus mistrust; autonomy versus shame and doubt;

initiative versus guilt; industry versus inferiority; identity versus role confusion; intimacy versus isolation; generativity versus self-absorption and stagnation; and ego integrity versus despair.

readability   The level of reading difficulty at which printed teaching tools are written. A measure of those elements in a given text of printed material that influence with what degree of success a group of readers will be able to read and understand the information; the ease, or, conversely, the difficulty, with which a person can understand or comprehend the style of writing of a selected printed passage.

readiness to learn   The time when the learner is receptive to learning and is willing and able to participate in the learning process; preparedness or willingness to learn.

reading   Also known as word recognition, it is the process of transforming letters into words and being able to pronounce them correctly.

realia   The most concrete form of stimuli that can be used to deliver information. Example: a real person or a model being used to demonstrate a procedure such as breast self-examination.

REALM (Rapid Estimate of Adult Literacy in Medicine)   A reading skills test to measure a patient's ability to read medical and health-related vocabulary.

receptive aphasia   An absence or impairment of the ability to comprehend what is read or heard due to a dysfunction in the Wernicke's area of the brain, which controls sensory abilities. Although hearing is unimpaired, the person is unable to understand the significance of the spoken word and is unable to communicate verbally.

reflective observation   A term used by Kolb to describe a dimension of processing; known as the "watching" mode.

rehabilitation   The relearning of previous skills, which often requires an adjustment to altered functional abilities and altered lifestyle.

repetition   A technique that strengthens learning by aiding in retention of information of new or difficult material through reinforcement of important points.

replica   A facsimile constructed to scale that resembles the features or substance of the original object. It may be examined or manipulated by the learner to get an idea of how something works. Example: resuscitation dolls.

respondeat superior   A legal term referring to the employer being responsible for a wrongdoing committed by an employee. A master-servant rule meaning "let the master respond and answer."

respondent conditioning   Emphasizes the importance of stimulus conditions and the associations formed in the learning process whereby, without thought or awareness, learning takes place when a newly conditioned stimulus (CS) becomes associated with a conditioned response (CR); also termed classical or Pavlovian conditioning.

return demonstration   A traditional instructional method by which the learner attempts to perform a psychomotor skill, with cues or prompting as needed from the teacher.

SAM (Suitability Assessment of Materials)   An evaluation instrument designed to measure the appropriateness of print materials, illustrations, and video- and audiotaped instructions for a given patient population.

selective attention   The process of recognizing and selecting appropriate and inappropriate stimuli.

self-composed instructional materials   Printed instructional materials composed by individual instructors for the purposes of supplementing teaching.

Self-Efficacy Theory   A framework that describes the belief that one is capable of accomplishing a specific behavior.

sensing-intuition (SN)   Describes how individuals perceive the world, either directly through the five senses or indirectly by way of the unconscious; one of four dichotomous preference dimensions in the Myers-Briggs Typology.

sensorimotor period   As defined by Piaget, this is the first key milestone in the cognitive development of children in the age group of infancy to toddlerhood when learning is enhanced through movement and manipulation of objects in the environment via visual, auditory, tactile, olfactory, taste, and motor stimulation.

sensory deficits   A category of common physical disabilities that includes, in particular, hearing and visual impairments.

silent epidemic   A term used to describe the literacy problem in the United States; also known as the silent barrier or silent disability.

simulation   A nontraditional method of instruction whereby an artificial or hypothetical experience is created that engages the learner in an activity reflecting real-life conditions but with out the risk-taking consequences of an actual situation.

simulation laboratory   A type of learning laboratory that contains real equipment in a lifelike setting, but that allows the learner to practice manipulating and using this equipment as a prelude to performing a task in a real-life situation. Frequently used to supplement the learning of psychomotor skills.

SMOG formula   A relatively easy to use, popular, valid test of readability based on 100% comprehension of printed material from grade 4 to college level.

social cognition   An aspect of cognitive theory that highlights the influence of social factors on perception, thought, motivation, and behaviors.

social learning   One of five major learning theories, this theory is seen as a mixture of behaviorist, cognitive, and psychodynamic influences; much of learning is a social process that occurs by observation and watching other people's behavior to see what happens to them. Role modeling is a central concept of this theory, with cognitive or psychodynamic aspects of internal processing and motivation sometimes considered in the learning process.

socioeconomic status (SES)   Variation in health status, health behavior, or learning abilities among individuals of different social and economic levels.

software   Computer programs and other instructional materials such as videotapes and overhead transparencies.

spatial intelligence A term used by Gardner to describe children who learn by images and pictures.

spontaneous recovery A response, which appears to be extinguished, reappears at any time (even years later), especially when stimulus conditions are similar to those in the initial learning experience.

Stages of Change Model A model developed by Prochaska that informs the phenomenon of health behaviors of the learner, particularly applied to addictive and problem behaviors, and includes the six distinct stages of change: precontemplation, contemplation, preparation, action, maintenance, and termination.

stereotyping An oversimplified conception, opinion, or belief about some aspect of an individual or group.

Suitability Assessment of Materials See *SAM.*

summative evaluation Systematic assessment of the degree to which individuals have learned or objectives have been met as a result of education intervention; also referred to as outcome evaluation.

support system Resources and significant others, such as family and friends, on whom the patient relies or is dependent for information or assistance in managing activities of daily living and who may serve as a positive or negative influence on teaching efforts.

syllogistic reasoning The ability of school-aged children to consider two premises and draw a logical conclusion from them.

symbol A type of model that conveys a message to the learner through the use of abstract constructs, like words, that stand for the real thing. Cartoons and printed materials are examples of symbolic forms of a message.

symbolic representations Numbers and words, symbols written and spoken to convey ideas or represent objects, which are the most common form of communication and yet are the most abstract types of messages.

tailoring Coordinating a patient's treatment regimens into their daily schedules by allowing new tasks to be associated with old behaviors.

task characteristics One of the three major variables defined by the behavioral objectives in the cognitive, affective, and psychomotor domains of learning, which must be considered when making appropriate choices of instructional materials.

taxonomic hierarchy See *taxonomy.*

taxonomy A form of hierarchical classification of cognitive, affective, and psychomotor domains of behaviors according to their degree or level of complexity.

teachable moment   As defined by Havighurst, that point in time when the learner is most receptive to a teaching situation; it can occur at any hour that a patient, family member, staff member, or nursing student has a question or needs information.

teaching   As one component of the educational process, it is a deliberate, intentional act of communicating information to the learner in response to identified learning needs with the objective of producing learning to achieve desired behavioral outcomes.

teaching method   A traditional or nontraditional technique or approach used by the teacher to bring the learner into contact with the content to be learned; a way or a process to communicate and share information with the learner.

teaching plan   Overall blueprint or outline for instruction clearly defining the relationship between the essential components of behavioral objectives, instructional content, teaching methods and tools, time frame for teaching, and methods of evaluation that fit together in a logical pattern of flow to achieve a predetermined goal.

teaching role   An expected and legally mandated standard of practice by the nurse that supports, encourages, and

assists the learner to acquire behaviors (knowledge, skills, and attitudes) and put them into meaningful parts and wholes to reach an optimum potential of functioning.

teaching strategy   An overall plan of action for instruction that anticipates barriers and resources of the learning experience to achieve specific behavioral objectives.

telecommunications   Technological devices for the deaf (TDD) as a resource for patient education.

telecommunications resources   Instructional tools used to help convey information via electrical energy from one place to another such as telephones, televisions, and computers.

Therapeutic Alliance Model   An interpersonal provider-patient model that addresses the continuum of compliance, adherence, and collaboration in therapeutic relationships.

thinking-feeling (TF)   An approach used by individuals to arrive at judgments through impersonal, logical, subjective, or empathetic processes; one of four dichotomous preference dimensions in the Myers-Briggs Typology.

TOFHLA   Defined as Test of Functional Health Literacy in Adults, it is a relatively new instrument for measuring patients' literacy level by using actual hospital materials, such as prescription labels, appointment slips, and informed consent documents, to determine their reading and numeracy skills.

tools   See *instructional materials/tools*.

transcultural nursing   A formal area of study and practice comparing and analyzing different cultures and subcultures with respect to cultural care, health practices, and illness beliefs with the goal of using these insights to provide culture-specific and culture-universal care to diverse groups of people.

transfer of learning   The effects of learning one skill on the subsequent performance of another related skill.

Usenet   A global discussion system made up of a cooperative network of computers that distribute and archive messages posted to topic-specific electronic discussion groups called newsgroups.

variable costs   Not predictable, volume-related expenses.

veracity   Truth telling; honesty.

visual impairment   A reduction or complete loss of vision due to infection, accident, poisoning, or congenital degeneration of the eye(s). See *legally blind*.

World Wide Web   A computer network of information servers around the world that are connected to the Internet; it is a technology-based educational resource that was created as a virtual space for the display of information.

WRAT (Wide Range Achievement Test) technique   A word recognition screening test used to assess a person's ability to recognize and pronounce a list of words out of context as a criterion for measuring comprehension of written materials. Level I test is designed for children ages 5 to 12 years; level II is intended to test persons over 12 years of age.

INDEX